Musculoskeletal Disorders and Injuries: Diagnosis and Therapeutic Strategies

Musculoskeletal Disorders and Injuries: Diagnosis and Therapeutic Strategies

Edited by Joel Reynolds

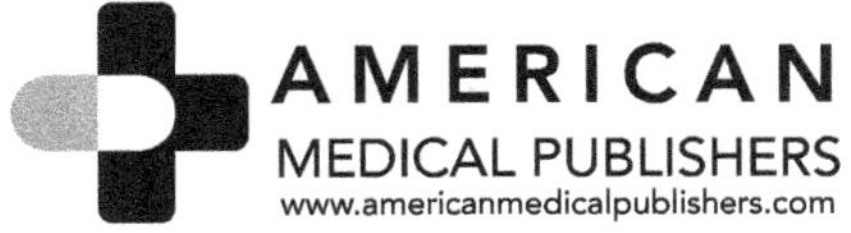

American Medical Publishers,
41 Flatbush Avenue,
1st Floor, New York,
NY 11217, USA

Visit us on the World Wide Web at:
www.americanmedicalpublishers.com

ISBN: 978-1-63927-400-0

Cataloging-in-Publication Data

Musculoskeletal disorders and injuries : diagnosis and therapeutic strategies / edited by Joel Reynolds.
p. cm.
Includes bibliographical references and index.
ISBN 978-1-63927-400-0
1. Musculoskeletal system--Diseases. 2. Musculoskeletal system--Wounds and injuries.
3. Musculoskeletal system. I. Reynolds, Joel.
RC925 .D57 2022
616.74--dc23

Table of Contents

Preface

The musculoskeletal system is an organ system which facilitates movement and provides support, form and stability to the body. It is comprised of the bones of the skeleton, muscles, tendons, cartilage, ligaments, joints and other connective tissue that bind tissues and organs together. The disorders of the musculoskeletal system encompass motion discrepancies or functional disorders. As several other body systems such as the nervous, vascular and integumentary systems are correlated with the musculoskeletal system, disorders within these systems also affect the musculoskeletal system. Articular disorders are the most common musculoskeletal disorder. The disorders of the muscles of a different body system can cause respiratory dysfunction, bladder malfunction and impairment of ocular motion. Muscular dysfunctions, such as paresis, ataxia or paralysis can arise due to infections or toxin exposure. The level of impairment caused by these disorders depends on the condition and its severity. The musculoskeletal system can also be injured due to acute traumatic events, repeated exposure to awkward posture, force or vibration. This book is a valuable compilation of topics, ranging from the basic to the most complex disorders and injuries of the musculoskeletal system. Some of the diverse topics covered in this book address the assessment and management of musculoskeletal disorders and trauma. For all those who are interested in orthopedics, this book can prove to be an essential guide.

The information contained in this book is the result of intensive hard work done by researchers in this field. All due efforts have been made to make this book serve as a complete guiding source for students and researchers. The topics in this book have been comprehensively explained to help readers understand the growing trends in the field.

I would like to thank the entire group of writers who made sincere efforts in this book and my family who supported me in my efforts of working on this book. I take this opportunity to thank all those who have been a guiding force throughout my life.

Editor

1

A retrospective analysis of bone mineral status in patients requiring spinal surgery

Tobias Schmidt[1,2*†], Katharina Ebert[1†], Tim Rolvien[1,2], Nicola Oehler[2], Jens Lohmann[3], Luca Papavero[3], Ralph Kothe[3], Michael Amling[1], Florian Barvencik[1] and Haider Mussawy[1,2]

Abstract

Background: Impaired bone quality is associated with poor outcome of spinal surgery. The aim of the study was to assess the bone mineral status of patients scheduled to undergo spinal surgery and to report frequencies of bone mineral disorders.

Methods: We retrospectively analyzed the bone mineral status of 144 patients requiring spinal surgery including bone mineral density by dual-energy X-ray absorptiometry (DXA) as well as laboratory data with serum levels of 25-hydroxyvitamin D (25-OH-D), parathyroid hormone, calcium, bone specific alkaline phosphate, osteocalcin, and gastrin. High-resolution peripheral quantitative computed tomography (HR-pQCT) was additionally performed in a subgroup of 67 patients with T-Score below − 1.5 or history of vertebral fracture.

Results: Among 144 patients, 126 patients (87.5%) were older than 60 years. Mean age was 70.1 years. 42 patients (29.1%) had suffered from a vertebral compression fracture. 12 previously undiagnosed vertebral deformities were detected in 12 patients by vertebral fracture assessment (VFA). Osteoporosis was present in 39 patients (27.1%) and osteopenia in 63 patients (43.8%). Only 16 patients (11.1%) had received anti-osteoporotic therapy, while 54 patients (37.5%) had an indication for specific anti-osteoporotic therapy but had not received it yet. The majority of patients had inadequate vitamin D status (73.6%) and 34.7% of patients showed secondary hyperparathyroidism as a sign for a significant disturbed calcium homeostasis. In a subgroup of 67 patients, severe vertebral deformities were associated with stronger deficits in bone microarchitecture at the distal radius compared to the distal tibia.

Conclusions: This study shows that bone metabolism disorders are highly prevalent in elderly patients scheduled for spinal surgery. Vertebral deformities are associated with a predominant deterioration of bone microstructure at the distal radius. As impaired bone quality can compromise surgical outcome, we strongly recommend an evaluation of bone mineral status prior to operation and anti-osteoporotic therapy if necessary.

Keywords: Osteoporosis, Vitamin D deficiency, Secondary hyperparathyroidism, Hypochlorhydria, Anti-osteoporotic medication

Background

Osteoporosis is a progressive disease that is characterized by a decrease in bone mass density and structures changes in trabecular and cortical bone leading to an increased risk of fractures. It is estimated that over 200 million people worldwide suffer from osteoporosis [1]. Moreover, it has been predicted that the lifetime risk of osteoporotic fractures in the United States is approximately 30–50% in women and 15–30% in men and that more than 40% of postmenopausal women will suffer one or more fragility fractures in their remaining lifetime [2].

Vertebral compression fractures are the most common complication of osteoporosis and strongly affect patients' overall health. The presence of a vertebral fracture increases the risk of a new vertebral fracture by five-fold [3] and patients with vertebral fractures often suffer from severe pain that can lead to long-term care and hospitalization which is associated with further

* Correspondence: to.schmidt@uke.de
†Equal contributors
[1]Department of Osteology and Biomechanics, University Medical Center Hamburg-Eppendorf, Lottestraße 59, 22529 Hamburg, Germany
[2]Department of Orthopedic Surgery, University Medical Center Hamburg-Eppendorf, Martinistrasse 52, 20246 Hamburg, Germany
Full list of author information is available at the end of the article

complications [4]. Furthermore, patients with vertebral fractures are at much greater risk for developing changes in spine structure as kyphotic deformities and spinal stenosis due to sagittal imbalance and degenerative changes [5].

Osteoporosis can be diagnosed by low bone density measured by dual-energy X-ray absorptiometry (DXA) or by a fragility fracture. Although DXA is the gold standard to measure areal bone mineral density (aBMD), it cannot be used to gain insights into three-dimensional bone architecture changes or distinguish between the cortical and trabecular compartments. In addition, it is well known that fractures often occur in patients with a T-score above − 2.5, who therefore do not meet the World Health Organization (WHO) criteria of osteoporosis [6]. These limitations of DXA are important because patients with vertebral fractures not only often have degenerative bone changes that influence the correct interpretation of the lumbar BMD, but in such cases DXA-measured aBMD at the lumbar spine may yield false high values.

In patients with vertebral fractures, the vertebral bodies are characterized by reduced bone volume tissue and the loss of trabeculae [7]. Interestingly, similar deficits are also observed in peripheral bone [8, 9]. This could explain why these patients are at particular risk of vertebral and peripheral fractures in the future [10, 11]. It also suggests that one way to improve the diagnosis of vertebral fractures is by assessing the peripheral bone architecture via high-resolution peripheral quantitative computed tomography (HR-pQCT) [12]. Indeed, several studies show that HR-pQCT measurements of the peripheral bone microstructure are predictive of osteoporosis-related fractures [13, 14].

In the recent years there have been significant advances in the management of osteoporosis. Many studies have investigated the effect of vitamin D and calcium supplements on osteoporosis and fracture risk [15]. Low circulating levels of 25-hydroxyvitamin D (25-OH-D) may lead to increased secretion of parathyroid hormone (PTH) which in turn induces bone loss through increased bone resorption. Despite the importance of vitamin D for maintaining balanced calcium homeostasis, deficiency is highly prevalent in Europe population particularly in northern Europe countries like Germany, where in contrast to Scandinavia food fortification with vitamin D is still lacking [16, 17].

In this study, we collected data of bone mineral status and bone quality in patients scheduled for spine surgery and report rates of untreated osteoporosis, vitamin D deficiency and hyperparathyroidism in a patient cohort in northern Germany.

Methods

Study group

Since early 2015 to the end of 2016 a total of 144 consecutive adult patients (> 50 years of age), who were scheduled for spine surgery in a single center in north Germany, were examined at our institution and included in this retrospective cross-sectional study. All patients were interviewed for previous fractures, medical treatment including anti-osteoporotic treatment and vitamin D supplementation, and associated diseases. Patients with diabetes mellitus type 1, treatment with glucocorticoids lasting over 3 months or tumors were excluded. Patients whose vertebral fractures were the result of major trauma were also excluded. Indication for specific anti-osteoporotic treatment was determined by using the evidence-based (S3) guidelines of German Association of Osteology (DVO). This guideline currently recommends the use of denosumab, raloxifene, bazedoxifene, estrogens, alendronate, risedronate, ibandronate, zoledronic acid, teriparatide and strontium ranelate as specific anti-osteoporotic treatment medication. Informed consent was obtained from all patients for the retrospective and anonymized database studies. This study was performed in accordance with the Declaration of Helsinki. The local ethics committee of the University Medical Center Hamburg-Eppendorf approved this retrospective study (PV5271).

Dual-energy X-ray absorptiometry (DXA)

All patients underwent aBMD measurements by DXA (iDXA, GE Healthcare, UK). Three skeletal areas, the both proximal femur and the lumbar spine (L1–L4), were measured by DXA. The patients were placed in the supine position and scanned according to the manual supplied by the manufacturer. The detected aBMD of the projected bone area was expressed in grams per square centimeter (g/cm2), and the corresponding T-, and Z-Score was calculated using the reference database provided by the manufacturer. DXA measurement at lumbar spine had to be excluded due to degenerative osteoproliferative changes in 25 patients and DXA measurement at proximal femur was not possible due to bilateral hip replacement in 13 patients. Yet, all patient in this study had at least one representative DXA measurement. The vertebral fractures were confirmed with vertebral fracture assessment (VFA) by DXA (Fig. 1a-c). Vertebral deformity severity was measured using VFA by DXA followed by grading of the vertebrae according to the semiquantitative method of Genant. Moderate deformity was defined as reduction of 25–40% in anterior, middle, and/or posterior vertebral height, while severe deformity was defined as a reduction in any of these heights by more than 40% [18].

High-resolution peripheral quantitative computed tomography (HR-pQCT)

The patients ($n = 67$) with a T-score below − 1.5 or a history of a vertebral fracture received additional assessment of peripheral bone structure by HR-pQCT (XtremeCT®, Scanco Medical AG, Brüttisellen). HR-pQCT scans of the

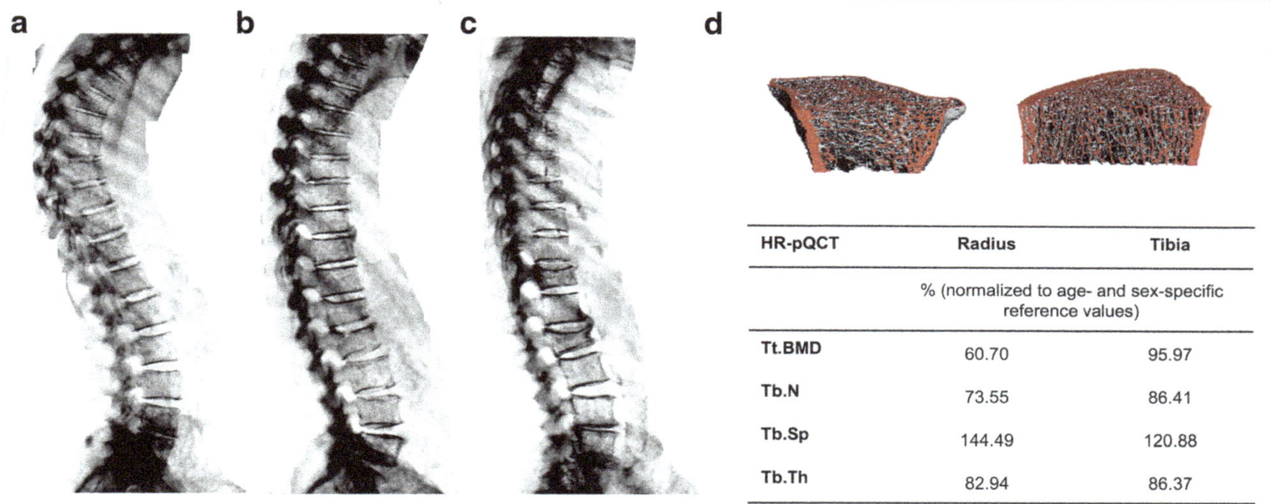

HR-pQCT	Radius	Tibia
	% (normalized to age- and sex-specific reference values)	
Tt.BMD	60.70	95.97
Tb.N	73.55	86.41
Tb.Sp	144.49	120.88
Tb.Th	82.94	86.37

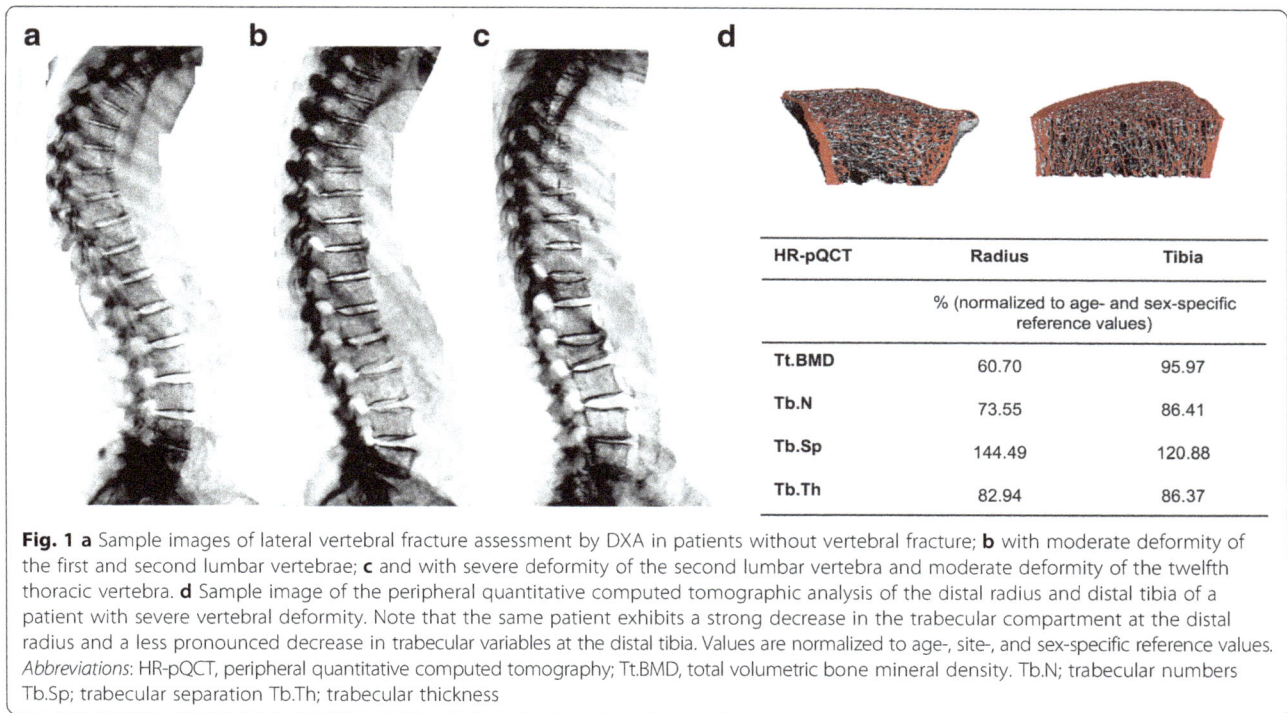

Fig. 1 **a** Sample images of lateral vertebral fracture assessment by DXA in patients without vertebral fracture; **b** with moderate deformity of the first and second lumbar vertebrae; **c** and with severe deformity of the second lumbar vertebra and moderate deformity of the twelfth thoracic vertebra. **d** Sample image of the peripheral quantitative computed tomographic analysis of the distal radius and distal tibia of a patient with severe vertebral deformity. Note that the same patient exhibits a strong decrease in the trabecular compartment at the distal radius and a less pronounced decrease in trabecular variables at the distal tibia. Values are normalized to age-, site-, and sex-specific reference values. *Abbreviations*: HR-pQCT, peripheral quantitative computed tomography; Tt.BMD, total volumetric bone mineral density. Tb.N; trabecular numbers Tb.Sp; trabecular separation Tb.Th; trabecular thickness

non-dominant distal radius (in cases of previous fracture, the contralateral limb was scanned) and the distal tibia were analyzed. The measured region was manually defined by a trained operator by placing a reference line at the endplate of the radius and tibia on a preliminary performed scout view. The same operator generated semiautomatic contours around the periosteal surface and the entire volume of interest is thereafter automatically separated into a cortical and trabecular region. A quality scan for calibration of the CT system was performed each day by using a phantom provided by the manufacturer. The scanning settings used were 60 kV/40 keV at a current of 900 μA. Each image comprised 110 slices with an isotropic voxel size of 82 μm. The following variables were analyzed by using the HR-pQCT system: total, cortical and trabecular area, total, cortical and trabecular volumetric BMD, cortical thickness, trabecular number, trabecular thickness, and trabecular separation. HR-pQCT values were normalized to age-, site-, and sex-specific reference values [19] and are expressed as percentage of corresponding reference value.

Laboratory values

Biochemical analyses of bone metabolism markers including serum levels of alkaline phosphatase (ALP), bone specific alkaline phosphatase (BAP), 25-OH-D, calcium, parathyroid hormone (PTH) and urinary level of deoxypyridinoline (DPD) were assessed by routine lab tests for evaluating osteoporosis. Reference values were adapted from the local laboratory for each parameter. Vitamin D inadequacy was defined as a 25-OH-D level below 30 ng/ml and deficiency as levels less than 20 ng/ml. These values reflect those of widely accepted thresholds [20]. Calcium, gastrin, 25-OH-D and parathyroid hormone were measured in all patients, bone specific AP were only measured in 115 patients, osteocalcin in 111 patients and urinary levels of DPD in 107 patient.

Statistics

The IBM SPSS statistics 22 program was used for statistical analyses. Data are expressed as mean values ± SD. Normal distribution of the data was tested with the Kolmogorov–Smirnov test. To test the differences between the study groups, we used the unpaired two-sided t-test and one-way ANOVA and post hoc Bonferroni test on the normally distributed data and the Mann–Whitney U test and Kruskal Wallis test for non-normally distributed data. *P* values of < 0.05 were considered as statistically significant.

Results

Study population characteristics

A total of 144 consecutive adult patients older than 50 years were included in this retrospective study. All patients were scheduled for spine surgery. The mean age and BMI was 70.1 ± 8.1 years and 26.2 ± 4.87 kg/m^2, respectively. Among 144 patients, 96 (66.4%) were females. 42 patients had suffered from a vertebral compression fracture in the past. Almost half of the patients (48.6%) had a diagnosis of lumbar spinal stenosis. Table 1 summarizes the characteristics of the study population.

Table 1 Demographic and laboratory data of of patients requiring spinal surgery

	Mean (± SD) or n (%)
n	144
Sex (no. of female, %)	96 (66.4)
Mean age in yr	70.1 (8.1)
Age (no. of patients)	
50–60 yr	18 (12.5%)
60–70 yr	55 (38.2%)
> 70 yr	71 (49.3%)
Weight (kg)	74.8 (14.4)
Height (cm)	168.0 (9.4)
Height change (cm)	3.7 (2.9)
Mean BMI (± SD)	26.2 (4.7)
History of a vertebral fracture	42 (29.1%)
Unknown vertebral deformity (Diagnosed by VFA)	12 (8.3%)
Proton pump inhibitor use	44 (30.6%)
Laboratory values	
25-OH-D (ng/ml)	24.3 (11.8)
Parathyroid hormone (ng/l)	84.3 (47.1)
Calcium (mmol/l)	2.23 (0.1)
Bone specific AP (µg/l) (*n* = 115)	13.6 (7.9)
Osteocalcin (µg/l) (*n* = 111)	18.9 (11.8)
Urine DPD (*n* = 107)	6.7 (2.8)
Elevated DPD	74 (69.2%)
Elevated Gastrin	20 (13.9%)

Bone densitometry

DXA was performed in all patients. However, DXA measurement in 25 patients at lumbar spine had to be excluded due to degenerative osteoproliferative changes. In 13 patients DXA measurement at the proximal femur was not possible due to bilateral hip replacement. Yet, all patient in this study had at least one representative DXA measurement. Osteoporosis at the lumbar spine was diagnosed in 27 of 119 patient (22.7%) whereas 22 of 131 patients (16.8%) showed T-scores below − 2.5 at the femur. Incidence of osteopenia was 34.5% at the lumbar spine and 45.8% at the femur. Table 2 shows the indication for spinal surgery and the corresponding T- and Z-scores for each subgroup. Patients requiring spinal surgery due to a compression fracture showed the lowest T- and Z-scores at the lumbar spine and at the femoral neck.

Deterioration of bone structure at the distal radius is associated with severity of vertebral fracture

Vertebral fracture assessment (VFA) of the spine revealed 12 previously unknown vertebral deformities in 12 different patients. Fig. 1a-c shows sample images of VFA by DXA in patients without vertebral deformity (a), moderate deformity (b) and severe deformity (c). In a subgroup of 67 patients with a T-score below − 1.5 or a history of fracture, we used HR-pQCT for further assessment of bone microstructure at the distal radius and distal tibia. 21 and 12 patients of this subgroup had moderate and severe vertebral fractures, respectively. The patients did not differ significantly in terms of age (mean 71.9 vs. 71.6), weight (72.7 kg vs. 78.4 kg), height (166 cm vs. 170 cm), or BMI (26.1 vs 26.9). Interestingly, when we compared patients with vertebral deformities to patients without deformities, the cases with severe vertebral deformity had significantly lower total volumetric BMD (17.75%) as well as trabecular and cortical microstructure parameters at the distal radius (Table 3). The tibial values demonstrated similar trends, albeit less pronounced and without achieving statistical significance (Table 3). Figure 1d demonstrates images of a patient with pronounced deterioration of bone microstructure at the distal radius.

Vitamin D status

25-OH-D and PTH were measured in all patients. Vitamin D inadequacy was defined as a 25-OH-D level below 30 ng/ml and deficiency as levels less than 20 ng/ml. The mean 25-OH-D concentration was 24.3 ng/ml. Values ranged from 4 to 60 ng/ml. The overall prevalence of vitamin D inadequacy was 73.6% and that of deficiency was 36.8% (Fig. 2a). Severe deficiency (25-OH-D < 10 ng/ml) was present in 17 patients (11.6%). 50 (35.4%) patients showed elevated PTH levels. While 12 of these patients showed hypocalcemic hyperparathyroidism, 38 patients displayed elevated PTH levels with normocalcemia. One patient showed elevated calcium and PTH levels

Table 2 T-scores and Z-scores of the DXA measurements in patients with different indication for spinal surgery (mean ± SD)

	n	T-Score lumbar spine	Z-Score lumbar spine	T-Score femoral neck	Z-Score femoral neck
All patients	144	−1.23 (1.4)	- 0.1 (1.5)	- 1.4 (1.0)	- 0.08 (1.1)
Indication for spinal surgery					
Lumbar spinal stenosis	70	−1.29 (1.73)	0.07 (1.56)	−1.62(1.15)	−0.04 (1.08)
Degenerative spondylolisthesis	35	−1.14 (1.45)	− 0.20 (1.38)	− 1.16 (0.98)	0.12 (1.10)
Herniation of lumbar disc	31	−0.77 (1.21)	−0.04 (1.41)	−1.06 (0.88)	0.32 (1.38)
Compression fracture	8	−2.6 (1.3)	−1.27 (0.91)	−1.72 (1.07)	−0.13 (1.05)

Table 3 Differences in bone microarchitecture between the patients with moderate/severe vertebral deformity and the patients without vertebral fractures

	No Deformity	Moderate Deformity		Severe Deformity	
n	34	21		12	
Mean age, years	71	71.9		72	
HR-pQCT variables					
Radius (normalized to age- and sex-specific reference values)	%	%	Δ %	%	Δ %
Total bone area	109.8 (15.7)	113.4 (18.5)	+ 3.5	110.2 (30.7)	+ 0.35
Cortical area	88.8 (21.7)	78.3 (27.3)	−10.5	65.4 (19.5)	*−23.4**
Trabecular area	110.8 (20.4)	117.2 (24.4)	+ 6.2	116.7 (36.8)	+ 5.7
Total vBMD	94.9 (20.7)	87.2 (18.9)	−7.6	76.2 (12.5)	*−18.7**
Cortical vBMD	83.3 (7.0)	80.1 (8.4)	−3.1	77.7 (6.9)	−5.5
Trabecular vBMD	100.7 (20.7)	93.5 (25.7)	−7.3	79.7 (17.4)	*−21.0**
Cortical thickness	70.4 (18.9)	61.1 (24.4)	−9.4	50.8 (14.9)	*−19.6**
Trabecular numbers	106.8 (14.6)	102.4 (22.7)	−4.4	92.4 (16.9)	*−14.4**
Trabecular thickness	94.9 (13.1)	92.0 (17.3)	−2.8	87.1 (13.5)	*−7.8**
Trabecular separation	95.8 (15.8)	105.3 (32.2)	+ 9.5	116.8 (28.1)	*+ 20.9**
Tibia (normalized to age- and sex-specific reference values)	%	%	Δ %	%	Δ %
Total bone area	112.1 (17.5)	115.5 (21.3)	+ 3.4	109.8 (19.5)	−2.3
Cortical area	90.7 (15.2)	91.6 (18.5)	+ 0.9	81.7 (15.7)	−9.0
Trabecular area	98.3 (15.4)	99.4 (22.6)	+ 1.1	95.6 (20.7)	−2.6
Total vBMD	90.7 (15.2)	91.6 (18.4)	+ 0.9	81.7 (15.7)	−9.0
Cortical vBMD	85.8 (8.8)	86.4 (8.9)	+ 0.6	82.7 (7.9)	−3.1
Trabecular vBMD	98.5 (18.9)	98.5 (23.6)	−0.0	87.8 (18.2)	−10.6
Cortical thickness	67.7 (21.5)	68.9 (26.0)	+ 1.2	58.8 (23.8)	−8.8
Trabecular numbers	110.1 (18.5)	105.8 (25.4)	−4.3	102.9 (22.1)	−7.1
Trabecular thickness	90.6 (15.7)	93.2 (12.4)	+ 2.6	87.0 (19.1)	−3.6
Trabecular separation	94.1 (19.6)	101.5 (29.6)	+ 7.4	104.9 (28.9)	+ 10.8

Abbreviations: HR-pQCT, peripheral quantitative computed tomography; vBMD, volumetric bone mineral density
The data are normalized to age- and sex-specific reference values. The differences (Δ) that are shown are relative to the non-fracture group.
* = Statistically significant ($p < 0.05$) differences to the non-fracture group

and was consequently diagnosed with primary hyperparathyroidism and were treated surgically with parathyroidectomy after preoperative localization of parathyroid adenoma. 44 (30.6%) patients used proton pump inhibitors and 20 (13.9%) of these patient showed elevated levels of gastrin suggesting PPI induced hypochlorhydria.

Anti-osteoporotic treatment

57 patients used vitamin D supplementation. However, only 28 of these patients had 25-OH-D levels above 30 ng/ml suggesting adequate vitamin D supplementation (Table 4). Patients with vitamin D supplementation were divided into two groups by daily intake of vitamin D. While patients with 500–1000 I.E. of vitamin D intake per week showed mainly vitamin D inadequacy, patients with higher intake mostly showed adequate levels (Fig. 2b). However, PTH levels did not differ significantly between these groups. Patients with no vitamin D supplementation had significantly higher level of PTH (Fig. 2b). While only 16 patients (11.1%) were previously treated with specific anti-osteoporotic medication, 54 patients (37.5%) had not received specific anti-osteoporotic treatment as recommended by the evidence-based (S3) guidelines of German Association of Osteology (Table 4) despite having an indication.

Recommendation for anti-osteoporotic treatment

Figure 3 summarizes the major findings and implication for anti-osteoporotic treatment in the patient cohort. Vitamin D supplementation was suggested in dependence of 25-OH-D levels. Patients with hypochlorhydria due to PPI use were recommended to use calcium gluconate supplementation to improve calcium absorption [21, 22]. Indication for specific anti-osteoporotic treatment was established by using the current official recommendation of the German Association of Osteology. The choice

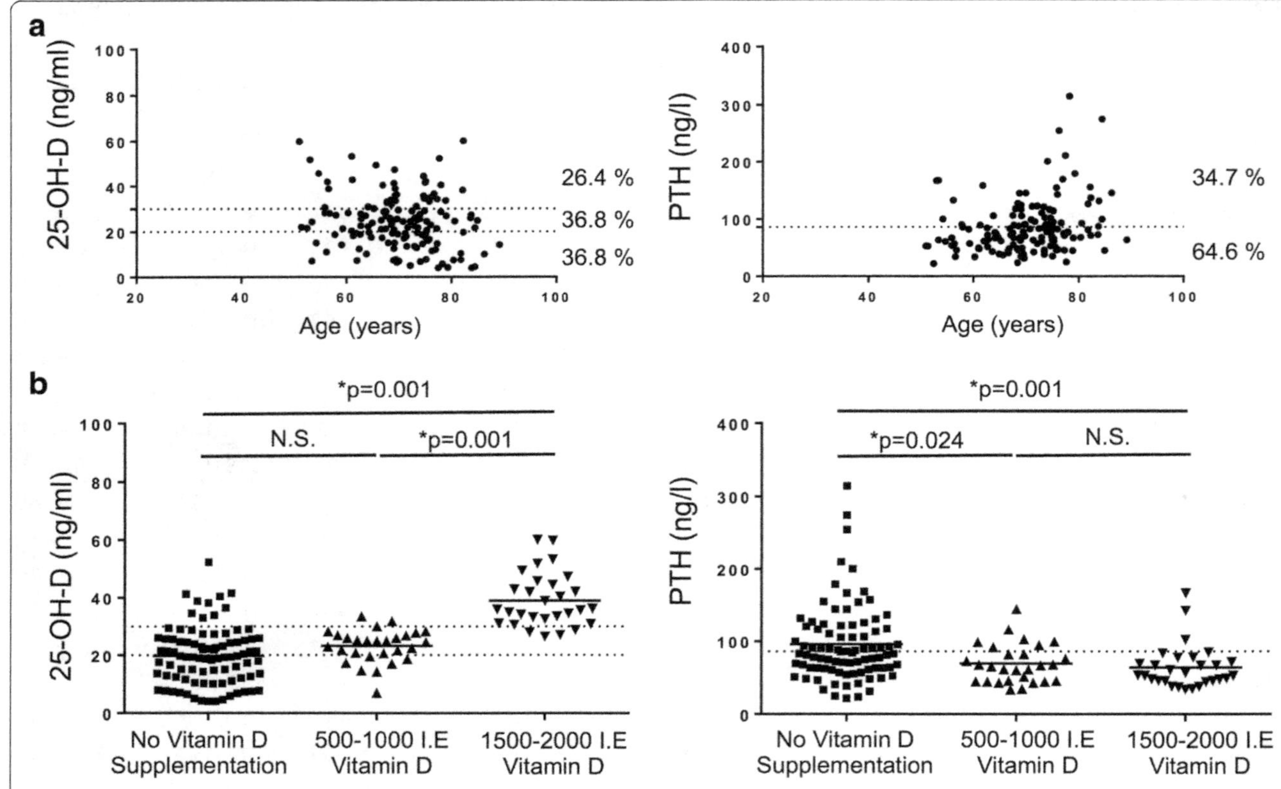

Fig. 2 a Prevalence of 25-OH-D deficiency and secondary hyperparathyroidism in 144 patients scheduled for spine surgery. **b** Levels of 25-OH-D (ng/ml) and parathyroid hormone (ng/l) in patients in dependence of daily vitamin D intake. * $p < 0.05$

Table 4 Anti-osteoporotic treatment in patients undergoing spinal surgery prior and recommendation after evaluation of bone mineral status

	Prior to Evaluation n (%)	Recommendation n (%)
Basic therapy		
Vitamin D supplementation	57 (39.6%)	144 (100%)
Adequate vitamin D supplementation (25-OH-D within recommended range)	28 (19.4%)	
Calcium supplementation	31 (21.5%)	20 (13.9%)
Specific anti-osteoporotic treatment	16 (11.1%)	70 (48.6%)
Bisphosphonate (oral)	8 (5.6%)	26 (18%)
Bisphosphonate (intravenous)	0 (0%)	14 (9.7%)
Denosumab	8 (5.6%)	25 (17.3%)
Teriparatide	0 (0%)	5 (3.5%)
Indication for specific treatment without therapy	54 (37.5%)	

of medication was based on an individualized decision taking risk factors and current bone mineral status and turnover into account.

Discussion

In this study we analysed the bone health of patients requiring spinal surgery. We found a high prevalence of untreated osteoporosis, vitamin D deficiency and parathyroid hormone elevations arising from vitamin D deficiency.

Many studies suggest that BMD is one of the main factors related to poor surgical outcome of patients undergoing spine fusion operations with instrumentation [23]. The ability of screws to resist pullout from bone is directly related to BMD [24]. Moreover, longer fusion constructs are recommended for patients with an osteoporotic spine resulting in longer operative time and increased postoperative time to recovery [25]. Hence, assessment of bone quality prior to operation is crucial finding the optimal surgical strategy to proactively plan for best surgical outcomes.

According to World Health Organization (WHO) recommendations every postmenopausal women and patients with high number of osteoporosis risk factors should undergo bone mineral density screening [26]. Prevalence of osteopenia and osteoporosis for patients requiring spine

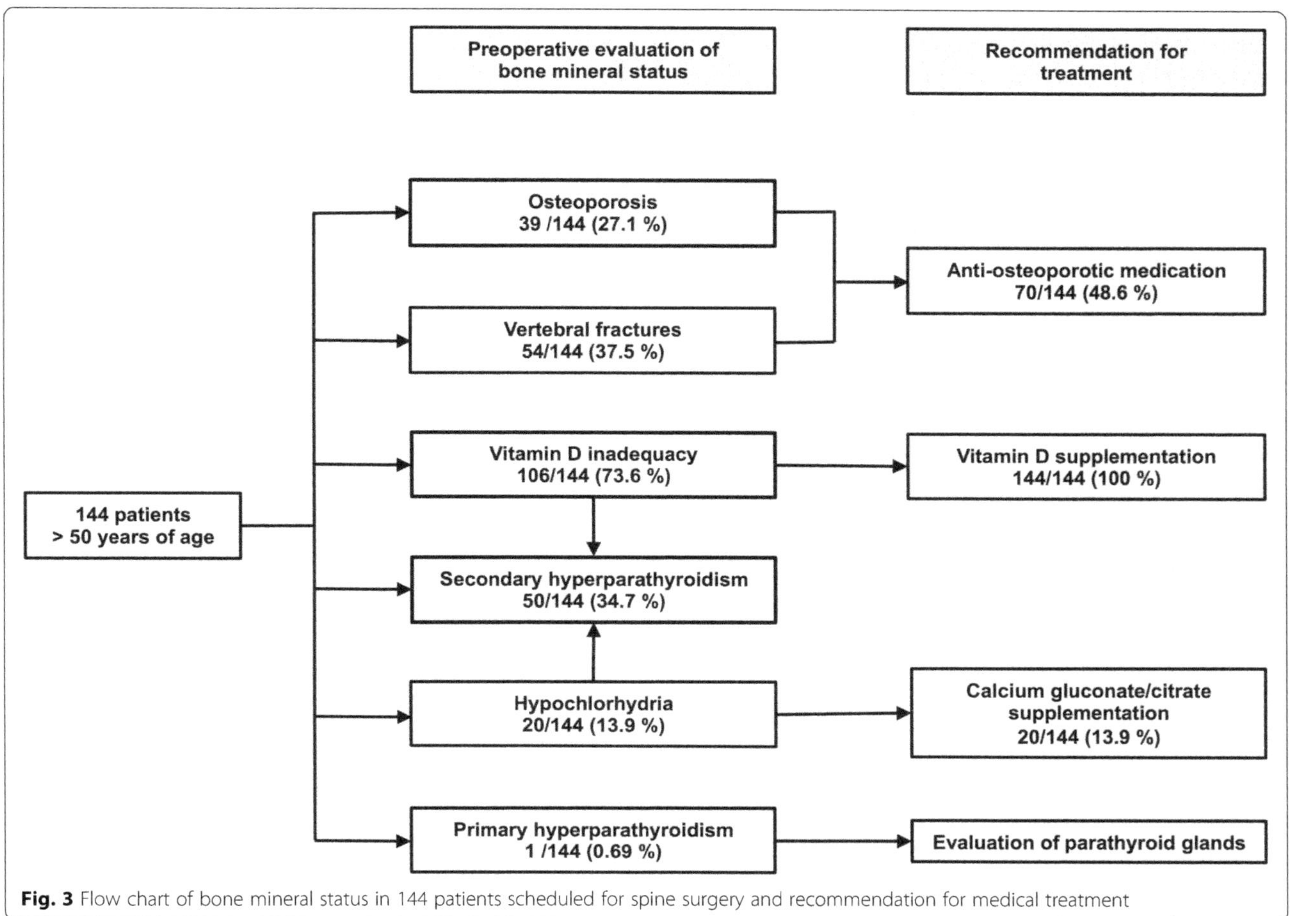

Fig. 3 Flow chart of bone mineral status in 144 patients scheduled for spine surgery and recommendation for medical treatment

surgery have been shown to be high with 46% and 31% for patients older than 50 years [27], respectively. While DXA is the gold standard to measure aBMD, it has been frequently reported that fractures often occur in patients with a T-score above – 2.5 [6] and that women with osteopenia and a prevalent fracture have the same fracture risk as women with osteoporosis [28]. In this context, it has been shown that other factors such as vitamin D deficiency or a predominant cortical bone loss are independently associated with increased fracture risk [29, 30]. Hence, to prevent future fractures and to archive better surgical outcome, it is important to identify and treat patients with reduced bone quality. It would be desirable that in elderly patients (> 50 years) scheduled to undergo elective spine surgery, bone mineral status including DXA measurement and biochemical assessment for reversible risk factors should be determined routinely and appropriate medical treatment including vitamin D supplementation initiated if necessary. In patients with a previous fracture and osteopenia or T-score within the normal range, assessment of peripheral bone structure by HR-pQCT can give useful additional information about the bone quality.

In this study, we found that patients with vertebral deformities had strong deficits in the cortical and trabecular compartments of the distal radius compared to patients without vertebral deformities. We also observed that these deficits at the radius were particularly pronounced in patients with severe vertebral deformity. Thus, the bone microarchitecture at the distal radius seems to reflect vertebral fragility better than the bone architecture at the distal tibia. Yet, it is important to mention that in our study the overall peripheral bone microstructure was only assessed in patients with a T-score below – 1.5. Thus, the patients without vertebral deformities in this study were also in the range of osteopenia or osteoporosis regarding DXA T-score. There are only a few clinical studies that have compared patients with and without vertebral fractures in terms of peripheral changes in the trabecular and cortical compartments. These studies have reported conflicting results in differences observed only at the radius (31), or at the radius and tibia [31–33]. However, studies that reported similar differences at the radius and the tibia compared healthy control patients to osteopenic or osteoporotic patients with vertebral deformities

[31, 34]. Furthermore, studies on patients with various kinds of fragility fractures support the notion that deterioration in bone microstructure plays an important role in the pathogenesis of fractures in general, and that such bone alterations are particularly pronounced at the distal radius [35, 36]. This may be partially explained be the protective effect of weight-bearing on bone microstructure [8, 37]. Moreover, both primary and secondary hyperparathyroidism have been associated with a predominant deterioration of bone microstructure at the distal radius [38, 39]. The possibility that peripheral bone structure can predict the severity of vertebral fracture is of high clinical interest because severe fracture cases have a higher risk of developing changes in spine structure such as kyphotic deformities and spinal stenosis due to sagittal imbalance and degenerative changes. These degenerative alterations falsify aBMD measurement at the spine. Moreover, patients with spinal fusion and/or spinal degeneration in combination with hip joint replacement are not measureable with DXA. In these patients the assessment of the peripheral bone structure at the distal radius could be a useful tool to evaluate and monitor skeletal fragility.

Vitamin D plays an essential role in bone remodelling and is crucial for adequate uptake of calcium. Vitamin D deficiency has been identified as an important risk factor for stress fractures in several studies [15, 40]. Correcting vitamin D deficiency can significantly increase bone mass in elderly people [41]. Nevertheless, a number of studies have reported high prevalence of deficient or inadequate vitamin D levels in patients requiring spinal surgery. Stoker et al. found that nearly 85% of adult patients undergoing spinal fusion showed deficient or inadequate 25-OH-D levels in the United States [20]. This is an even higher rate of insufficiency than in our study with 73.6% of patients showing inadequate vitamin D status. Other studies report similarly rates of vitamin D insufficiency comparable to the vitamin D status of the general population [16, 42].

Vitamin D deficiency often result in secondary hyperparathyroidism causing increased bone resorption. In our study 35.4% of patients showed elevated PTH levels. Some studies suggest that levels of 20 ng/ml are sufficient to avoid secondary hyperparathyroidism, while other studies argue for higher minimum threshold (30 ng/ml) to maintain skeletal health [43]. In our study, patients who received more than 1500–2000 I.E. vitamin D per day mostly reached levels of 25-OH-D > 30 ng/ml, while patients with lower intake (daily 1000 I.E.) showed levels between 20 and 30 ng/ml. However, PTH did not differ between these groups suggesting that levels above 20 ng/ml are generally enough to avoid secondary hyperparathyroidism. Nevertheless, we think based on the current literature and own previous studies it is reasonable to recommend higher intake to reach 25-OH-D levels above 30 ng/ml for optimal osteoid mineralization [43]. Most importantly, with proper treatment patients can have secondary hyperparathyroidism reversed in relatively short time before undergoing elective spinal surgery.

As gastric calcium solubility has been shown to be pH-dependent, hypochlorhydria which is defined by reduced stomach acid production can induce calcium malabsorption which negatively affects bone mineralization [21]. Therefore, patients with hypochlorhydria which can be caused by long term use of proton pump inhibitors (PPI) display higher prevalence for osteoporosis and increased fracture risk [44]. As calcium gluconate or citrate have been shown to be very effective in correcting calcium malabsorption in patients with reduced stomach acid production [21], we recommend calcium gluconate or citrate supplementation in patients with permanent use of PPI.

Prevention is the most important principle in the management of osteoporosis. This is especially important for patient with previous fragility fractures. However, recent studies suggest that there is a large gap between patients with fragility fractures and those receiving appropriate anti-osteoporotic therapy [45]. While the availability of acute surgical treatment for vertebral fractures is considered excellent in Germany, many studies show a deficient in postoperative medical management of patients underlying low BMD resulting in high prevalence of untreated osteoporosis ranging from 30 to 70% [46, 47]. In our study, we found that 37.5% of patients had not received anti-osteoporotic treatment despite having an indication.

Our study has several limitations due to its retrospective design. Firstly, it has to be taken into account that the mean age in our study group was 70.1 years, an age where prevalence of osteoporosis is dramatically increasing. In fact the prevalence of osteoporosis in women > 70 years-old is 13–26% according to prior studies [48]. Secondly, compression fractures of the spine composed a large portion of patients which elevates the prevalence of osteoporosis and increases the number of patients in need of specific anti-osteoporotic therapy. Thirdly, regarding vitamin D status geographic differences has to be considered as northern European population generally has a higher risk to develop vitamin D deficiency and secondary hyperparathyroidism due to reduced sun light exposure.

Conclusion

This study shows that despite recent advances in the diagnosis and treatment of osteoporosis, elderly people scheduled for spinal surgery often show diminished bone mineral density, inadequate vitamin D status, elevated PTH levels and frequently have no anti-osteoporotic therapy. Future studies should aim to investigate the outcome of spinal surgery with regard to the preoperative bone mineral status and the effects of accurately timed preoperative anti-osteoporotic treatment. Considering the potential negative effects of low BMD and vitamin D deficiency for surgical outcome, preoperative screening and initiation of therapy for elderly patients is highly recommended.

Abbreviations

25-OH-D: 25-hydroxyvitamin D; ALP: Alkaline phosphatase; BAP: Bone specific alkaline phosphatase; BMD: Bone mineral density; DPD: Deoxypyridinoline; DXA: Dual-energy X-ray absorptiometry; HR-pQCT: High-resolution peripheral quantitative computed tomography; PTH: Parathyroid hormone; WHO: World Health Organization

Acknowledgements

Not applicable.

Funding

No funding was obtained for this study.

Authors' contributions

Study design: TS, JL, LP, RK, MA, FB, HM. Study conduct: TS, KE, TR, NO, JL, LP, RK, HM. Data collection: TS, KE, TR, NO, HM. Data analysis: TS. Drafting manuscript: TS, KE, TR, HM. Approving final version of manuscript: TS, KE, TR, NO, JL, LP, RK, MA, FB, HM.

Consent for publication

Not applicable.

Competing interests

T.S., K.E., T.R., N.O., J.L., R.K., L.P., M.A., F.B., H.M. declare that they have no conflict of interest. F.B. receives speaker and consultant fees from Alexion, Lilly, MSD, and Pfizer.

Author details

[1]Department of Osteology and Biomechanics, University Medical Center Hamburg-Eppendorf, Lottestraße 59, 22529 Hamburg, Germany. [2]Department of Orthopedic Surgery, University Medical Center Hamburg-Eppendorf, Martinistrasse 52, 20246 Hamburg, Germany. [3]Clinic for Spinal Surgery, Schoen Klinik Eilbek, Denhaide 120, 22081 Hamburg, Germany.

References:

1. Reginster JY, Burlet N. Osteoporosis: a still increasing prevalence. Bone. 2006;38(2 Suppl 1):S4–9.
2. Melton LJ 3rd, Chrischilles EA, Cooper C, Lane AW, Riggs BL. Perspective. How many women have osteoporosis? J Bone Miner Res. 1992;7(9):1005–10.
3. Cummings SR, Melton LJ. Epidemiology and outcomes of osteoporotic fractures. Lancet. 2002;359(9319):1761–7.
4. Lin JT, Lane JM. Nonmedical management of osteoporosis. Curr Opin Rheumatol. 2002;14(4):441–6.
5. Keller TS, Harrison DE, Colloca CJ, Harrison DD, Janik TJ. Prediction of osteoporotic spinal deformity. Spine (Phila Pa 1976). 2003;28(5):455–62.
6. Schuit SC, van der Klift M, Weel AE, de Laet CE, Burger H, Seeman E, Hofman A, Uitterlinden AG, van Leeuwen JP, Pols HA. Fracture incidence and association with bone mineral density in elderly men and women: the Rotterdam study. Bone. 2004;34(1):195–202.
7. Genant HK, Delmas PD, Chen P, Jiang Y, Eriksen EF, Dalsky GP, Marcus R, San Martin J. Severity of vertebral fracture reflects deterioration of bone microarchitecture. Osteoporos Int. 2007;18(1):69–76.
8. Stein EM, Liu XS, Nickolas TL, Cohen A, Thomas V, McMahon DJ, Zhang C, Yin PT, Cosman F, Nieves J, et al. Abnormal microarchitecture and reduced stiffness at the radius and tibia in postmenopausal women with fractures. J Bone Miner Res. 2010;25(12):2572–81.
9. Stein EM, Liu XS, Nickolas TL, Cohen A, McMahon DJ, Zhou B, Zhang C, Kamanda-Kosseh M, Cosman F, Nieves J, et al. Microarchitectural abnormalities are more severe in postmenopausal women with vertebral compared to nonvertebral fractures. J Clin Endocrinol Metab. 2012;97(10):E1918–26.
10. Klotzbuecher CM, Ross PD, Landsman PB, Abbott TA, 3rd, Berger M: Patients with prior fractures have an increased risk of future fractures: a summary of the literature and statistical synthesis. J Bone Miner Res 2000, 15(4):721–739.
11. Roux C, Fechtenbaum J, Kolta S, Briot K, Girard M. Mild prevalent and incident vertebral fractures are risk factors for new fractures. Osteoporos Int. 2007;18(12):1617–24.
12. Geusens P, Chapurlat R, Schett G, Ghasem-Zadeh A, Seeman E, de Jong J, van den Bergh J. High-resolution in vivo imaging of bone and joints: a window to microarchitecture. Nat Rev Rheumatol. 2014;10(5):304–13.
13. Boutroy S, Van Rietbergen B, Sornay-Rendu E, Munoz F, Bouxsein ML, Delmas PD. Finite element analysis based on in vivo HR-pQCT images of the distal radius is associated with wrist fracture in postmenopausal women. J Bone Miner Res. 2008;23(3):392–9.
14. Melton LJ, 3rd, Riggs BL, van Lenthe GH, Achenbach SJ, Muller R, Bouxsein ML, Amin S, Atkinson EJ, Khosla S: Contribution of in vivo structural measurements and load/strength ratios to the determination of forearm fracture risk in postmenopausal women. J Bone Miner Res 2007, 22(9):1442–1448.
15. Chapuy MC, Arlot ME, Duboeuf F, Brun J, Crouzet B, Arnaud S, Delmas PD, Meunier PJ. Vitamin D3 and calcium to prevent hip fractures in the elderly women. N Engl J Med. 1992;327(23):1637–42.
16. Chapuy MC, Preziosi P, Maamer M, Arnaud S, Galan P, Hercberg S, Meunier PJ. Prevalence of vitamin D insufficiency in an adult normal population. Osteoporos Int. 1997;7(5):439–43.
17. Brown J, Sandmann A, Ignatius A, Amling M, Barvencik F. New perspectives on vitamin D food fortification based on a modeling of 25(OH)D concentrations. Nutr J. 2013;12(1):151.
18. Genant HK, Wu CY, van Kuijk C, Nevitt MC. Vertebral fracture assessment using a semiquantitative technique. J Bone Miner Res. 1993;8(9):1137–48.
19. Burt LA, Liang Z, Sajobi TT, Hanley DA, Boyd SK. Sex- and Site-Specific Normative Data Curves for HR-pQCT. J Bone Miner Res. 2016;31(11):2041–7.
20. Stoker GE, Buchowski JM, Bridwell KH, Lenke LG, Riew KD, Zebala LP. Preoperative vitamin D status of adults undergoing surgical spinal fusion. Spine (Phila Pa 1976). 2013;38(6):507–15.
21. Krause M, Keller J, Beil B, van Driel I, Zustin J, Barvencik F, Schinke T, Amling M. Calcium gluconate supplementation is effective to balance calcium homeostasis in patients with gastrectomy. Osteoporos Int. 2015;26(3):987–95.
22. Schinke T, Schilling AF, Baranowsky A, Seitz S, Marshall RP, Linn T, Blaeker M, Huebner AK, Schulz A, Simon R, et al. Impaired gastric acidification negatively affects calcium homeostasis and bone mass. Nat Med. 2009;15(6): 674–81.
23. Ponnusamy KE, Iyer S, Gupta G, Khanna AJ. Instrumentation of the osteoporotic spine: biomechanical and clinical considerations. Spine J. 2011;11(1):54–63.
24. Galbusera F, Volkheimer D, Reitmaier S, Berger-Roscher N, Kienle A, Wilke HJ. Pedicle screw loosening: a clinically relevant complication? Eur Spine J. 2015;24(5):1005–16.
25. Dodwad SM, Khan SN. Surgical stabilization of the spine in the osteoporotic patient. The Orthopedic clinics of North America. 2013;44(2):243–9.
26. Lane JM, Nydick M. Osteoporosis: current modes of prevention and treatment. The Journal of the American Academy of Orthopaedic Surgeons. 1999;7(1):19–31.
27. Chin DK, Park JY, Yoon YS, Kuh SU, Jin BH, Kim KS, Cho YE. Prevalence of osteoporosis in patients requiring spine surgery: incidence and significance of osteoporosis in spine disease. Osteoporos Int. 2007;18(9):1219–24.
28. Pasco JA, Seeman E, Henry MJ, Merriman EN, Nicholson GC, Kotowicz MA. The population burden of fractures originates in women with osteopenia, not osteoporosis. Osteoporos Int. 2006;17(9):1404–9.
29. Szulc P, Boutroy S, Vilayphiou N, Chaitou A, Delmas PD, Chapurlat R. Cross-sectional analysis of the association between fragility fractures and bone microarchitecture in older men: the STRAMBO study. J Bone Miner Res. 2011;26(6):1358–67.
30. Pasco JA, Henry MJ, Kotowicz MA, Sanders KM, Seeman E, Pasco JR, Schneider HG, Nicholson GC. Seasonal periodicity of serum vitamin D and

parathyroid hormone, bone resorption, and fractures: the Geelong osteoporosis study. J Bone Miner Res. 2004;19(5):752–8.

31. Melton LJ 3rd, Riggs BL, Keaveny TM, Achenbach SJ, Kopperdahl D, Camp JJ, Rouleau PA, Amin S, Atkinson EJ, Robb RA, et al. Relation of vertebral deformities to bone density, structure, and strength. J Bone Miner Res. 2010;25(9):1922–30.
32. Liu XS, Wang J, Zhou B, Stein E, Shi X, Adams M, Shane E, Guo XE. Fast trabecular bone strength predictions of HR-pQCT and individual trabeculae segmentation-based plate and rod finite element model discriminate postmenopausal vertebral fractures. J Bone Miner Res. 2013;28(7):1666–78.
33. Sornay-Rendu E, Cabrera-Bravo JL, Boutroy S, Munoz F, Delmas PD. Severity of vertebral fractures is associated with alterations of cortical architecture in postmenopausal women. J Bone Miner Res. 2009;24(4):737–43.
34. Wang J, Stein EM, Zhou B, Nishiyama KK, Yu YE, Shane E, Guo XE. Deterioration of trabecular plate-rod and cortical microarchitecture and reduced bone stiffness at distal radius and tibia in postmenopausal women with vertebral fractures. Bone. 2016;88:39–46.
35. Boutroy S, Bouxsein ML, Munoz F, Delmas PD. In vivo assessment of trabecular bone microarchitecture by high-resolution peripheral quantitative computed tomography. J Clin Endocrinol Metab. 2005;90(12):6508–15.
36. Stein EM, Kepley A, Walker M, Nickolas TL, Nishiyama K, Zhou B, Liu XS, McMahon DJ, Zhang C, Boutroy S, et al. Skeletal structure in postmenopausal women with osteopenia and fractures is characterized by abnormal trabecular plates and cortical thinning. J Bone Miner Res. 2014;29(5):1101–9.
37. Sornay-Rendu E, Boutroy S, Munoz F, Delmas PD. Alterations of cortical and trabecular architecture are associated with fractures in postmenopausal women, partially independent of decreased BMD measured by DXA: the OFELY study. J Bone Miner Res. 2007;22(3):425–33.
38. Trombetti A, Stoermann C, Chevalley T, Van Rietbergen B, Herrmann FR, Martin PY, Rizzoli R. Alterations of bone microstructure and strength in end-stage renal failure. Osteoporos Int. 2013;24(5):1721–32.
39. Hansen S, Beck Jensen JE, Rasmussen L, Hauge EM, Brixen K. Effects on bone geometry, density, and microarchitecture in the distal radius but not the tibia in women with primary hyperparathyroidism: a case-control study using HR-pQCT. J Bone Miner Res. 2010;25(9):1941–7.
40. Burgi AA, Gorham ED, Garland CF, Mohr SB, Garland FC, Zeng K, Thompson K, Lappe JM. High serum 25-hydroxyvitamin D is associated with a low incidence of stress fractures. J Bone Miner Res. 2011;26(10):2371–7.
41. Grados F, Brazier M, Kamel S, Duver S, Heurtebize N, Maamer M, Mathieu M, Garabedian M, Sebert JL, Fardellone P. Effects on bone mineral density of calcium and vitamin D supplementation in elderly women with vitamin D deficiency. Joint Bone Spine. 2003;70(3):203–8.
42. Kim TH, Lee BH, Lee HM, Lee SH, Park JO, Kim HS, Kim SW, Moon SH. Prevalence of vitamin D deficiency in patients with lumbar spinal stenosis and its relationship with pain. Pain Physician. 2013;16(2):165–76.
43. Priemel M, von Domarus C, Klatte TO, Kessler S, Schlie J, Meier S, Proksch N, Pastor F, Netter C, Streichert T, et al. Bone mineralization defects and vitamin D deficiency: histomorphometric analysis of iliac crest bone biopsies and circulating 25-hydroxyvitamin D in 675 patients. J Bone Miner Res. 2010;25(2):305–12.
44. Zhou B, Huang Y, Li H, Sun W, Liu J. Proton-pump inhibitors and risk of fractures: an update meta-analysis. Osteoporos Int. 2016;27(1):339–47.
45. Dipaola CP, Bible JE, Biswas D, Dipaola M, Grauer JN, Rechtine GR. Survey of spine surgeons on attitudes regarding osteoporosis and osteomalacia screening and treatment for fractures, fusion surgery, and pseudoarthrosis. Spine J. 2009;9(7):537–44.
46. Freedman BA, Potter BK, Nesti LJ, Giuliani JR, Hampton C, Kuklo TR. Osteoporosis and vertebral compression fractures-continued missed opportunities. Spine J. 2008;8(5):756–62.
47. Vestergaard P, Rejnmark L, Mosekilde L. Osteoporosis is markedly underdiagnosed: a nationwide study from Denmark. Osteoporos Int. 2005;16(2):134–41.
48. Looker AC, Melton LJ, 3rd, Borrud LG, Shepherd JA: Lumbar spine bone mineral density in US adults: demographic patterns and relationship with femur neck skeletal status. Osteoporos Int 2012, 23(4):1351–1360.

2

Routine versus on demand removal of the syndesmotic screw: a protocol for an international randomised controlled trial (RODEO-trial)

S. A. Dingemans[1], M. F. N. Birnie[1], F. R. K. Sanders[1], M. P. J. van den Bekerom[2], M. Backes[1], E. van Beeck[3], F. W. Bloemers[4], B. van Dijkman[5], E. Flikweert[6], D. Haverkamp[7], H. R. Holtslag[1], J. M. Hoogendoorn[8], P. Joosse[9], M. Parkkinen[10], G. Roukema[11], N. Sosef[12], B. A. Twigt[13], R. N. van Veen[14], A. H. van der Veen[15], J. Vermeulen[12], J. Winkelhagen[16], B. C. van der Zwaard[17], S. van Dieren[1], J. C. Goslings[2] and T. Schepers[1*]

Abstract

Background: Syndesmotic injuries are common and their incidence is rising. In case of surgical fixation of the syndesmosis a metal syndesmotic screw is used most often. It is however unclear whether this screw needs to be removed routinely after the syndesmosis has healed. Traditionally the screw is removed after six to 12 weeks as it is thought to hamper ankle functional and to be a source of pain. Some studies however suggest this is only the case in a minority of patients. We therefore aim to investigate the effect of retaining the syndesmotic screw on functional outcome.

Design: This is a pragmatic international multicentre randomised controlled trial in patients with an acute syndesmotic injury for which a metallic syndesmotic screw was placed. Patients will be randomised to either routine removal of the syndesmotic screw or removal on demand. Primary outcome is functional recovery at 12 months measured with the Olerud-Molander Score. Secondary outcomes are quality of life, pain and costs. In total 194 patients will be needed to demonstrate non-inferiority between the two interventions at 80% power and a significance level of 0.025 including 15% loss to follow-up.

Discussion: If removal on demand of the syndesmotic screw is non-inferior to routine removal in terms of functional outcome, this will offer a strong argument to adopt this as standard practice of care. This means that patients will not have to undergo a secondary procedure, leading to less complications and subsequent lower costs.

Keywords: Syndesmosis, Syndesmotic screw, Routine removal, Removal on demand, Functional outcome

* Correspondence: t.schepers@amc.nl
[1]Department of Surgery, Trauma Unit, Academic Medical Centre, University of Amsterdam, P.O. Box 22660, 1100 DD Amsterdam, The Netherlands
Full list of author information is available at the end of the article

Background

Ankle fractures are among the most common fractures. It is estimated that the incidence of ankle fractures ranges from about 25,000 in the Netherlands to more than five million people in the United States annually and the incidence is rising [1, 2]. Both young and elderly people are at risk for these fractures. In general, younger people are more at risk as a result of a more active lifestyle and elderly people because of poorer bone quality [3, 4]. Approximately half of the patients with an ankle fracture require surgical treatment because of joint instability. In approximately 20% of these fractures there is a concomitant injury of the syndesmosis and syndesmotic repair is indicated [5]. After anatomical reduction a syndesmotic 'positioning screw' is placed through the fibula into the tibia to maintain this reduction and allow the syndesmotic ligaments to heal. Extensive research has been conducted regarding the technical aspects of the placement of the syndesmotic screw. For example, the number of screws, their diameter, the level of placement and whether they should engage three or four cortices have been investigated thoroughly [6–10]. After a period of 8 – 10 weeks the syndesmosis will generally be healed and the screw will lose its function. It is an ongoing discussion whether the syndesmotic screw needs to be removed subsequently. Most surgeons advocate its removal because of suspected impaired range of motion and chance of breakage of the screw [9, 11–13]. During normal ambulation the fibula moves and the syndesmosis widens [14, 15]. The positioning screw is thought to restrict this movement and the screw is therefore removed. However, several case series have shown similar outcomes in patients in which the syndesmotic screw was retained compared to patients in whom the syndesmotic screw was removed [16–18]. The positioning screw is most likely not causing complaints in patients with retained screws because of loosening or breakage of the screw [16, 17, 19, 20]. In a recent systematic review there seemed to be no significant difference in functional outcome between patients undergoing routine removal and patients in whom the syndesmotic screw was only removed in case of symptomatic implants. [21] However, this was only based on one underpowered RCT and several low quality case-series and therefore high-quality evidence on this subject is desirable.

We therefore initiated a randomized controlled trial in which we aim to investigate the effect of 'removal of demand' of the syndesmotic screw(s) compared to 'routine removal' on functional outcome. Furthermore we will investigate the economic effect of leaving the syndesmotic screw(s) in place.

Design

This pragmatic international multicentre randomised controlled trial will randomise between routine- and on demand removal of the syndesmotic screw(s) after placement for a traumatic syndesmotic injury (both isolated syndesmotic injuries and concomitant syndesmotic injuries in ankle fractures). Both teaching and non-teaching hospitals will participate in this study including three academic Level 1 trauma centres in Europe. An overview of participating centres is shown in Table 1.

Participants

The eligible study population will consist of consecutive adult patients with a traumatic syndesmotic injury.

Inclusion criteria

- Placement of one or two metallic syndesmotic screw(s) for an unstable ankle fracture with a syndesmotic injury or an isolated syndesmotic injury
- Syndesmotic screw(s) placed within 2 weeks of the trauma
- Physical condition allows the patient to undergo an elective second procedure (i.e. removal of the screw)

Exclusion criteria

- ISS score > 15
- Injuries to the ipsi- and contralateral side which may hamper rehabilitation
- Other medical conditions which hamper physical rehabilitation (i.e. musculoskeletal disabilities or severe psychological conditions)

Table 1 Participating centres

Academic Medical Centre[a]	Amsterdam, the Netherlands
Bovenij Hospital	Amsterdam, the Netherlands
Catharina Hospital	Eindhoven, the Netherlands
Deventer Hospital	Deventer, the Netherlands
Flevo Hospital	Almere, the Netherlands
Haaglanden MC	The Hague, the Netherlands
Helsinki University Hospital[a]	Helsinki, Finland
Jeroen Bosch Hospital	's-Hertogenbosch, the Netherlands
Maasstad Hospital	Rotterdam, the Netherlands
Noordwest Hospital Group	Alkmaar, the Netherlands
OLVG	Amsterdam, the Netherlands
Slotervaart Hospital	Amsterdam, the Netherlands
Spaarne Hospital	Amsterdam, the Netherlands
VU University Medical Centre[a]	Amsterdam, the Netherlands
Westfries Hospital	Hoorn, the Netherlands

[a]level 1 trauma centres

- Insufficient understanding of the Dutch or English language

Interventions

Patients will be informed about the study by their treating physician following the procedure in which the syndesmotic screw was placed. After this, patients are contacted by the coordinating investigator to request participation in the study. After obtaining signed informed consent patients will be randomly assigned in a 1:1 allocation ratio to one of the following groups:

1) Control group: Routine removal of the syndesmotic screw(s) 8 – 12 weeks following the index procedure

or

2) Intervention group: On demand removal of the syndesmotic screw(s)

Patients in the control group will undergo routine removal of the syndesmotic screw 8 – 12 weeks postoperatively (according to the preference of the treating surgeon). Patients will not undergo routine removal in case of 1) a contra-indication for undergoing a second procedure for example due to a (new) medical condition or 2) explicit request of the patient after consultation of their treating surgeon. In the intervention group the screw will only be removed in case of symptomatic implants, defined as: 1) implants causing pain, 2) implants (suspected of) causing restricted range-of-motion 3) explicit request of the patient 4) an infection or 5) other problems related to the screw such as protruding screw-head. The screw will only be removed after a consultation of the treating surgeon (except in patients who wish to no longer participate in the study). In patients in the control group in whom the syndesmotic screw brakes prior to planned removal, the screw will be left in place and only removed in case of symptoms.

Study procedures

This study is a pragmatic trial, which implies physicians are allowed to follow local guidelines concerning the treatment of these injuries apart from the intervention investigated. Participating centres are however informed that the preferred surgical technique is a tricortical 3.5 mm diameter screw between 2 and 4 cm of the pilon. If a large reduction clamp is used, the preferred technique is the use of a temporary K-wire as 'glide path' [22]. Besides this, participating centres are allowed to choose their own postoperative treatment routine: for example in the use of a cast, non-weight bearing regime and timing of syndesmotic screw removal (within the predefined time window). At 3 months following the index procedure, patients are assessed at the outpatient clinic. Patients are instructed to visit the outpatient clinic sooner in case of any signs of a POWI: warmth, redness, pain, drainage or a fever above 38.5 degrees Celsius. During the visit to the outpatient clinic the patients are seen by their treating physician and the coordinating investigator. The coordinating investigator will document signs of POWI and will determine its presence or any special findings on physical examination. Furthermore patients are requested to fill out several questionnaires (Table 1). At the six and 12 months follow-up, patients are requested to fill out the same questionnaires and the range-of-motion is measured. Follow-up will take place within a window of 2 weeks of the projected follow-up moment.

Randomisation

Randomisation will be stratified by centre and age category (i.e. ≥ 60 years and < 60 years). Randomisation will be blocked within strata. Randomisation sequence is generated by a dedicated computer randomisation software program (CASTOR®, Amsterdam, The Netherlands), ensuring allocation concealment. Randomisation will mostly be performed at the outpatient clinic by coordinating investigator using a dedicated, password protected, SSL–encrypted website.

Primary Outcome

The primary outcome parameter is functional outcome 12 months following the index procedure measured with the Olerud-Molander ankle score (OMAS) (Table 2).

To be able to assess the Minimally Clinical Important Difference of the OMAS, anchor questions will be added to the OMAS at six and 12 months as described by Walenkamp et al. [23].

Secondary outcomes

Secondary outcome measures of the study are:

- Functional outcome with the American Orthopedic Foot and Ankle Hindfoot Score (AOFAS) [24]
- Pain as measured by a ten-point Visual Analog Scale.
- Range of motion, both absolute and as a percentage compared with the uninjured side.
- Postoperative wound infections classified using the criteria as defined by The Centers for Disease Control and Prevention (CDC-criteria) [25]
- Synostosis or recurrent diastasis (as seen on radiographs made in case of symptoms)
- Health-related quality of life as measured by the EQ-5D-5 L questionnaire [26].
- Health care resources utilization (including amongst others; number of visits to the general practitioner

Table 2 Time table and follow-up schedule

RODEO-trial	Enrollment	Randomization / Allocation	Follow-up		
TIMEPOINT	Post-operatively	8 – 12 weeks post-operatively	3 months Post-operatively	6 months Post-operatively	12 months Post-operatively
Enrollment					
Eligibility screening	X				
Informed Consent	X				
Intervention					
Removal of syndesmotic screw (according to randomization)		X			
Assessment					
Plain radiographs	X		X		
OMAS			X	X	X
Visual analogue pain scale (VAS)			X	X	X
Range-of-Motion			X	X	X
POWI			X		
AOFAS			X	X	X
EQ-5D-5 L			X	X	X
i-MCQ			X	X	X
i-PCQ			X	X	X

and use of home care organizations) as measured by way of a combination of the Dutch/English iMTA Medical Consumption Questionnaire (iMCQ) and iMTA Productivity Cost Questionnaire (iPCQ) (only applicable for the Dutch study population).

- Costs (economic evaluation including budget impact analysis): the economic evaluation of the RODEO-trial will be performed as a cost-effectiveness (CEA) as well as a cost-utility (CUA) analysis (only applicable for the Dutch study population).

Furthermore general demographics will be assessed such as age, gender, body mass index, co-morbidities, American Society of Anesthesiologists (ASA) classification, substance abuse, level of activity, bone mineral density (when available), fracture characteristics, surgical characteristics, duration of non-weight bearing period and use of physiotherapy.

Sample size

We based our sample size calculation on a non-inferiority design. The Olerud-Molander score (OMAS) will serve as primary outcome measure. We have used the results from an earlier study on this subject for our sample size calculation [27]. For the sample size calculation we hypothesized an equal OMAS between the two groups. Using a one-sided significance level (α) of 0.025 and a power (ß) of 90% with a standard deviation (SD) of 19 points (derived from the study mentioned before) and setting our non-inferiority limit at 10 a total of 76 patients are needed in each study arm. Taking a 10% loss to follow-up into account, a total number of 167 subjects will be needed to demonstrate non-inferiority between the two treatment strategies. Furthermore we performed a sample size calculation for a subgroup analysis based on age. We hypothesize that the SD will be lower in these subgroups due to increased homogeneity, therefore we have used an SD of 16 for the sample size calculation of the subgroups. Using a significance level (α) of 0.05 and a power (ß) of 90% 88 patients are needed in each subgroup to prove non-inferiority. Taking 10% loss to follow-up into account a total of 193 patients need to be randomized.

Statistical analysis

The primary endpoint will be analysed according to the intention-to-treat and the per-protocol principle, non-inferiority will only be declared if both types of analysis prove non-inferiority. The primary endpoint will be analysed using a one sided test for non-inferiority with an alpha of 0.025. Descriptive methods will be used to assess quality of data, homogeneity of treatment groups and endpoints. Normality of the data will be analysed by visually inspecting the histograms. Secondary outcomes will be analysed using either a t-test or Mann-Whitney U test for continuous data according to the distributing of the data and a Chi Square test for categorical data. Missing data will be handled through multiple imputation with predictive mean matching. All analyses will be performed using the standard statistical software.

Separate analyses will be performed on subgroups based on age. A multivariable analysis will be performed to identify predictors of worse functional outcome.

The CEA and CUA will be performed on the intention to treat data, with a time horizon of 12 months and from a societal perspective. The primary economic outcomes are the costs per quality adjusted life year (QALY) and the costs per point functional recovery improvement. Moreover a budget impact analysis (BIA) will be performed with a time horizon of 4 years. The questionnaires estimating the secondary outcome measures 'resources utilization' and 'costs' will only be used in patients included in the Netherlands due to practical feasibility and to ensure a valid outcome.

Recruitment and consent

The patient will be informed about the RODEO-trial following placement of a syndesmotic screw or when he or she visits the outpatient clinic following surgery and is provided with the patient information letter. Patients will have a minimum of 2 days to decide whether they want to participate or not in the study. For patients recruited directly postoperatively this means they can be included upon their first visit at the outpatient clinic. For patients who are informed for the first time at the outpatient clinic the coordinating investigator will contact them by phone (if the patient agrees to be contacted by phone by the coordinating investigator). Randomisation will take place after they have returned the signed informed consent forms.

Benefits and risks assessment, group relatedness

A recent systematic review suggests that our intervention is safe and has similar functional outcome compared to the routine removal [21]. Subjects will not undergo additional investigations and interventions due to participation in the RODEO-trial and therefore risks to subjects involved in this trial are at least similar to current practice. Potential benefits for subjects in the investigational treatment arm could be a lower risk of surgical site infections and not having to undergo a secondary procedure.

Indemnities

The institutional review board at the AMC has waived liability insurance, because no additional risk can be attributed to participation in this study.

Publication plan

The principal investigator, the study designer and the study coordinator will be named author. All others will obtain group authorship in the study group. All authors including group members are allowed to present the results after approval of the principle investigator.

Discussion

Displayed above is the protocol for an adequately powered study investigating the difference in routine removal versus removal on demand of the syndesmotic screw in ankle injuries. This will be the first RCT able to prove whether a statistically significant and clinically relevant difference exists.

Since this is a pragmatic trial, surgeons are allowed to choose their own postoperative treatment routine. This, combined with the 15 participating centres will result in a variation in for example the use of a cast, the duration of non-weight bearing mobilisation and a minor variation in the timing of the removal of the syndesmotic screw. However, we believe that this situation accurately reflects daily practice, considering that slight variations in post-operative treatment regimens are inevitable.

The inclusion of the University Hospital Helsinki makes this trial international. This greatly improves the external validity of the trial. Not all secondary outcome measures can be used in an international setting. The budget impact analysis and the health care resources utilization for example can only be used for patients in the Netherlands. This is due to practical feasibility but also to ensure a valid outcome. When the same (translated) questionnaire would be used in patients in Finland, results would not be extractable since the costs of healthcare (e.g. a surgical procedure or a visit to the physiotherapist) will not likely be the same as in the Netherlands. However, the participation of a hospital outside of the Netherlands will give us more insight in how to implement the results not just in the Netherlands, but in the rest of Europe as well.

If this trial proves that removal on demand is indeed non-inferior to routine removal of the syndesmotic screw(s) in terms of functional outcome, this will offer a strong argument to adopt this as standard practice of care. It would mean that patients will not have to undergo a secondary procedure, leading to less complications and subsequent lower costs.

Abbreviations

CEA: Cost-effectiveness analysis; CUA: Cost-utility analysis; EQ-5D: EuroQuality of Life-5D; iMCQ: iMTA medical consumption questionnaire; iPCQ: MTA productivity cost questionnaire; N: Number; NA: Not available; POWI: Postoperative wound infection; QALY: Quality adjusted life year; RCT: Randomised controlled trial

Acknowledgements

Not applicable

Funding

Funding for this study was received from ZonMw (Programma Doelmatigheid grant number: 843002705).

Authors' contributions

SD designed the study and drafted the manuscript, MFNB and FRKS participated in drafting the manuscript and are involved in the acquisition of data. MPJB participated in the design of the study, helped the draft and critically revised the manuscript, MB, EB, HRH, SvD and JCG participated in the design of the study and critically revised the manuscript, TS designed the study, helped the draft and critically revised the manuscript. FWB, BD, EF, DH, JMH, PJ, GR, NS, BAT, RNV, AHV, JV, JW, BCZ and MP are involved in the acquisition of data and have critically revised the manuscript for intellectual content. All authors read and approved the final manuscript.

Consent for publication

Not applicable

Competing interests

The authors declare that they have no competing interests.

Author details

[1]Department of Surgery, Trauma Unit, Academic Medical Centre, University of Amsterdam, P.O. Box 22660, 1100 DD Amsterdam, The Netherlands. [2]Department of Orthopedic Surgery, OLVG, P.O. Box 95500, 1090 HM Amsterdam, The Netherlands. [3]Department of Public Health, Erasmus MC, P.O. Box 2040, 3000 CA Rotterdam, The Netherlands. [4]Department of Surgery, Trauma Unit, VU University Medical Centre, P.O. Box 7057, 1007 MB Amsterdam, The Netherlands. [5]Department of Surgery, Flevo Hospital, P.O. Box 3005, 1300 EG Almere, The Netherlands. [6]Department of Surgery, Deventer Hospital, P.O. Box 5001, 7400 GC Deventer, The Netherlands. [7]Department of Surgery, Slotervaart Hospital, P.O. Box 90440, 1006BK Amsterdam, The Netherlands. [8]Department of Surgery, Haaglanden MC, P.O. Box 432, 2501 CK The Hague, The Netherlands. [9]Department of Surgery, Noordwest Hospital Group, P.O. Box 501, 1815 JD Alkmaar, The Netherlands. [10]Department of Orthopaedics and Traumatology, Helsinki University Hospital, Topeliuksenkatu 5, 00260 Helsinki, Finland. [11]Department of Surgery, Maasstad Hospital, P.O. Box 9100, 3007 AC Rotterdam, The Netherlands. [12]Department of Surgery, Spaarne Hospital, P.O. Box 770, 2130 AT Hoofddorp, The Netherlands. [13]Department of Surgery, BovenIJ Hospital, P.O. Box 37610, 1030 BD Amsterdam, The Netherlands. [14]Department of Surgery, OLVG, P.O. Box 95500, 1090 HM Amsterdam, The Netherlands. [15]Department of Surgery, Catharina Hospital, P.O. Box 1350, 5602 ZA Eindhoven, The Netherlands. [16]Department of Surgery, Westfries Hospital, P.O. Box 600, 1620 AR Hoorn, The Netherlands. [17]Department of Orthopaedics, Jeroen Bosch Hospital, P.O. Box 90153, 5200 ME 's-Hertogenbosch, The Netherlands.

References

1. De Boer a S, Schepers T, Panneman MJ, et al. Health care consumption and costs due to foot and ankle injuries in the Netherlands, 1986-2010. BMC Musculoskelet Disord. 2014;15(1):128. https://doi.org/10.1186/1471-2474-15-128.
2. Daly PJ, Fitzgerald RH Jr, Melton LJ, Ilstrup DM. Epidemiology of ankle fractures in Rochester, Minnesota. Acta Orthop Scand. 1987;58(5):539. https://doi.org/10.3109/17453678709146395.
3. Kannus P, Palvanen M, Niemi S, Parkkari J, Järvinen M. Stabilizing incidence of low-trauma ankle fractures in elderly people Finnish statistics in 1970-2006 and prediction for the future. Bone. 2008;43(2):340–2. https://doi.org/10.1016/j.bone.2008.04.015.
4. Robertson GAJ, Wood AM, Aitken SA, et al. Increasing number and incidence of low-trauma ankle fractures in elderly people: Finnish statistics during 1970-2000 and projections for the future. Foot ankle Int. 2002;35(3): 430–3. https://doi.org/10.1177/1071100714546548.
5. van den Bekerom MPJ, Lamme B, Hogervorst M, Bolhuis HW. Which ankle fractures require syndesmotic stabilization? J Foot Ankle Surg. 46(6):456–63. https://doi.org/10.1053/j.jfas.2007.08.009.
6. Schepers T. Acute distal tibiofibular syndesmosis injury: a systematic review of suture-button versus syndesmotic screw repair. Int Orthop. 2012;36(6): 1199–206. https://doi.org/10.1007/s00264-012-1500-2.
7. Schepers T, Van Der Linden H, Van Lieshout EMM, Niesten DD, Van Der Elst M. Technical aspects of the syndesmotic screw and their effect on functional outcome following acute distal tibiofibular syndesmosis injury. Injury. 2014;45(4):775–9. https://doi.org/10.1016/j.injury.2013.09.035.
8. van den Bekerom MPJ, Hogervorst M, Bolhuis HW, van Dijk CN. Operative aspects of the syndesmotic screw: review of current concepts. Injury. 2008; 39(4):491–8. https://doi.org/10.1016/j.injury.2007.11.425.
9. Schepers T, Van Zuuren WJ, Van Den Bekerom MPJ, Vogels LMM, Van Lieshout EMM. The management of acute distal tibio-fibular syndesmotic injuries: results of a nationwide survey. Injury. 2012;43(10):1718–23. https://doi.org/10.1016/j.injury.2012.06.015.
10. Schepers T, Dingemans SA, Rammelt S. Recent developments in the treatment of acute syndesmotic injuries. Fuß Sprunggelenk. 2016;14(2):66–78. https://doi.org/10.1016/j.fuspru.2016.02.004.
11. Schatzker JTM. Fractures of the ankle. In: The rationale of operative fracture care. New York: Springer-Verlag; 2005.
12. Bell DP, Wong MK. Syndesmotic screw fixation in Weber C ankle injuries-should the screw be removed before weight bearing? Injury. 2006;37(9): 891–8. https://doi.org/10.1016/j.injury.2006.02.003.
13. Heim U, Pfeiffer K. Periphere Osteosynthesen. Berlin: Springer-Verlag; 1988.
14. Grath GB. Widening of the ankle mortise. A clinical and experimental study. Acta Chir Scand Suppl. 1960;Suppl 263:1–88.
15. Close JR. Some applications of the functional anatomy of the ankle joint. J Bone Joint Surg Am. 1956;38-A(4):761–81.
16. Manjoo A, Sanders DW, Tieszer C, MacLeod MD. Functional and radiographic results of patients with syndesmotic screw fixation: implications for screw removal. J Orthop Trauma. 2010;24(1):2–6. https://doi.org/10.1097/BOT.0b013e3181a9f7a5.
17. Weening B, Bhandari M. Predictors of functional outcome following transsyndesmotic screw fixation of ankle fractures. J Orthop Trauma. 2005; 19(2):102–8.
18. de Souza LJ, Gustilo RB, Meyer TJ. Results of operative treatment of displaced external rotation-abduction fractures of the ankle. J Bone Joint Surg Am. 1985;67(7):1066–74.
19. Hamid N, Loeffler BJ, Braddy W, et al. Outcome after fixation of ankle fractures with an injury to the syndesmosis: the effect of the syndesmosis screw. J Bone Joint Surg Br. 2009;91(8):1069–73. https://doi.org/10.1302/0301-620X.91B8.22430.
20. Kaftandziev I, Spasov M, Trpeski S, Zafirova-Ivanovska B, Bakota B. Fate of the syndesmotic screw-search for a prudent solution. Injury. 2015;46:S125–9. https://doi.org/10.1016/j.injury.2015.10.062.
21. Dingemans SA, Rammelt S, White TO, Goslings JC, Schepers T. Should syndesmotic screws be removed after surgical fixation of unstable ankle fractures?: a systematic review. Bone Joint J. 2016;98-B(11):1497–504. https://doi.org/10.1302/0301-620X.98B11.BJJ-2016-0202.R1.
22. Needleman RL. Accurate reduction of an ankle syndesmosis with the "glide path" technique. Foot Ankle Int. 2013;34(9):1308–11. https://doi.org/10.1177/1071100713485740.
23. Walenkamp MMJ, de Muinck Keizer R-J, Goslings JC, Vos LM, Rosenwasser MP, Schep NWL. The minimum clinically important difference of the patient-rated wrist evaluation score for patients with distal radius fractures. Clin Orthop Relat Res. 2015;473(10):3235–41. https://doi.org/10.1007/s11999-015-4376-9.
24. Kitaoka HB, Alexander IJ, Adelaar RS, Nunley JA, Myerson MS, Sanders M. Clinical rating systems for the ankle-hindfoot, midfoot, hallux, and lesser toes. Foot ankle Int. 1994;15(7):349–53.
25. Berríos-Torres SI, Umscheid CA, Bratzler DW, et al. Centers for Disease Control and Prevention guideline for the prevention of surgical site infection, 2017. JAMA Surg. 2017; https://doi.org/10.1001/jamasurg.2017.0904.
26. Rabin R, de Charro F. EQ-5D: a measure of health status from the EuroQol group. Ann Med. 2001;33(5):337–43.
27. Boyle MJ, Gao R, Frampton CM, Coleman B. Removal of the syndesmotic screw after the surgical treatment of a fracture of the ankle in adult patients does not affect one-year outcomes: a randomised controlled trial. Bone Joint J. 2014;96-B(12):1699–705. https://doi.org/10.1302/0301-620X.96B12.34258.

3

Reconstruction of iliac crest defect after autogenous harvest with bone cement and screws reduces donor site pain

Jing Zhang[1†], Yuxuan Wei[1†], Yue Gong[2], Yang Dong[1*] and Zhichang Zhang[1*]

Abstract

Background: The iliac crest is the most common autogenous bone graft donor site, although associated with postoperative pain, functional disability, cosmesis, morphology and surgical satisfaction. We assessed each aspect above by comparing iliac crest reconstruction with bone cement and screws following harvest with no reconstruction.

Methods: We evaluated patients who underwent large iliac crest harvesting, including ten patients who underwent iliac crest defect reconstruction with bone cement and cancellous screws (R group) and ten randomly matched patients without reconstruction (NR group) were evaluated prospectively in the same period. Local pain, cosmesis and other complications were assessed postoperatively at 1 week, 6 weeks, 3 months and 6 months.

Results: Pain, cosmesis and satisfaction of patients significantly differed between the two groups. The R group exhibited less complications and lower pain visual analogue scores at postoperative 1 week ($p < 0.001$), 6 weeks ($p < 0.001$) and 3 months ($p < 0.01$) but not at 6 months, at which time patients reported almost no pain. One patient reported pain for more than 1 year in the NR group. The R group exhibited better cosmesis, morphology and satisfaction than the NR group. In the NR group, one patient suffered pain when sitting up and another when wearing a belt.

Conclusion: Postoperative pain can be reduced and cosmesis can be improved through reconstructing the iliac crest defects after autogenous harvesting with bone cement and cancellous screws. The technique is simple, safe and easy to implement.

Keywords: Iliac crest bone graft, Morbidity, Reconstruction of donor site, Bone cement

Background

Autogenous bone grafts are widely used in clinical orthopedics due to their biological and nonimmunologic properties compared with other materials. The iliac crest is the most common donor site because of its easy access, low morbidity and ability to provide sufficient quantities of both cortical and cancellous bone [1]. However, complication rates following iliac crest bone harvesting have been reported from 2 to 49%. Most patients suffer from pain which has an effect on sleep within 1 month after surgery, and even 13 to 20% of the patients experience chronic pain [2, 3]. The most common complication is pain at the donor site after that less frequently complications including secondary fracture, superficial numbness, infection, abdominal hernia and gait abnormality [4–6]. In addition, harvesting a large graft from iliac crest bone leads to some problems such as depression of surgical area, poor cosmetic appearance, having influence on walking, recreation, household chores and so on [2].

Some studies have indicated that reconstruction of iliac crest defects after harvesting can reduce complications [7–10]. Various implantation materials and techniques have been used to rebuild iliac defects. Burton and colleagues [11] reconstructed the iliac crest with a hydroxyapatite-calcium triphosphate

* Correspondence: dongyang6405@163.com; zzc_sjtu@sjtu.edu.cn
†Jing Zhang and Yuxuan Wei contributed equally to this work.
[1]Department of Orthopaedic Surgery, Shanghai Jiao Tong University Affiliated Sixth People's Hospital, Shanghai 200233, China
Full list of author information is available at the end of the article

biphasic compound, which improved the body's ability to reform new bone but did not alleviate the pain. Furthermore, the technique is only suitable for harvesting parts of cancellous bones. Other studies have been carried out for the repair of iliac crest defects using autogenous bone [7], bovine cancellous grafts [9], polymethyl methacrylate bone cement [12] and allografts fixed with cannulated screws [10]. Although such studies provided some options to reduce the donor site pain, we still try to find a more simple and effective method.

In this study, we used a new technique with bone cement and screws to repair large iliac bicortical bone defects after autogenous harvesting for bone tumors, such as giant cell tumors of bone or other benign tumors. The purpose of this study was to evaluate the benefits of this new method.

Methods

Study population

Patients who underwent autogenous iliac crest grafting to repair a bone defect or nonunion after primary bone tumor excision in 2016 were selected for inclusion in this trial. The following inclusion criteria were utilized for patient selection: surgical treatment with a large iliac crest graft for repair of a bone defect or nonunion association with primary bone tumor excision; harvest of more than 40 mm × 30 mm of iliac crest; and patients aged between 18 and 60 years old. Patients with osteoporosis or who could not tolerate the surgery for iliac crest reconstruction were not included. That patients were asked whether they wanted to receive conventional procedures or the new method prior the study took place and that the control group was matched after the study population for the new method was gathered.

Twenty patients were included in this study. Ten patients who conducted reconstruction were allocated to the reconstructed group (R group) and were compared with 10 patients whose iliac crest defect was not reconstructed (NR group). All surgical procedures were performed by the same chief surgeon.

Operation technique

Both groups underwent the same procedure of the harvest. The volume of the bone graft depended on the volume of the tumor. The iliac crest graft harvest was on the same side as the bone tumor. In supine position, a skin incision was made along iliac crest contour. We dissected soft tissue and harvested the required amount of iliac crest using an osteotome from 3 cm posterior to the anterior superior iliac spine (Fig. 1a). In the R group, according to the harvesting size, three or more cancellous screws were implanted leaving 2—3 cm of head end out of the bone as an anchor providing support and adhesion for the bone cement (Fig. 1b). The defect area was filled with bone cement which was formed into the shape of the iliac crest contour (Fig. 1c). Careful attention was paid to ensure that the cement did not extend beyond the original shape of the bone to avoid discomfort. After the bone cement had solidified, a drainage tube was placed, and the incision was closed. The only difference between the two groups was that the defect of the iliac crest was reconstructed in the R group, whereas no reconstruction was performed in the NR group.

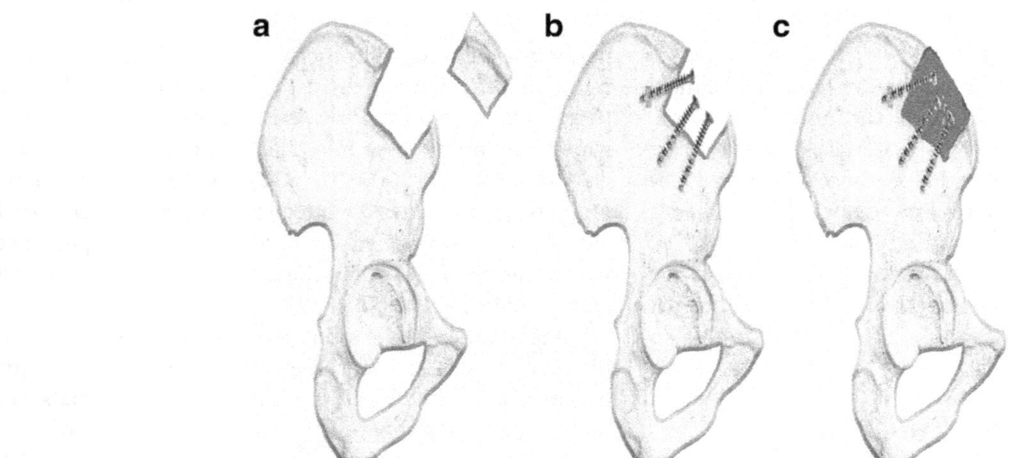

Fig. 1 The procedure of reconstruction of the iliac crest after autografting. **a** the defect after the iliac crest harvesting. **b** Cancellous screws were implanted leaving 2—3 cm of head out of the bone as an anchor. **c** Filled bone cement into the defect and shaped them into the shape of the iliac crest contour making ensure that the cement did not extend beyond the original shape

Table 1 The clinical assessment contents and criteria

Pain VAS	Range of 0 to 10(0 indicates no pain, 10 indicates the worst pain imaginable)
Function disability	Sitting up
	Wearing a belt
	Sleep on the operation side
Cosmesis of the operated side	Range of 0 to 10 (10 indicates that the appearance is almost no different from the contralateral side. 0 means very bad)
Depression of the defect	The same as the contralateral side (depression < 1 cm, normal)
	Depressed compared with the contralateral side(> 1 cm, depression)
Surgical satisfaction scale	Range of 0 to 10(10 indicates it' s very satisfied. 0 indicates it' s not satisfied at all)

Assessment

Postoperative pain was evaluated using the pain visual analog scale (pain VAS) in both groups at 1 week, 6 weeks, 3 months and 6 months after the surgery. Functional disability was evaluated based on the pain of the patients reported when they performed 3 daily activities: sitting up, wearing a belt, and sleeping on the operation side. Cosmesis of the operated site, morphology of the defect, and surgical satisfaction scale (SSS) were only assessed at 6 months (Table 1). Complications were recorded during the follow-up and a radiologic evaluation was performed using posterior-anterior radiograph images of the pelvis at 1 week, 6 weeks, 3 months and 6 months after the surgery.

Differences between groups were analyzed using Student's t-test and Fisher's exact test. All statistical analyses were performed using SPSS 20.0 software (SPSS Inc., Chicago, IL). $P < 0.05$ was considered as statistically significant.

Results

The demographic data between the two groups had no significant differences, as presented in Table 2. The pain VAS of the R group was 1.1 ± 0.53, markedly lower than that of the NR group of 4.3 ± 0.48 ($p < 0.001$) at 1 week after surgery. Similarly, the VAS score showed significant differences between the two groups at 6 weeks (0.3 ± 0.46 vs 1.8 ± 0.42, $p < 0.001$) and 3 months (0 vs 0.8 ± 0.63, $p < 0.01$). In comparison to the R group where no patient suffered from pain after 6 months ($p = 0.29$, Fig. 2). However, one patient suffered from pain for more than 1 year in the NR group.

Complications in the R group included one patient who reported thigh numbness and one who reported slight pain when wearing a waist belt during the first 6 months postoperatively, which were alleviated by the sixth month. On the other hand, two patients reported numbness on the outside of the thigh in the NR group. One patient suffered pain when wearing a waist belt and another patient reported ache when sitting up.

There was a significant difference between the two groups in cosmesis assessment. The mean score of cosmesis was 9.6 in the R group, which was significantly higher than that of the NR group of 7.5 ($p < 0.001$). The result of SSS was consistent with the cosmesis score (Fig. 3). The morphology of the two groups was also significantly different. In the R group, there was no depression, whereas 9 cases of depression appeared in the NR group ($p < 0.001$, Table 2).

Posterior-anterior radiograph images of the pelvis were assessed postoperatively during the 6 months. There was no secondary fracture of bone or dislocation or fractured bone cement in both groups (Fig. 4).

Discussion

The iliac crest remains the most frequently site for autogenous grafts with many advantages compared with other sites such as distal radius and artificial bone. However, postoperative pain and poor cosmesis are major deterrents in harvesting bone from the iliac crest. Different methods have been used to solve these problems, such as injection of local anesthetic which have achieved different levels of success [1, 13]. However, the results were still not satisfying because of the problems mentioned above. Therefore, some researchers have attempted to reconstruct the iliac crest after harvesting bone and discovered that it could alleviate donor site pain and access good cosmesis [8, 10, 14, 15].

In our study, we used bone cement and cancellous screws to reconstruct the defect of the iliac crest after

Table 2 The demographic data of all patients

	R group	NR group	*P* values
Number of patients	10	10	
Age(years)	38.7 ± 14.2(18–59)	36 ± 10.2(24–53)	$p = 0.634$
Sex (F:M)	5:5	6:4	$P = 1$
Average size of iliac crest defect(cm^2)	14.55 ± 2.0	13.5 ± 1.6	$p = 0.297$

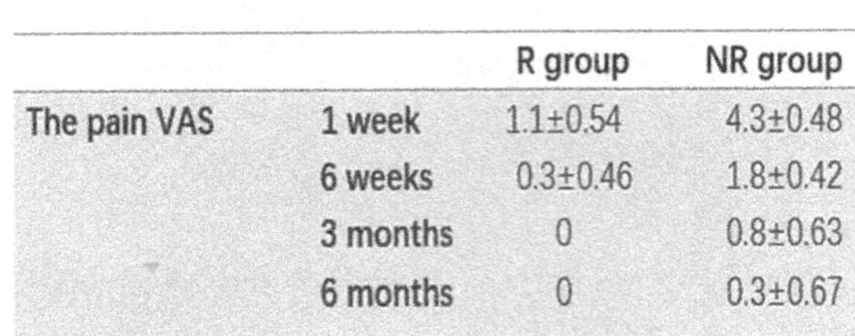

		R group	NR group
The pain VAS	1 week	1.1±0.54	4.3±0.48
	6 weeks	0.3±0.46	1.8±0.42
	3 months	0	0.8±0.63
	6 months	0	0.3±0.67

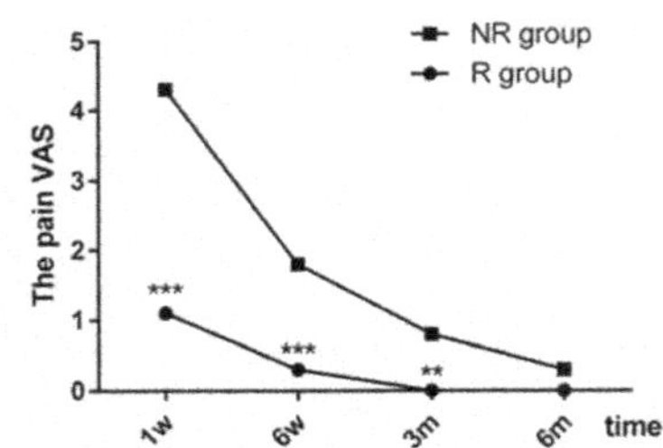

Fig. 2 The pain VAS scores between the two groups during the postoperative 6 months. The pain VAS between the R group and the NR group was 1.1 ± 0.53 vs 4.3 ± 0.48, 0.3 ± 0.46 vs 1.8 ± 0.42, 0 vs 0.8 ± 0.63 and 0 vs 0.3 ± 0.67 at 1 week, 6 weeks, 3 months and 6 months after surgery. ** $p < 0.01$, *** $p < 0.001$

harvesting. The result of this study revealed significant differences between the two groups at postoperative 1 week, 6 weeks and 3 months. No patient experienced chronic pain in the R group compared with the NR group. The results of other complications, cosmesis and satisfaction in the R group were better than those in the NR group.

Some researchers reconstructed the iliac crest after autografting using different methods and materials [10, 12]. Y-F Niu and colleagues shaped the allograft iliac crest to match the defect and reconstructed the anatomical contour, and then they fixed the allograft with hollow compression screws [10]. Jong Seong Lee and colleagues harvested a wedge of iliac crest with a bone burr on each wall and filled the defect with bone cement [12]. The results of theirs were similar in postoperative pain, cosmesis and additional complications. Both of them significantly reduced postoperative pain and yielded good cosmesis without increasing other adverse events.

Nonetheless, our method shows some improvements compared to the methods above. Bone cement is easier to obtain than matched iliac crest allografts which are difficult to acquire and carry exorbitant prices, often influencing some patients to refuse the reconstruction. Therefore, the surgery can be carried out in most hospitals. We were able to harvest autologous iliac crest grafts of different sizes and shapes because of the plasticity of bone cement. The surgical procedure is simple and generally takes less time. Compared to the research conducted by Jong Seong Lee et al., we added cancellous screws as a framework to provide an anchor for the bone cement and to prevent displacement and loosening; furthermore, bone cement is not limited to a particular shape.

The causes of postoperative pain after iliac crest harvesting are not clear, although we suspect that postoperative pain may be closely related to the following factors. The process of iliac crest harvesting causes damage to bone and soft tissue, and different sizes of autografts may lead to different degrees of pain [16]. The micromotion of the fracture, stimulation of the bone stump to the soft tissue, and adhesion and scarring of soft tissue are the main causes of postoperative pain. In our study, the decrease in pain may be related to the following factors. Firm fixation of the bone cement is the main reason, which can prevent micromotion of the fracture or between the bone cement and the walls of the bone defect. Bone cement reconstructs the anatomical shape of the iliac crest to reduce irritation to soft tissue. Careful separation of soft tissue and effective stitching can also prevent tissue adhesion and formation of scar.

Reconstruction of iliac crest donor site defects not only alleviates pain but also improves cosmesis and satisfaction. There was no collapse or displacement of implants, which could result in re-operation during the follow-up period, as reported by Jong Seong Lee et al. [12]. We believe that this method of reconstruction is

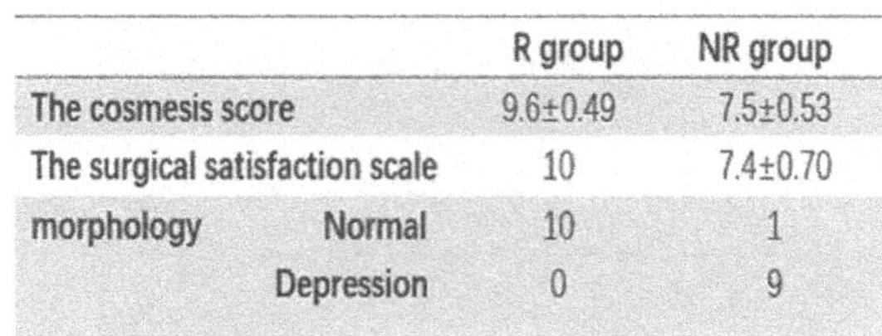

		R group	NR group
The cosmesis score		9.6±0.49	7.5±0.53
The surgical satisfaction scale		10	7.4±0.70
morphology	Normal	10	1
	Depression	0	9

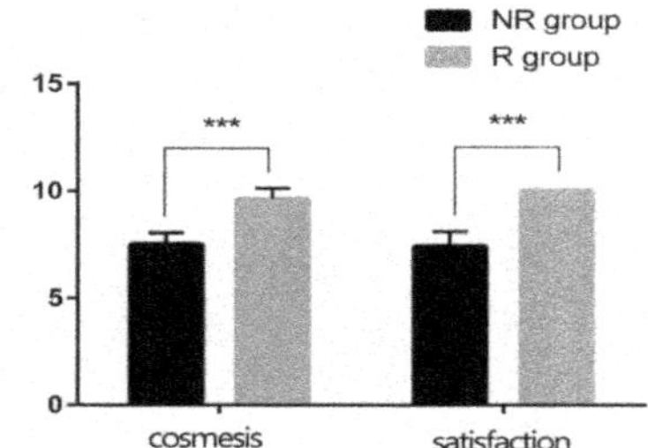

Fig. 3 Cosmesis and surgical satisfaction scale scores between the two groups at postoperative 6 months. The cosmesis score between R group and NR group was 9.6 ± 0.49 vs 7.5 ± 0.53 and the SSS was 10 vs 7.4 ± 0.70. *** $p < 0.001$

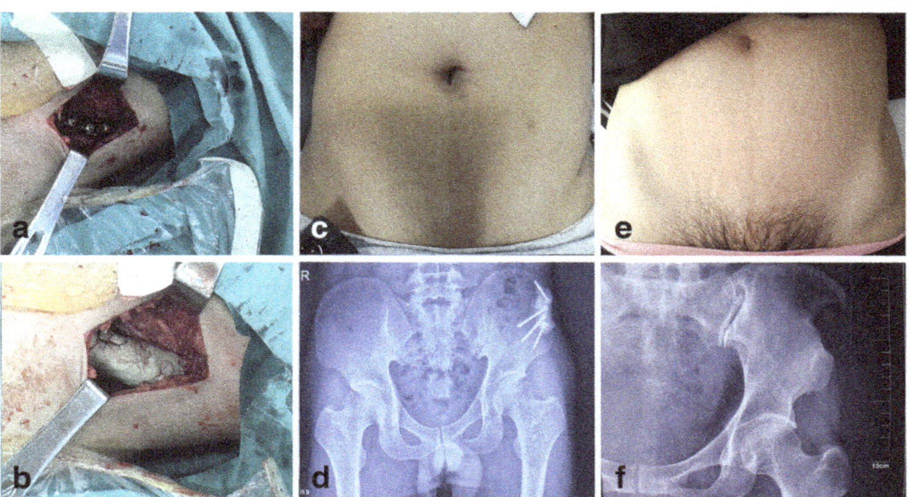

Fig. 4 A 40 years old male (**a, b, c, d**) in R group and a 47 years old female (**e, f**) in NR group, who were diagnosed with giant cell tumor of distal femur, experienced curettage of bone tumor and iliac crest graft. **a** The screws are implanted after iliac crest harvesting. **b** Bone cement is filled into the defect area. **c** The cosmesis and morphology of the surgical area compared with contralateral. **d** posterior-anterior radiograph images of the pelvis at 6 months after surgical reconstruction. **e** and **f**, The cosmesis of the surgical area compared with contralateral and posterior-anterior radiograph images of the pelvis at 1 year after surgery without reconstruction

more reliable which like a reinforced concrete structure, providing sufficient stability. In addition, this method could prevent some complications such as abdominal hernia theoretically.

This study still has some limitations. Although the results show that patients can benefit from reconstruction of the defect, the sample size was relatively small. Longer follow-up periods may discover additional differences, despite the reported advantages and disadvantages. More careful operation could avoid some complications, such as superficial numbness. In summary, a prospective randomized study with a larger sample and a longer follow-up are necessary. In addition, it should be considered whether pain is associated with the style of surgery that the patient underwent.

Conclusions

Postoperative pain can be reduced and cosmesis can be improved through reconstructing the iliac crest defects after autogenous harvesting with bone cement and cancellous screws. The technique is simple, safe and easy to be implanted, making it possible to be performed in most hospitals. However, a larger sample of patients and a prospective, controlled study are necessary to verify and extend our results.

Abbreviations

NR group: The not reconstructed group; pain VAS: The pain visual analog scale; R group: The reconstructed group; SSS: Surgical satisfaction scale

Acknowledgements

The authors would like to thank all patients who participated in the study.

Funding

No funding was obtained for this study.

Authors' contributions

Conception and design: ZZ, YD and JZ. Performed the surgery: ZZ. Development of methodology: JZ, YW and YG. Acquisition of data: JZ and YW. Analysis and interpretation of data: JZ, YW and YG. Writing, review, and/or revision of manuscript: ZZ, YD, JZ, YW and YG. Study supervision: ZZ, YD. All authors read and approved the final manuscript.

Consent for publication

Participators agreed to publication and signed the consent.

Competing interests

The authors declare that they have no competing interest.

Author details

[1]Department of Orthopaedic Surgery, Shanghai Jiao Tong University Affiliated Sixth People's Hospital, Shanghai 200233, China. [2]Department of Breast Surgery, Key Laboratory of Breast Cancer in Shanghai, Fudan University Shanghai Cancer Center, Fudan University, Shanghai 200032, China.

References

1. Zenner J, Hitzl W, Mayer M, Koller H. Analysis of postoperative pain at the anterior iliac crest harvest site: a prospective study of the intraoperative local administration of ropivacaine. Asian Spine J. 2015;9(1):39–46.
2. Kim DH, Rhim R, Li L, Martha J, Swaim BH, Banco RJ, Jenis LG, Tromanhauser SG. Prospective study of iliac crest bone graft harvest site pain and morbidity. Spine J. 2009;9(11):886–92.
3. Armaghani SJ, Even JL, Zern EK, Braly BA, Kang JD, Devin CJ. The evaluation of donor site pain after harvest of Tricortical anterior iliac crest bone graft for spinal surgery: a prospective study. Spine (Phila Pa 1976). 2016;41(4): E191–6.
4. Willcox MJ. Lumbar herniation of kidney following iliac crest bone harvest. Case Rep Surg. 2016;2016:5365647.
5. Fasolis M, Boffano P, Ramieri G. Morbidity associated with anterior iliac crest bone graft. Oral Surg Oral Med Oral Pathol Oral Radiol. 2012;114(5):586–91.

6. Zermatten P, Wettstein M. Iliac wing fracture following graft harvesting from the anterior iliac crest: literature review based on a case report. Orthop Traumatol Surg Res. 2012;98(1):114–7.
7. Defino HL, Rodriguez-Fuentes AE. Reconstruction of anterior iliac crest bone graft donor sites: presentation of a surgical technique. Eur Spine J. 1999;8(6): 491–4.
8. Chau AM, Xu LL, van der Rijt R, Wong JH, Gragnaniello C, Stanford RE, Mobbs RJ. Reconstruction versus no reconstruction of iliac crest defects following harvest for spinal fusion: a systematic review: a review. J Neurosurg Spine. 2012;16(6):565–72.
9. Makridis KG, Ahmad MA, Kanakaris NK, Fragkakis EM, Giannoudis PV. Reconstruction of iliac crest with bovine cancellous allograft after bone graft harvest for symphysis pubis arthrodesis. Int Orthop. 2012;36(8):1701–7.
10. Niu YF, An XF, Wu DJ, Xu SG, Zhang CC, Li M. Anatomical reconstruction of donor site after large iliac crest graft harvest with equivalent iliac crest allograft. A prospective controlled study. Eur Rev Med Pharmacol Sci. 2013; 17(14):1951–7.
11. Burton DC, Carlson BB, Johnson PL, Manna BJ, Riazi-Kermani M, Glattes RC, Jackson RS. Backfilling of iliac crest defects with hydroxyapatite-calcium triphosphate biphasic compound: a prospective, randomized computed tomography and patient-based analysis. Spine J. 2013;13(1):54–61.
12. Lee JS, Park YJ, Wang L, Chang YS, Shetty GM, Nha KW. Modified iliac crest reconstruction with bone cement for reduction of donor site pain and morbidity after open wedge high Tibial osteotomy: a prospective study. Knee Surg Relat Res. 2016;28(4):277–82.
13. O'Neill KR, Lockney DT, Bible JE, Crosby CG, Devin CJ. Bupivacaine for pain reduction after iliac crest bone graft harvest. Orthopedics. 2014;37(5): e428–34.
14. Resnick DK. Reconstruction of anterior iliac crest after bone graft harvest decreases pain: a randomized, controlled clinical trial. Neurosurgery. 2005; 57(3):526–9. discussion 526-529
15. Bapat MR, Chaudhary K, Garg H, Laheri V. Reconstruction of large iliac crest defects after graft harvest using autogenous rib graft: a prospective controlled study. Spine (Phila Pa 1976). 2008;33(23):2570–5.
16. Pirris SM, Nottmeier EW, Kimes S, O'Brien M, Rahmathulla G. A retrospective study of iliac crest bone grafting techniques with allograft reconstruction: do patients even know which iliac crest was harvested? Clinical article. J Neurosurg Spine. 2014;21(4):595–600.

4

Distribution of ossified spinal lesions in patients with severe ossification of the posterior longitudinal ligament and prediction of ossification at each segment based on the cervical OP index classification: a multicenter study (JOSL CT study)

Takashi Hirai[1,23*], Toshitaka Yoshii[1,23], Narihito Nagoshi[2], Kazuhiro Takeuchi[3,23], Kanji Mori[4,23], Shuta Ushio[1,23], Akio Iwanami[2], Tsuyoshi Yamada[1,23], Shoji Seki[5,23], Takashi Tsuji[6,23], Kanehiro Fujiyoshi[7,23], Mitsuru Furukawa[8,23], Soraya Nishimura[2,9,23], Kanichiro Wada[10,23], Takeo Furuya[11,23], Yukihiro Matsuyama[12,23], Tomohiko Hasegawa[12,23], Katsushi Takeshita[13,23], Atsushi Kimura[13,23], Masahiko Abematsu[14,23], Hirotaka Haro[15,23], Tetsuro Ohba[15,23], Masahiko Watanabe[16,23], Hiroyuki Katoh[16,23], Kei Watanabe[17,23], Hiroshi Ozawa[18,23], Haruo Kanno[19,23], Shiro Imagama[20,23], Kei Ando[20,23], Shunsuke Fujibayashi[21,23], Masao Koda[22,23], Masashi Yamazaki[22,23], Morio Matsumoto[2], Masaya Nakamura[2], Atsushi Okawa[1,23] and Yoshiharu Kawaguchi[5,23]

Abstract

Background: In patients with ossification of the posterior longitudinal ligament (OPLL) in the cervical spine, it is well known that the thoracic ossified lesions often coexist with the cervical lesions and can cause severe myelopathy. However, the prevalence of OPLL at each level of the thoracic and lumbar spinal segments is unknown. The aims of this study were to investigate how often OPLL occurs at each level in the thoracolumbar spine in patients with a radiological diagnosis of cervical OPLL and to identify the spinal levels most likely to develop ossification.

Methods: Data were collected from 20 institutions in Japan. Three hundred and twenty-two patients with a diagnosis of cervical OPLL were included. The OPLL index (OP index), defined as the sum of the vertebral body and intervertebral disc levels where OPLL is present, was used to determine disease severity. An OP index ≥20 was defined as severe OPLL. The prevalence of OPLL at each level of the thoracic and lumbar spinal segments was calculated.

(Continued on next page)

* Correspondence: hirai.orth@tmd.ac.jp
[1]Department of Orthopedic Surgery, Tokyo Medical and Dental University, 1-5-45 Yushima, Bunkyo-ku, Tokyo 113-8519, Japan
[23]Japanese Organization of the Study for Ossification of Spinal Ligament (JOSL), 1-5-45 Yushima, Bunkyo-ku, Tokyo 113-8519, Japan
Full list of author information is available at the end of the article

(Continued from previous page)

Results: Women were more likely to have ossified lesions in the thoracolumbar spine than men. Severe OPLL was significantly more common in women than in men (20% vs. 4.5%). For thoracic vertebral OPLL, the most frequently affected was the T1 segment in both men and women, followed by the T1/2 and T3/4 intervertebral levels in men and women, respectively. Ossified lesions were frequently seen at the intervertebral and vertebral levels around the cervicothoracic and thoracolumbar junctions in men with severe OPLL, whereas OPLL was more diffusely distributed in the thoracic spine in women with severe OPLL.

Conclusion: Thoracolumbar OPLL occurred most often at T1 in men and at T3/4 in women. In severe OPLL cases, although ossified lesions were frequently seen at the intervertebral and vertebral levels around the cervicothoracic and thoracolumbar junctions in men, OPLL could be observed more diffusely in the thoracic spine in women.

Keywords: OPLL, Computed tomography, Whole spine, Ossification predisposition, Prevalence,

Background

Ossification of the spinal ligaments is a form of heterotopic ossification that occurs throughout the spine. Ossification of the posterior longitudinal ligament (OPLL) involves the spinal canal and often leads to myelopathy [1, 2]. Cervical OPLL, which can be detected easily on plain radiographs, has been investigated in detail as far back as the nineteenth century [3]. Ossified lesions in the thoracic spine sometimes coexist with cervical OPLL and cause severe symptoms. However, it is difficult to diagnose pathologic conditions of the thoracic spine on radiographs alone, so the prevalence of thoracic OPLL remains unclear [4]. Recently, multidetector computed tomography (CT) has been found to be the most suitable modality for identifying ossification in the thoracic spine, regardless of any superimposed thoracic complexities. Nevertheless, there is no detailed multicenter research on the prevalence of thoracolumbar OPLL. The purpose of this study was to investigate the prevalence of ossified lesions in the thoracolumbar spine in patients with cervical OPLL at multiple institutions. We also investigated how frequently OPLL occurred at each spinal level and attempted to clarify which levels of the spine are more predisposed to OPLL lesions.

Methods

Patients and methods

The study included patients with a radiographic diagnosis of OPLL involving the cervical spine as well as symptoms, such as neck pain, numbness in the upper and/or lower extremities, and clumsiness or gait disturbance. Each patient underwent whole-spine CT imaging at any one of the 20 institutions where members of the research team worked. Patients who had undergone anterior decompression surgery for OPLL and patients younger than 15 years of age were excluded. Four hundred and fifty-six patients with OPLL were identified, of whom only 322 had full demographic and anthropometric data available for analysis (Fig. 1). The study involved

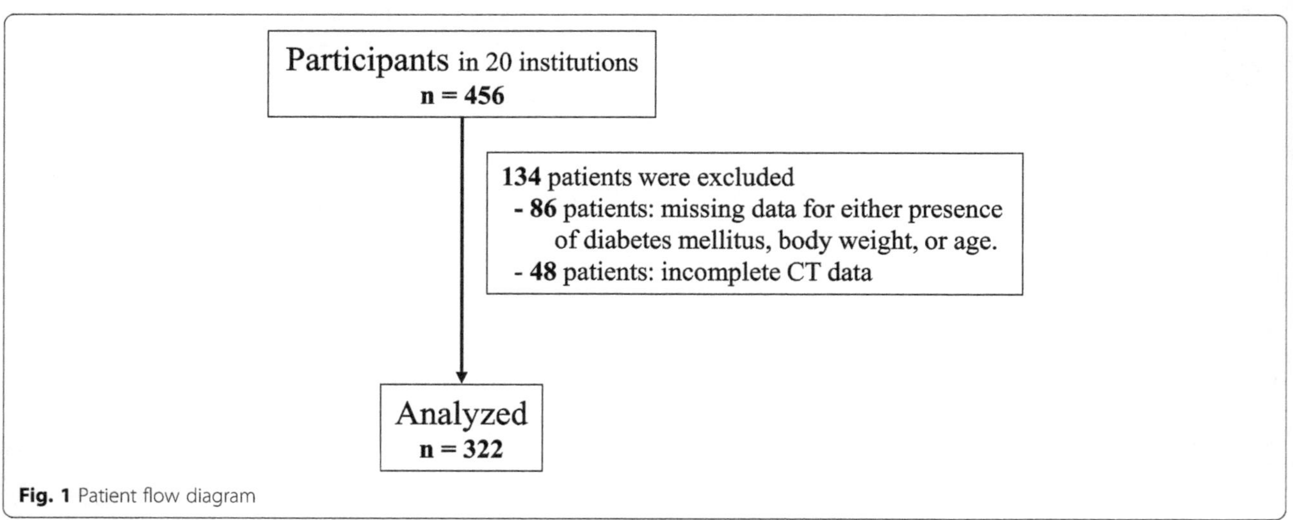

Fig. 1 Patient flow diagram

Table 1 Demographics of male and female patients

	Male + Female ($n = 322$)	Male ($n = 242$)	Female ($n = 80$)	P (M vs F)
Age (years old)	64.7 ± 11.2	64.7 ± 11.6	64.6 ± 10.0	0.90
Diabetes Mellitus (%)	31.7%	31.8%	31.3%	0.92
BMI	25.7 ± 4.8	25.8 ± 4.8	25.5 ± 4.7	0.62
JOSL CT classification				
Grade 1 (1 < cervical OP-index≤5)	169 (52.5%)	125 (51.7%)	44 (55%)	–
Grade 2 (6 < cervical OP-index ≤9)	107 (33.2%)	83 (34.3%)	24 (30%)	–
Grade 3 (10 < cervical OP-index)	46 (14.3%)	34 (14.0%)	12 (15%)	–
Cervical OP-index	5.83 ± 2.9	5.86 ± 2.9	5.75 ± 3.0	0.78
OP-index	9.21 ± 6.8	8.24 ± 5.5	12.1 ± 9.0	< 0.01
No. of patients with OP-index of > = 20 (%)	27 (8.3%)	11 (4.5%)	16 (20%)	< 0.01

Data are expressed as the mean ± standard deviation; *BMI* body mass index, *OP-index* ossification index of OPLL

242 men and 80 women with a mean age of 64.6 (range 30–93) years. The study was approved by the institutional review board at each institution. Informed consent was obtained from all patients before enrollment in the study.

Evaluations

Basic clinical data were collected for all patients, including for age, sex, presence of diabetes, and body mass index (BMI). CT images of the cervical, thoracic, and lumbosacral spine, from the occipital bone to the sacrum, were obtained in each patient. The prevalence of OPLL in the cervical spine from the clivus to C7 and in other spinal regions from T1 to S1 was evaluated on mid-sagittal CT images. The analysis was independently performed by five senior spine surgeons (TH, KT, KM, AI, TY). Prior to reviewing the images for this study, all of the readers interpreted the same images for 20 patients to check interobserver agreement. The average kappa coefficient was 0.76 (0.71–0.81), which indicated good agreement and was consistent with the findings of a previous study [5]. Ossified lesions were recorded at each vertebral body and at the intervertebral disc level. An OPLL index (OP index) [5], defined as the sum of the vertebral body and intervertebral disc levels where OPLL is present, was calculated according to the method described in a previous report [5]. Patients with an OP index ≥20 were deemed to have severe OPLL. We also defined the sum of the levels at which OPLL was present in the cervical spine as the cervical OP index. Using a previously reported method [6], we divided patients into three groups according to their cervical OP index values, namely, grade 1 (≤5), grade 2 (6–9), and grade 3 (≥10). The physical and radiologic data were compared between the male and female patient populations. Furthermore, we investigated whether there was an association between the cervical

Table 2 Incidence of ossified lesion in each level

Incidence	Male + Female		Male		Female	
Segment	total	OS>20	total	OS>20	total	OS>20
C1	10.2%	7.4%	11.6%	0.0%	6.3%	12.5%
C2	41.6%	74.1%	43.0%	72.7%	37.5%	75.0%
C2-3	40.7%	77.8%	40.1%	63.6%	42.5%	87.5%
C3	57.5%	85.2%	59.1%	81.8%	52.5%	87.5%
C3-4	42.2%	63.0%	41.7%	81.8%	43.8%	50.0%
C4	72.7%	85.2%	73.1%	81.8%	71.3%	87.5%
C4-5	37.0%	63.0%	36.4%	72.7%	38.8%	56.3%
C5	79.5%	85.2%	82.2%	90.9%	71.3%	81.3%
C5-6	41.9%	81.5%	41.3%	90.9%	43.8%	75.0%
C6	71.7%	92.6%	71.5%	100.0%	72.5%	87.5%
C6-7	32.3%	74.1%	31.8%	100.0%	33.8%	56.3%
C7	36.3%	81.5%	36.4%	100.0%	36.3%	68.8%
C7-T1	19.6%	74.1%	17.8%	100.0%	25.0%	56.3%
T1	18.0%	74.1%	14.9%	72.7%	27.5%	75.0%
T1-2	17.7%	74.1%	13.6%	81.8%	30.0%	68.8%
T2	11.2%	59.3%	7.9%	54.5%	21.3%	62.5%
T2-3	15.5%	81.5%	10.7%	81.8%	30.0%	81.3%
T3	9.9%	63.0%	4.5%	54.5%	23.8%	68.8%
T3-4	17.7%	81.5%	12.4%	81.8%	33.8%	81.3%
T4	8.4%	55.6%	5.0%	54.5%	18.8%	56.3%
T4-5	18.0%	88.9%	13.2%	72.7%	32.5%	100.0%
T5	8.1%	44.4%	3.7%	18.2%	21.3%	62.5%
T5-6	16.5%	70.4%	11.6%	45.5%	31.3%	87.5%
T6	6.2%	40.7%	2.1%	18.2%	18.8%	56.3%
T6-7	14.9%	59.3%	11.6%	36.4%	25.0%	75.0%
T7	6.2%	33.3%	2.5%	18.2%	17.5%	43.8%
T7-8	14.3%	63.0%	9.9%	54.5%	27.5%	68.8%
T8	5.3%	29.6%	2.1%	18.2%	15.0%	37.5%
T8-9	11.5%	48.1%	8.7%	36.4%	20.0%	56.3%
T9	4.7%	33.3%	1.7%	18.2%	13.8%	43.8%
T9-10	11.5%	48.1%	9.1%	36.4%	18.8%	56.3%
T10	3.1%	14.8%	2.1%	9.1%	6.3%	18.8%
T10-11	8.7%	33.3%	6.2%	18.2%	16.3%	43.8%
T11	3.4%	18.5%	1.7%	18.2%	8.8%	18.8%
T11-12	11.5%	48.1%	8.7%	54.5%	20.0%	43.8%
T12	4.0%	33.3%	2.9%	36.4%	7.5%	31.3%
T12-L1	17.7%	70.4%	14.5%	54.5%	27.5%	81.3%
L1	7.1%	40.7%	5.8%	45.5%	11.3%	37.5%
L1-2	11.5%	48.1%	9.1%	45.5%	18.8%	50.0%
L2	6.5%	40.7%	5.0%	45.5%	11.3%	37.5%
L2-3	13.7%	55.6%	10.7%	54.5%	22.5%	56.3%
L3	3.1%	22.2%	1.7%	18.2%	7.5%	25.0%
L3-4	8.1%	29.6%	5.0%	27.3%	17.5%	31.3%
L4	0.9%	11.1%	0.4%	9.1%	2.5%	12.5%
L4-5	9.0%	25.9%	7.4%	18.2%	13.8%	31.3%
L5	1.6%	11.1%	0.8%	9.1%	3.8%	12.5%
L5-S1	12.1%	48.1%	10.7%	45.5%	16.3%	50.0%
S1	0.3%	3.7%	0.4%	9.1%	0.0%	0.0%

low more significant different ($0.01 < p < 0.05$)
moderate more significant different ($0.001 < p < 0.01$)
high more significant different ($p < 0.001$)

OP index grade and the prevalence of thoracolumbar OPLL at each level.

Statistical analysis

Student's unpaired t test was used to identify statistically significant differences in age, BMI, and the OP index for the cervical spine between men and women. Chi-squared test was used to test for a sex-related difference in the presence of diabetes. Tukey's post hoc test was applied to compare the three groups classified according to cervical OP grade. A forward stepwise logistic regression model was used to investigate whether the cervical OP grade could predict the presence of OPLL in the thoracolumbar spine and the prevalence of patients with an OP index of ≥20 [7]. All statistical analyses were performed using SPSS for Windows version 22.0 (IBM Corp., Armonk, NY). All data are expressed as the mean ± standard deviation. A p-value < 0.05 was considered to be statistically significant.

Results

Demographic data

Patient demographic characteristics are summarized in Table 1. Mean patient age was 64.7 years. Mean BMI was 25.7 and 31.7% (102/233 patients) of the patients had diabetes mellitus. Using the CT classification, the cervical OP index was grade 1 in 169 patients (52.5%), grade 2 in 107 patients (33.2%), and grade 3 in 46 patients (14.3%). The mean cervical and whole-spine OP index values were 5.83 and 9.21, respectively. Twenty-seven patients (8.3%) had an OP index ≥20. Severe OPLL was significantly more common in women than in men (16 patients, 20% vs. 11 patients, 4.5%, $p < 0.01$). There was no significant sex-related difference in age, prevalence of diabetes mellitus, or BMI. Interestingly, the OP index for the whole spine was significantly higher in women than in men (9.2 vs. 8.2, $p < 0.01$). However, there was no statistically significant sex-related difference in the cervical OP index.

Pattern of distribution of ossified lesions throughout the spine in patients with severe OPLL

The prevalence of OPLL at each level of the spine is shown in Table 2. Thoracic OPLL occurred most often at T1 (14.9%) and at T1/2 (13.6%) in men and at T1 (27.5%) and T3/4 (33.8%) in women. Lumbar OPLL was most common at L1 (5.8%) and T12/L1 (14.5%) in men and at L1 and L2 (both 11.3%) and T12/L1 (27.5%) in women.

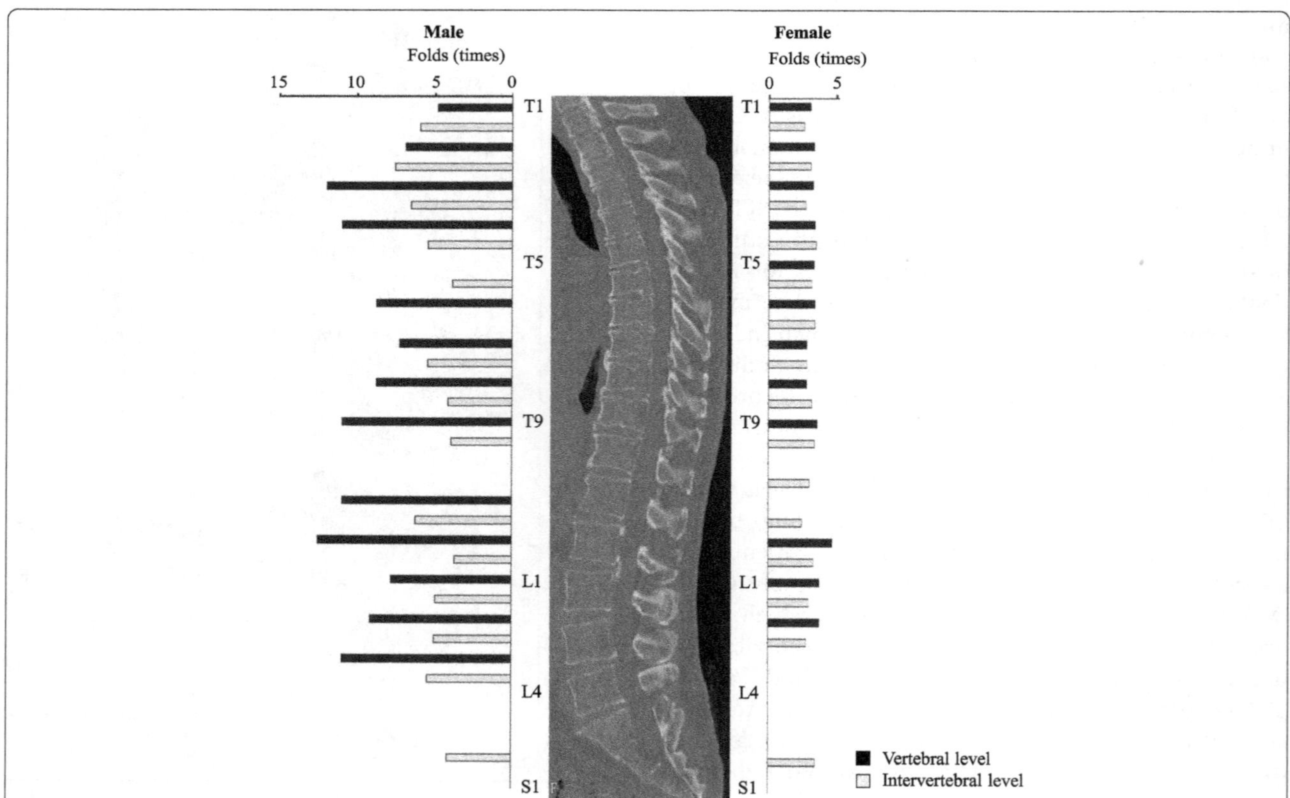

Fig. 2 Hazard ratios for the prevalence of ossified lesions at each spinal level in patients with severe OPLL compared with patients with OPLL of any grade. OPLL, ossification of the posterior longitudinal ligament

We then compared the prevalence of OPLL at each level in all patients and that in patients with an OP index ≥20. Overall, the patients with severe OPLL were more likely to have OPLL at the level of the upper cervical spine and at levels from the lower cervical spine to the upper lumbar spine. In men with severe OPLL, ossified lesions were frequently seen at the intervertebral and vertebral levels from C6/7 to T4/5 and from T11/12 to L3/4. However, severe OPLL appeared to be distributed more diffusely in the thoracic spine in women. There were no statistically significant differences in the prevalence of thoracic OPLL at T5, T6/7, T10, and T10/11 in men or at T8, T10, T11, and T11/12 in women. Interestingly, the only significant difference in prevalence of OPLL in the area from the lower lumbar spine to the sacrum was at L5/S1 in both sexes. We also investigated the fold difference in prevalence of ossified lesions at each spinal segment (Fig. 2, Table 3). The prevalence of severe OPLL in the thoracic spine was 3.9–12.6 fold higher in men and 2.3–4.2 fold higher in women. Of note, in men with OPLL affecting the upper thoracic spine, there was a 12.0 fold increase in likelihood at T3 and a 7.6 fold increase at T2/3, and in those with lower thoracic OPLL, there was a 12.6 fold increased likelihood at T12 and a 6.3fold increase at T11/12. Interestingly, although thoracic OPLL had a bimodal distribution in men, the distribution was uniform in women. The distribution pattern in the lumbar spine was very similar between the sexes. However, the prevalence of ossified lesions increased to a greater extent in men (by 4.25–11.0 fold) than in women (by 2.5–3.3 fold). In the lumbosacral region, there was a significantly increased prevalence of ossified lesions only at L5/S1 in both men (4.2 fold) and women (3.1 fold).

Prevalence of OPLL at each level according to cervical OP index grade

The cervical OP index classification was originally designed to categorize cervical OPLL into three grades of severity according to the sum of all ossifications in the cervical spine. The prevalence of OPLL was investigated at each vertebral and intervertebral segment according to grade to evaluate the usefulness of this classification for prediction of the prevalence of OPLL at each segment in the thoracic and lumbar spines (Table 4). Overall, the prevalence of ossified lesions in the upper thoracic spine and at the thoracolumbar junction increased significantly with increasing grade of severity. The distribution of prevalence of OPLL was similar in men and women. A weak or no association between the prevalence of OPLL and the cervical OP index classification was found in the middle thoracic spine in men. However, statistically significant differences were observed at T4/5, T5/6, T6, T6/7, T8/9, and T9/10 in women. A significant correlation was found at the thoracolumbar junction, except at L2 in men and at T11, L1, L1/2, and L2 in women.

Table 3 Hazard ratio of the incidence of ossified lesion at each level in patients with OP-index ≧20 compared to total patients

	Male		Female	
Segment	Folds change	p	Folds change	p
T1	4.9	0	2.7	0.0008
T1–2	6.0	0	2.3	0.0079
T2	6.9	0	2.9	0.0023
T2–3	7.6	0	2.7	0.0004
T3	12.0	0	2.9	0.0012
T3–4	6.6	0	2.4	0.0012
T4	11.0	0	3.0	0.0044
T4–5	5.5	0	3.1	0
T5	–	0.1224	2.9	0.0023
T5–6	3.9	0.005	2.8	0.0001
T6	8.8	0.0246	3.0	0.0044
T6–7	–	0.0505	3.0	0.0003
T7	7.3	0.0424	2.5	0.0469
T7–8	5.5	0.0001	2.5	0.0039
T8	8.8	0.0246	–	0.0794
T8–9	4.2	0.0127	2.8	0.0068
T9	11.0	0.0121	3.2	0.0141
T9–10	4.0	0.0161	3.0	0.0044
T10	–	0.628	–	0.2477
T10–11	–	0.3488	2.7	0.0327
T11	11.0	0.0121	–	0.455
T11–12	6.3	0	–	0.0871
T12	12.6	0	4.2	0.0219
T12-L1	3.8	0.0019	3.0	0.0001
L1	7.9	0	3.3	0.0237
L1–2	5.0	0	2.7	0.0186
L2	9.2	0	3.3	0.0237
L2–3	5.1	0.0001	2.5	0.0148
L3	11.0	0.0121	–	0.1003
L3–4	5.5	0.0159	–	0.3594
L4	–	0.1505	–	0.2534
L4–5	–	0.4713	–	0.1779
L5	–	0.2926	–	0.4113
L5-S1	4.2	0	3.1	0.0081
S1	–	0.1505	–	–

JOSL-CT grading system for prediction of prevalence of OPLL at each thoracolumbar spinal level

We further investigated the hazard ratios for the prevalence of OPLL at each spinal level where there was a

Table 4 Incidence of ossified lesion in each level according to cervical OP-index grading system

Incidence	Male + Female			Male			Female		
Segment	Grade 1	Grade 2	Grade 3	Grade 1	Grade 2	Grade 3	Grade 1	Grade 2	Grade 3
T1	4.8%*	21.5*	58.7*	2.4*	13.1*	34.8*	2.4*	7.5*	15.2*
T1-2	7.1*%	21.5*	47.8*	3.6*	13.1*	26.1*	3.6*	8.4*	15.2*
T2	4.2%*	11.2*	37.0*	1.8*	5.6*	21.7*	2.4*	5.6*	10.9*
T2-3	8.9%*	14.0*	41.3*	4.8*	6.5*	21.7*	4.2*	7.5*	15.2*
T3	3.6%*	10.3*	28.3*	1.2*	3.7*	10.9*	2.4*	6.5*	13.0*
T3-4	10.1%*	19.6*	37.0*	4.8*	12.1*	17.4*	5.4*	7.5*	15.2*
T4	5.4%*	8.4*	19.6*	2.4	3.7	8.7	3.0*	4.7*	8.7*
T4-5	11.9%*	17.8*	39.1*	7.7	10.3	15.2	4.2*	7.5*	19.6*
T5	6.0%*	7.5*	17.4*	1.8	2.8	6.5	4.2	3.7	8.7
T5-6	11.9%*	16.8*	30.4*	7.1	8.4	13.0	4.8*	7.5*	13.0*
T6	3.0%*	6.5*	17.4*	0.0*	1.9*	6.5*	3.0*	3.7*	8.7*
T6-7	10.1	17.8	23.9	5.4	12.1	10.9	4.8*	5.6*	10.9*
T7	4.8*	4.7*	15.2*	1.2	0.9	6.5	3.6	3.7	6.5
T7-8	10.1*	15.9*	23.9*	4.8	9.3	10.9	5.4	5.6	10.9
T8	4.2*	2.8*	15.2*	1.2	0.0	6.5	3.0	2.8	6.5
T8-9	6.5*	13.1*	23.9*	4.2	7.5	10.9	2.4*	5.6*	10.9*
T9	3.6	3.7	10.9	0.6	0.9	4.3	3.0	2.8	4.3
T9-10	8.3*	12.1*	19.6*	5.4	7.5	8.7	3.0*	4.7*	8.7*
T10	1.8	3.7	6.5	0.6	2.8	2.2	1.2	0.9	2.2
T10-11	6.5	8.4	15.2	3.6	5.6	4.3	3.0*	2.8*	8.7*
T11	1.8*	2.8*	10.9*	0.0*	1.9*	4.3*	1.8	0.9	4.3
T11-12	4.8*	15.0*	28.3*	2.4*	9.3*	15.2*	2.4*	5.6*	10.9*
T12	1.2*	4.7*	13.0*	0.6*	2.8*	6.5*	0.6*	1.9*	4.3*
T12-L1	8.9*	25.2*	32.6*	6.0*	15.0*	17.4*	3.0*	8.4*	13.0*
L1	3.6*	9.3*	15.2*	1.8*	6.5*	8.7*	1.8	2.8	4.3
L1-2	5.4*	17.8*	19.6*	3.0*	10.3*	13.0*	2.4	6.5	6.5
L2	3.6	10.3	8.7	1.8	5.6	6.5	1.8	4.7	2.2
L2-3	6.0*	19.6*	28.3*	3.6*	10.3*	19.6*	2.4*	9.3*	6.5*
L3	1.2*	3.7*	8.7*	0.0*	1.9*	4.3*	1.2	1.9	4.3
L3-4	5.4	12.1	8.7	1.8	5.6	6.5	3.0	5.6	2.2
L4	0.6	0.0	4.3	0.0	0.0	2.2	0.6	0.0	2.2
L4-5	8.9	8.4	8.7	6.5	4.7	4.3	2.4	3.7	4.3
L5	0.6	1.9	4.3	0.6	0.0	2.2	0.0	1.9	2.2
L5-S1	8.9	15.9	15.2	6.5	10.3	10.9	2.4	4.7	4.3
S1	0.0	0.0	2.2	0.0	0.0	2.2	0.0	0.0	0.0

low more significant different ($0.01 < p < 0.05$)
moderate more significant different ($0.001 < p < 0.01$)
high more significant different ($p < 0.001$)

significant correlation between the prevalence of OPLL and the cervical OP index grade (Fig. 3, Table 5). The hazard ratio was 2.1–5.0 in the upper thoracic spine, 6.5 at T6 in the middle thoracic spine in men, and 2.0–4.3 from T4/5 to T6/7 in women. At the thoracolumbar junction in men, the hazard ratio was 2.0–5.0 at both the intervertebral and vertebral segments, but not at the L2 vertebral level. However, a significant correlation (2.1–3.7-fold) was found at T10/11, T11/12, T12, T12/L1, and L2/3 in women.

Discussion

Various studies [5, 8–10] have reported high concomitance rate in spinal ligament ossification. In this study, we identified the prevalence of OPLL in the thoracic and lumbar spines in patients with cervical OPLL. Kawaguchi et al. [5] demonstrated that more than 50% of patients with cervical OPLL also had OPLL at the thoracic and/or lumbar spine. The prevalence of thoracic OPLL in the general population is reported to be 1.6–1.9% in Japan [4, 8]. This finding suggests that patients with

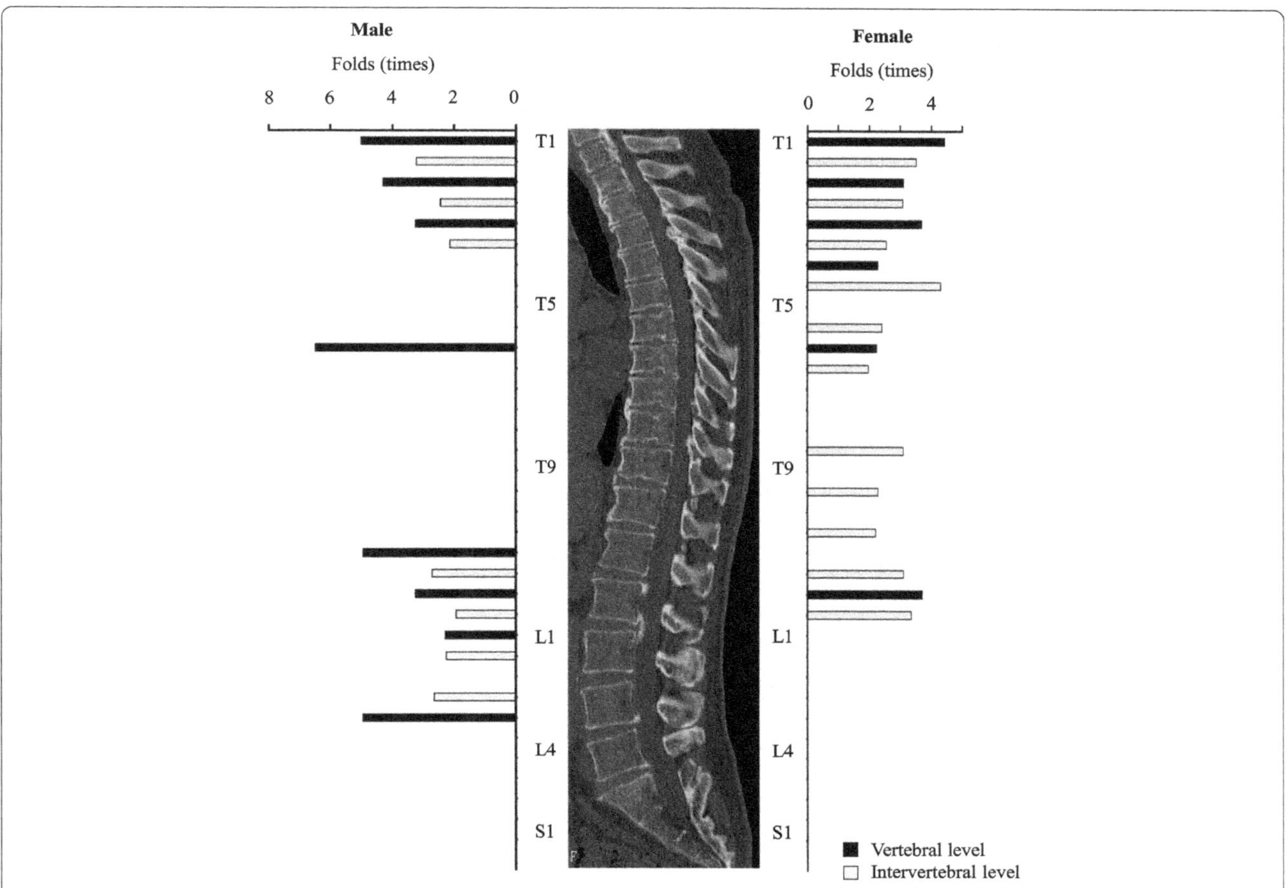

Fig. 3 Logistic regression model showing a significant correlation between cervical OP index grade and prevalence of ossification of the posterior longitudinal ligament at different thoracic and lumbar spinal levels

cervical OPLL have a predisposition to hyperostosis in the posterior longitudinal ligament throughout the spine. Therefore, when an ossified lesion is detected in the cervical spine, a whole-spine CT study should be performed to detect lesions in other spinal segments.

Several studies [11–13] have demonstrated that the most frequently involved thoracic site on plain radiography is T6. However, Fujimori et al. [8] reviewed whole-spine CT data for 1500 patients who underwent positron emission tomography and CT (PET-CT) and concluded that the most frequently affected level was T1/2 in men and T5/6 in women. Mori et al. [4] reviewed ossified lesions in patients undergoing chest CT and found that thoracic OPLL was identified most often at T3/4. Our study also demonstrated that thoracic OPLL was most common at T1/2 in men and at T3/4 in women. The likely explanation for the discrepancy between the results of conventional radiographs and those of CT images is that information about the upper thoracic spine is often masked by the superposed bony structures such as the shoulders and ribs. Furthermore, it is known that the posterior longitudinal ligament is thickest and widest in the transitional portion of the cervicothoracic junction [14], so ossification may occur in the upper thoracic spine.

We found that approximately 70–100% of ossified lesions in men with severe OPLL occurred at the cervicothoracic junction, whereas approximately 70–100% of ossified lesions in women with severe OPLL occurred in the middle thoracic spine and approximately 55–75% occurred at the cervicothoracic and thoracolumbar junctions. Furthermore, in women with severe OPLL, ossified lesions tended to occur consistently from the upper thoracic spine to the lumbar spine at a rate approximately 2–3 times that in women with OPLL of any grade. However, the prevalence of ossified lesions in men with severe OPLL was relatively higher at the T3 and T8 vertebral levels and at the thoracolumbar junction (Fig. 2, Table 3). These findings indicate that the presence of ossified lesions at the T3, T8 and thoracolumbar junction might be rare in men (Table 2).

In this study, we categorized patients with cervical OPLL into three groups according to the number of

Table 5 Increased risk of OPLL in each level according to cervical OP-index grading system

Grade 1+	Male		Female	
Segment	Odds ratio	p	Odds ratio	p
T1	5.0	0	4.5	0
T1–2	3.2	0	3.5	0.001
T2	4.3	0	3.1	0.003
T2–3	2.5	0.001	3.1	0.002
T3	3.3	0.005	3.7	0.001
T3–4	2.1	0.004	2.6	0.006
T4	–	0.07	2.3	0.027
T4–5	–	0.133	4.3	0
T5	–	0.12	–	0.111
T5–6	–	0.24	2.4	0.01
T6	6.5	0.013	2.3	0.034
T6–7	–	0.084	2.0	0.045
T7	–	0.077	–	0.169
T7–8	–	0.089	–	0.075
T8	–	0.09	–	0.123
T8–9	–	0.078	3.1	0.003
T9	–	0.104	–	0.312
T9–10	–	0.359	2.3	0.027
T10	–	0.25	–	0.234
T10–11	–	0.628	2.2	0.043
T11	5.0	0.036	–	0.153
T11–12	2.7	0.001	3.1	0.003
T12	3.3	0.023	3.7	0.024
T12-L1	2.0	0.007	3.4	0.001
L1	2.3	0.021	–	0.101
L1–2	2.3	0.006	–	0.08
L2	–	0.07	–	0.465
L2–3	2.7	0	2.1	0.041
L3	5.0	0.036	–	0.189
L3–4	–	0.07	–	0.763
L4	–	0.993	–	0.46
L4–5	–	0.449	–	0.381
L5	–	0.47	–	0.118
L5-S1	–	0.24	–	0.312
S1	5.0	0.993	–	–

segments at which cervical OPLL could be confirmed. In a previous study [6], we demonstrated that this classification could predict not only the presence but also the degree of hyperostosis in the whole spine. Therefore, we investigated whether there was a correlation between this classification system and the prevalence of ossified lesions at each segment in the thoracolumbar spine. The prevalence of OPLL in the thoracic and lumbar spines increases with increasing severity of cervical hyperostosis. Although OPLL in the upper thoracic spine is generally able to be detected on CT sagittal images, which are often reconstructed, ossification in the thoracolumbar junction cannot be found when patients with cervical OPLL are examined. Park et al. [9] reported coexistence of cervical and thoracic OPLL (tandem calcification) in 33.8% of patients with cervical OPLL, 8.9% of whom subsequently underwent surgery for deterioration of thoracic OPLL. Thoracic stenosis attributable to OPLL is often not recognized or misdiagnosed as lumbar canal stenosis, especially in patients with myelopathic symptoms mainly involving the lower extremities [15]. These reports suggest that patients with a high cervical OP index value are at increased risk of ossified lesions that can cause a spinal disorder. Therefore, whole-spine CT screening is recommended for a patient with cervical OPLL who presents with severe gait disturbance.

Cervical OPLL has occasionally been reported to coexist with not only thoracic OPLL but also ossification of the ligamentum flavum (OLF) [16, 17] and diffuse idiopathic skeletal hyperostosis (DISH) [18, 19]. Fujimori et al. investigated the concomitance of spinal ligament ossification in patients undergoing PET-CT and concluded that the frequencies in patients with cervical OPLL were 13, 34, and 36% for thoracic OPLL, OLF, and DISH, respectively. Mori et al. also reported prevalence of 36 and 8.7% for OLF and DISH in more than 3000 patients undergoing chest CT for investigation of pulmonary disease. There have also been some reports on the prevalence of ossification of other spinal ligaments in patients with cervical OPLL [5, 6]. Kawaguchi et al. reviewed the CT data for 178 patients with cervical OPLL and reported that 64.6% had OLF, while Nishimura et al. evaluated whole-spine CT images for 234 patients with cervical OPLL and found that the prevalence rate of DISH was 48.7%. Thus, ossification of each ligament may influence hyperostosis of each ligament.

This study does have some limitations in that it is based on CT examination of patients with cervical OPLL rather than being a population-based study. Further, we could not evaluate quantitative measurements of clinical symptoms. In addition, we did not determine the distribution of ossification in spinal ligaments other than the OPLL. However, in spite of these limitations, we believe that this study provides important epidemiological information for not only patients with cervical OPLL but also radiologists and spine surgeons.

Conclusion

This multi-institutional study represents the largest review of whole-spine CT images in patients with cervical

OPLL. The most frequent segment was T1 in both men and women for thoracic vertebral OPLL, and T1/2 and T3/4 intervertebral levels in men and women, respectively. Ossified lesions were frequently seen at the intervertebral and vertebral levels around the cervicothoracic and thoracolumbar junctions in men with severe OPLL, but could be observed more diffusely in the thoracic spine in their female counterparts.

Abbreviations

BMI: Body mass index; CT: Computed tomography; DISH: Diffuse idiopathic skeletal hyperostosis; JOSL: Japanese Organization of the study for ossification of spinal ligament; OLF: Ossification of ligamentum flavum; OPLL: Ossification of posterior longitudinal ligament; PET-CT: Positron emission tomography-computed tomography

Acknowledgements

This study was supported by the grant of the Ministry of Health, Labour and Welfare. We greatly thank to Nobuko Nakajima and Yukiko Oya for data collection.

Funding

This work was supported by Health and Labour Science Research Grants. No other financial associations that may be relevant or seen as relevant to the submitted manuscript.

Authors' contributions

TH, TY, KM, MM, MN, AO and YK designed the study; TH, TY, NN, KM, SU, AI, KT, TY, SS, TT, KF, MF, SN, KW, MK, TF, YM, TH, KT, AK, MA, HH, TO, MW, HK, KW, HO, HK, SI, KA, SF, MK, MY, MM, MN, and YK collected the data; KM, TY, TH, AI and KT analyzed and interpreted the data; KM and YK wrote the initial draft; TH, NN, KM and SU performed statistical analyses. KM, TY, TH, AI, KT, TY, SS, TT, KF, MF, SN, KW, MK, TF, YM, TH, KT, AK, MA, HH, TO, MW, HK, KW, HO, HK, SI, KA, SF, MK, MY, MM, MN, AO and YK participated in revising the manuscript. MM, MN, AO and YK supervise the study; MM and AO participated in acquisition of funding. All authors read and approved the final manuscript.

Ethics approval and consent to participate

Written informed consent was obtained from each participant before registration at each institution. The local ethics committee of each institute approved this study, namely, the ethics committees of Shiga University of Medical Science, Tokyo Medical and Dental University, Keio University, National Hospital Organization Okayama Medical Center, University of Toyama, Kitasato Institute Hospital, National Hospital Organization Murayama Medical Center, Hirosaki University Graduate School of Medicine, Chiba University Graduate School of Medicine, Hamamatsu University School of Medicine, Jichi Medical University, Kagoshima University, University of Yamanashi, Tokai University School of Medicine, Niigata University Medicine and Dental General Hospital, Tohoku Medical and Pharmaceutical University Tohoku University School of Medicine, Nagoya University Graduate School of Medicine, Kyoto University, and University of Tsukuba.

Consent for publication

Not applicable.

Competing interests

The authors declare that they have no competing interests.

Author details

[1]Department of Orthopedic Surgery, Tokyo Medical and Dental University, 1-5-45 Yushima, Bunkyo-ku, Tokyo 113-8519, Japan. [2]Department of Orthopedic Surgery, School of Medicine, Keio University, 35 Shinanomachi, Shinjuku-ku, Tokyo 160-8582, Japan. [3]Department of Orthopedic Surgery, National Hospital Organization Okayama Medical Center, 1711-1 Tamasu, Okayama, Okayama 701-1154, Japan. [4]Department of Orthopedic Surgery, Shiga University of Medical Science, Tsukinowa-cho, Seta, Otsu, Shiga 520-2192, Japan. [5]Department of Orthopedic Surgery, Faculty of Medicine, University of Toyama, 2630 Sugitani, Toyama, Toyama 930-0194, Japan. [6]Department of Orthopedic Surgery, Fujita Health University, 1-98 Dengakugakubo, Kutsukake, Toyoake, Aichi 470-1192, Japan. [7]Department of Orthopedic Surgery, National Hospital Organization Murayama Medical Center, 2-37-1 Gakuen, Musashimurayama, Tokyo 208-0011, Japan. [8]Department of Orthopedic Surgery, Shizuoka City Shimizu Hospital, 1231 Miyakami, Shimizu-ku, Shizuoka 424-8636, Japan. [9]Department of Orthopedic Surgery, Keiyu Hospital, 3-7-3 Minatomirai, Nishi-ku, Yokohama, Kanagawa 220-0012, Japan. [10]Department of Orthopedic Surgery, Hirosaki University Graduate School of Medicine, 53 Honcho, Hirosaki, Aomori 036-8203, Japan. [11]Department of Orthopedic Surgery, Chiba University Graduate School of Medicine, 1-8-1 Inohana, Chuo-ku, Chiba, Chiba 260-0856, Japan. [12]Department of Orthopedic Surgery, Hamamatsu University School of Medicine, 1-20-1 Handayama, Hamamatsu, Shizuoka 431-3125, Japan. [13]Department of Orthopedics, Jichi Medical University, 3311-1 Yakushiji, Shimotsuke, Tochugi 329-0498, Japan. [14]Department of Orthopedic Surgery, Graduate School of Medicine and Dental Science, Kagoshima University, 8-35-1 Sakuragaoka, Kagoshima, Kagoshima 890-8520, Japan. [15]Department of Orthopedic Surgery, University of Yamanashi, 1110 Shimokato, Chuo-ku, Yamanashi 409-3898, Japan. [16]Department of Orthopedic Surgery, Surgical Science, Tokai University School of Medicine, 143 Shimokasuya, Isehara, Kanagawa 259-1143, Japan. [17]Department of Orthopedic Surgery, Niigata University Medicine and Dental General Hospital, 1-754 Asahimachidori, Chuo-ku, Niigata, Niigata 951-8520, Japan. [18]Department of Orthopedic Surgery, Tohoku Medical and Pharmaceutical University, 4-4-1 Komatsushima, Aobaku, Sendai, Miyagi 981-8558, Japan. [19]Department of Orthopaedic Surgery, Tohoku University School of Medicine, 1-1 Seiryomachi, Aoba-ku, Sendai, Miyagi 980-8574, Japan. [20]Department of Orthopedic Surgery, Nagoya University Graduate School of Medicine, 65 Tsurumaicho, Showa-ku, Nagoya, Aichi 466-0065, Japan. [21]Department of Orthopedic Surgery, Graduate School of Medicine, Kyoto University, 54 Kawaharacho, Shogoin, Sakyo-ku, Kyoto, Kyoto 606-8507, Japan. [22]Department of Orthopedic Surgery, Faculty of Medicine, University of Tsukuba, 2-1-1 Amakubo, Tsukuba, Ibaraki 305-8576, Japan. [23]Japanese Organization of the Study for Ossification of Spinal Ligament (JOSL), 1-5-45 Yushima, Bunkyo-ku, Tokyo 113-8519, Japan.

References

1. Sakai K, Okawa A, Takahashi M, Arai Y, Kawabata S, Enomoto M, Kato T, Hirai T, Shinomiya K. Five-year follow-up evaluation of surgical treatment for cervical myelopathy caused by ossification of the posterior longitudinal ligament: a prospective comparative study of anterior decompression and fusion with floating method versus laminoplasty. Spine. 2012;37(5):367–76.
2. Matsumoto M, Toyama Y, Chikuda H, Takeshita K, Kato T, Shindo S, Abumi K, Takahata M, Nohara Y, Taneichi H, Tomita K, Kawahara N, Imagama S, Matsuyama Y, Yamazaki M, Okawa A. Outcomes of fusion surgery for ossification of the posterior longitudinal ligament of the thoracic spine: a multicenter retrospective survey: clinical article. J Neurosurg Spine. 2011; 15(4):380–5.
3. Key GA. On paraplegia depending on the ligament of the spine. Guy Hosp Rep. 1838;3:17–34.
4. Mori K, Imai S, Kasahara T, Nishizawa K, Mimura T, Matsusue Y. Prevalence, distribution, and morphology of thoracic ossification of the posterior longitudinal ligament in Japanese: results of CT-based cross-sectional study. Spine. 2014;39(5):394–9.
5. Kawaguchi Y, Nakano M, Yasuda T, Seki S, Hori T, Kimura T. Ossification of the posterior longitudinal ligament in not only the cervical spine, but also other spinal regions: analysis using multidetector computed tomography of the whole spine. Spine. 2013;38(23):E1477–82.
6. Hirai T, Yoshii T, Iwanami A, Takeuchi K, Mori K, Yamada T, Wada K, Koda M, Matsuyama Y, Takeshita K, Abematsu M, Haro H, Watanabe M, Watanabe K, Ozawa H, Kanno H, Imagama S, Fujibayashi S, Yamazaki M, Matsumoto M, Nakamura M, Okawa A, Kawaguchi Y. Prevalence and distribution of ossified lesions in the whole spine of patients with cervical ossification of the posterior longitudinal ligament a multicenter study (JOSL CT study). PLoS

One. 2016;11(8):e0160117.

7. Hicks GE, Fritz JM, Delitto A, McGill SM. Preliminary development of a clinical prediction rule for determining which patients with low back pain will respond to a stabilization exercise program. Arch Phys Med Rehabil. 2005;86(9):1753–62.
8. Fujimori T, Watabe T, Iwamoto Y, Hamada S, Iwasaki M, Oda T. Prevalence, concomitance, and distribution of ossification of the spinal ligaments: results of whole spine CT scans in 1500 Japanese patients. Spine. 2016; 41(21):1668–76.
9. Park JY, Chin DK, Kim KS, Cho YE. Thoracic ligament ossification in patients with cervical ossification of the posterior longitudinal ligaments: tandem ossification in the cervical and thoracic spine. Spine (Phila Pa 1976). 2008;33(13):E407–10.
10. Yamada T, Yoshii T, Yamamoto N, Hirai T, Inose H, Kato T, Kawabata S, Okawa A. Clinical outcomes of cervical spinal surgery for cervical Myelopathic patients with coexisting lumbar Spinal Canal stenosis (tandem spinal stenosis) a retrospective analysis of 297 cases. Spine (Phila Pa 1976). 2018;43(4):E234–41.
11. Ohtsuka K, Terayama K, Yanagihara M, et al. An epidemiological survey on ossification of ligaments in the cervical and thoracic spine in individuals over 50 years of age. Nihon Seikeigeka Gakkai Zasshi. 1986;60:1087–98.
12. Tsuyama N, Kurokawa T. Ossifi cation of the posterior longitudinal ligament in the thoracic and lumbar spine. Statistical report of ossification of the posterior longitudinal ligament for all of Japan (in Japanese). Rinsho Seikei Geka. 1977;12:337–9.
13. Akiyama N, Onari K, Kitao S, et al. Ossifi cation of the posterior longitudinal ligament of the thoracic spine; radiological study (in Japanese). Seikeigeka. 1981;32:1029–39.
14. Schuenke M, Schulte E, Schumacher U. THIEME atlas of anatomy general anatomy and musculoskeletal system. 1st ed. Stuttgart: Thieme; 2010. p. 76–117.
15. Epstein NE, Schwall G. Thoracic spinal stenosis: diagnostic and treatment challenges. J Spinal Disord. 1994;7(3):259–69.
16. Hou X, Sun C, Liu X, Liu Z, Qi Q, Guo Z, Li W, Zeng Y, Chen Z. Clinical features of thoracic spinal stenosis-associated myelopathy: a retrospective analysis of 427 cases. Clin Spine Surg. 2016;29(2):86–9.
17. Miyazawa N, Akiyama I. Ossification of the ligamentum flavum of the cervical spine. J Neurosurg Sci. 2007;51(3):139–44.
18. Guo Q, Ni B, Yang J, Zhu Z. Simultaneous ossification of the posterior longitudinal ligament and ossification of the ligamentum flavum causing upper thoracic myelopathy in DISH: case report and literature review. Eur Spine J. 2011;20(Suppl 2):S195–201.
19. Mori K, Yoshii T, Hirai T, Iwanami A, Takeuchi K, Yamada T, Seki S, Tsuji T, Fujiyoshi K, Furukawa M, Nishimura S, Wada K, Koda M, Furuya T, Matsuyama Y, Hasegawa T, Takeshita K, Kimura A, Abematsu M, Haro H, Ohba T, Watanabe M, Katoh H, Watanabe K, Ozawa H, Kanno H, Imagama S, Ito Z, Fujibayashi S, Yamazaki M, Matsumoto M, Nakamura M, Okawa A, Kawaguchi Y. Prevalence and distribution of ossification of the supra/interspinous ligaments in symptomatic patients with cervical ossification of the posterior longitudinal ligament of the spine: a CT-based multicenter cross-sectional study. BMC Musculoskelet Disord. 2016;17(1):492.

5

Epidemiology of paediatric presentations with musculoskeletal problems in primary care

Albert Tan[1], Victoria Y. Strauss[2], Joanne Protheroe[1*] and Kate M. Dunn[1]

Abstract

Background: Musculoskeletal disease is a common cause of morbidity, but there is a paucity of musculoskeletal research focusing on paediatric populations, particularly in primary care settings. In particular, there is limited information on population consultation frequency in paediatric populations, and frequency varies by age and sex. Few studies have examined paediatric musculoskeletal consultation frequency for different body regions. The objective was to determine the annual consultation prevalence of regional musculoskeletal problems in children in primary care.

Methods: Musculoskeletal codes within the Read morbidity Code system were identified and grouped into body regions. Consultations for children aged three to seventeen in 2006 containing these codes were extracted from recorded consultations at twelve general practices contributing to a general practice consultation database (CiPCA). Annual consultation prevalence per 10,000 registered persons for the year 2006 was determined, stratified by age and sex, for problems in individual body regions.

Results: Over 8 % (8.27%, 95% CI 7.86 to 8.68%) of the 16,862 children consulted with a musculoskeletal problem during 2006. Annual consultation prevalence for any musculoskeletal problem was significantly higher in males than females (male: female prevalence ratio 1.18, 95% CI 1.06 to 1.31). Annual consultation prevalence increased with age and the most common body regions consulted for were the foot, knee and back all of which had over 100 consultations (109, 104 and 101 respectively) per 10,000 persons per year.

Conclusions: This study provides new and detailed information on patterns of paediatric musculoskeletal consultations in primary care. Musculoskeletal problems in children are varied and form a significant part of the paediatric primary care workload. The findings of this study may be used as a resource for planning future studies.

Keywords: Musculoskeletal, Paediatric, Primary care

Background

Musculoskeletal problems are a common reason for healthcare consultation, with an estimated 24% of the population seeking primary healthcare from a General Practitioner (GP) each year [1]. Around 7% of children visit primary care for musculoskeletal problems each year [1], and yet the majority of musculoskeletal research has focused on adult populations. There is a paucity of musculoskeletal research investigating the paediatric population [2].

Population-based and school-based studies have demonstrated that pain is a common feature of childhood [3] and that that the majority of pain in childhood has a musculoskeletal cause. [4, 5] In children, pain is the most common symptom of a musculoskeletal problem, although other symptoms include limping, stiffness, muscle weakness and fatigue [6]. A systematic review of population-based studies in children and adolescents estimated the prevalence of musculoskeletal pain to be between 8.5% and 40% (recall periods from one week to six months) with the

* Correspondence: j.protheroe@keele.ac.uk
[1]Arthritis Research UK Primary Care Centre, Research Institute for Primary Care & Health Sciences, Keele University, Keele, Staffordshire ST5 5BG, UK
Full list of author information is available at the end of the article

knee, back and neck suggested as common sites of musculoskeletal pain [7].

There is limited information about consultations for paediatric musculoskeletal problems in primary care. Very few studies provide information broken down into more than two age-groups within the paediatric population (e.g. [8] and [6] use three age-groups), and given the rapid changes in musculoskeletal problems with age in general paediatric populations [9], this is a large gap. In addition, few studies provide comparable data for different body regions, which means comparisons of prevalence across different body regions is difficult, and there is limited international data (e.g. three of four studies identified in a search were Dutch [10–12] plus one from the UK [1].

The aim of this study was to describe the annual consultation prevalence of regional musculoskeletal problems for children aged three to 17 years in primary care. Particular objectives were to examine figures by age-group, sex and body region.

Methods

CiPCA

This was an analysis of all healthcare visits for musculoskeletal problems among children in a UK primary care medical record database. The study used the Consultations in Primary Care Archive (CiPCA), which is an ongoing primary care medical record database containing anonymised data on all consultations (contacts between patients and healthcare professionals) in 12 general practices in North Staffordshire, UK [13]. In the UK, general practice serves as the first point of contact for health care for over 95 % of the population.

All practices within CiPCA document consultations using the Read clinical classification system which provides Read codes and Read terms. This is a hierarchical coding system which contains between one and five characters and is commonly used in UK primary care. Each extra character represents more information regarding a consultation. For example, N is the chapter for musculoskeletal/connective tissue, "N07" is internal derangement of knee and "N071C" is the code for old tear of lateral meniscus. A healthcare professional may assign one or more Read codes to a consultation. Practices within CiPCA are required to code clinical consultations to a high standard and undergo an annual cycle of training and assessment in computerised morbidity coding. Data regarding consultations in the calendar year 2006 were examined and in this year, 97 % of GP consultations recorded in CiPCA had one or more morbidity codes assigned [14].

Ethical approval for CiPCA was granted by the North Staffordshire Research Ethics Committee. Separate ethical approval was not required for this study.

Study population and musculoskeletal problems definitions

The registered population as of 1st July 2006 was 100,758 patients. A total of 16,862 registered patients were aged between three and 17 years.

To define musculoskeletal presentations for this study, we used the same Read codes that were used in a previously published study by Jordan et al. in which they determined the annual consultation prevalence of regional musculoskeletal problems in primary care [1]. In the study by Jordan et al., all Read codes potentially related to pain or musculoskeletal disorders were identified, a total of 5098. Consultations for children aged three to 17 years occurring during the calendar year 2006 and containing any of these 5908 musculoskeletal Read codes were identified.

The majority of these 5908 codes come from the musculoskeletal diagnosis chapter (N) and injury chapter (S) for example, knee joint pain (N0946) and knee sprain (S54), respectively. They also contain musculoskeletal pain symptoms under the symptoms chapters of R and 1, e.g. general aches and pains (R00z2) and aching muscles (1DCC). The full list can be accessed by www.keele.ac.uk/mrr. We followed the same approach used in the study by Jordan et al. [1] in which the 5908 Read codes were each assigned to 48 body regions. In that study, a framework for allocation of codes to body regions was created using a sample of 100 codes. Four GPs were trained in these use of this and assigned codes to body regions. The term of unspecified was used when a region could not be assigned (for example aching muscles).

In this study, primary care consultations were included if they occurred at the practice, via home visit or were telephone consultations; this excluded secondary care appointments or accident and emergency visits, as this study focused on primary care appointments.

Statistical analysis

The study population was divided into four age-groups: pre-school (three to five years); school age (six to nine years); early adolescence (10 to 13 years); late adolescence (14 to 17 years). The division is based on that used previously [8], expanded to include 14 to 17 year olds.

Annual consultation prevalence was calculated for all musculoskeletal problems, for each body region, stratified by age-group and sex. Annual consultation prevalence was defined as the proportion of patients registered with contributing GP practices at mid-year (1st July) of 2006 who had at least one musculoskeletal consultation as defined above. Annual consultation prevalence for each body region was defined as the proportion of the patients who had at least one consultation in the year containing a Read code assigned to that body region.

To compensate for demographic differences between the CiPCA and the general population of England and Wales, standardised annual consultation prevalence figures were calculated and presented by weighting each age/sex-specific rate based on the proportion of age/sex group in the general population of England and Wales in 2006 [15]. Pearson's chi squared test was used to test the statistical significance of differences between age and sex groups in prevalence rates of regional and overall musculoskeletal consultation. In addition, a standardised prevalence ratio of the standardised prevalence rate in males to that in female. This standardised ratio was calculated by Negative binomial regression that was deemed to account for small prevalence in large sample sizes [16]. All analyses were conducted using STATA v12.0.

Results

Eight percent (8.27%; 95% CI 7.86 to 8.68%) of children consulted at least once with a musculoskeletal problem during 2006. The annual consultation prevalence for any musculoskeletal problem was significantly higher (p = 0.04) in males than females (male: female prevalence ratio 1.18, 95% CI 1.06 to 1.31). The annual consultation prevalence were similar in the two youngest age-groups, but then increased with age-group for both sexes (see Fig. 1).

Consultation prevalence by body region

The most common body regions for paediatric musculoskeletal consultations were the foot, knee and back (see Table 1), all of which had over 100 consultations (109, 104 and 101 respectively) per 10,000 persons per year.

Rates of consultation increased with increasing age-group for most body regions, with statistically significant age trends ($p < 0.05$) found in all regions described with the exception of the head and hip (see Tables 2 and 3). Back problems went from a relatively infrequent cause of musculoskeletal complaints in under nines to being the most common cause of musculoskeletal complains in the 14–17 year old age-group for both sexes (228 per 10,000 persons in males; 95% CI 178 to 293; 205 per 10,000 persons in females; 95% CI 157 to 268).

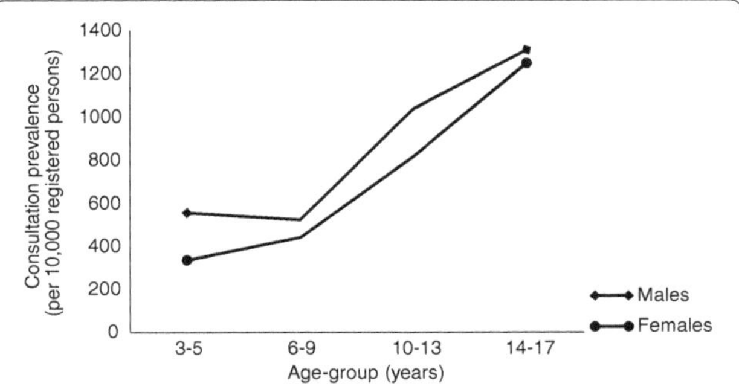

Fig. 1 Annual consultation prevalence for all musculoskeletal problems per 10,000 registered persons (aged 3 to 17 years) by sex and age-group

For both sexes consultations with a foot complaint increased sharply from the 6–9 age-group to the 10–13 age-group. The foot was the most common region of musculoskeletal problems in the 10–13 age group for both males (182 per 10,000 persons per year; 95% CI 134 to 245) and females (170 per 10,000 persons per year; 95% CI 124 to 232) before declining in the 14–17 year old age-group for both sexes.

Although a sex predisposition was suggested by the data for several body regions, the only body region for which a statistically significant sex trend was found for overall rates of consultation was the knee, which was more common in males (Rate ratio of males/females: 1.42 (95% CI: 1.05, 1.91)).

Discussion

This paper presents new data on the population-based annual primary care consultation prevalence of paediatric musculoskeletal problems, including figures stratified by age-group, sex and body region. In total, over 8% of the paediatric population consulted at least once with a musculoskeletal problem during the study year, and there was a clear rise in prevalence by age-group. Consultations were slightly (but significantly) more common among males than females. The most common body regions for paediatric musculoskeletal consultations were the foot, knee and back, each with around 1% of the sample population seeking healthcare.

The broad age-specific figures presented are similar to previous UK estimates of musculoskeletal annual consultation prevalence [1, 17, 18], and support the limited evidence on increasing musculoskeletal consultation rates with age [18–21]. However, our findings provide more detailed information on this trend through the use of four age-groups. This trend for increasing numbers of consultations with age parallels the reported increases in population prevalence of musculoskeletal problems by age in childhood [7, 9].

The overall sex trend in this study was a higher rate of primary care musculoskeletal consultations among boys than girls (male: female prevalence ratio 1.18 (95%CI 1.06 to 1.31). This differs from primary care figures from adults, which indicated that consultations were more common in females [1].

Sex trends for musculoskeletal consultations are conflicting in previous studies. Jordan et al. [1] demonstrated a higher rate of musculoskeletal consultation in males (75.6 per 1000 per year in boys aged zero to 14 compared to 59.7 per 1000 per year in girls). De Inocencio [6] demonstrated a higher rate of musculoskeletal consultation in females (187 per 1000 per year in girls compared to 148 per 1000 per year in boys). McCormick

Table 1 Standardised annual consultation prevalence per 10,000 registered persons (aged 3 to 17 years) for the 12 most common regional problems

Body region	Rate per 10,000 persons (95% CI) [a]		Male: female prevalence ratio (95% CI) [a]	
Foot	109	(93 to 124)	0.97	(0.72 to 1.29)
Knee	104	(89 to 119)	1.42	(1.05 to 1.91)
Back (any [b])	101	(86 to 115)	1.00	(0.75 to 1.35)
Chest	81	(67 to 94)	1.38	(0.98 to 1.93)
Head	72	(59 to 85)	1.32	(0.92 to 1.90)
Hand	49	(38 to 62)	1.37	(0.88 to 2.11)
Neck	45	(35 to 56)	0.97	(0.63 to 1.52)
Ankle	37	(28 to 46)	1.07	(0.66 to 1.76)
Pelvis	36	(27 to 45)	0.89	(0.54 to 1.46)
Hip	26	(18 to 33)	0.74	(0.41 to 1.34)
Wrist	19	(13 to 26)	0.77	(0.39 to 1.52)
Shoulder	13	(7 to 18)	0.46	(0.19 to 1.12)

[a] males and females; age sex-standardised based on population figures for England and Wales in 2006 [15]
[b] includes consultations coded as upper back, lower back or back

Table 2 Standardised annual consultation prevalence per 10,000 registered persons (aged 3 to 17 years) for each body region - males by age-group

Male (age-group in years) prevalence										
Region	Total [a]	3–5	(95% CI)	6–9	(95% CI)	10–13	(95% CI)	14–17	(95% CI)
Ankle	37	13	(4 to 49)	32	(15 to 66)	53	(30 to 93)	46	(26 to 80)
Back	48	7	(1 to 38)	18	(7 to 47)	22	(9 to 52)	110	(77 to 158)
Back (any [b])	101	13	(4 to 49)	27	(13 to 59)	93	(61 to 142)	228	(178 to 293)
Chest	81	0	(0 to 26)	77	(48 to 123)	93	(61 to 142)	167	(125 to 224)
Elbow	8	0	(0 to 26)	9	(2 to 33)	9	(2 to 32)	23	(10 to 50)
Foot	109	67	(36 to 123)	45	(25 to 83)	182	(134 to 245)	118	(83 to 167)
Hand	49	33	(14 to 78)	36	(18 to 72)	58	(34 to 98)	88	(58 to 131)
Head	72	114	(71 to 181)	73	(45 to 118)	89	(57 to 136)	65	(32 to 89)
Head/neck	12	27	(10 to 69)	14	(5 to 40)	4	(1 to 25)	11	(4 to 34)
Hip	26	7	(1 to 38)	23	(0 to 17)	31	(15 to 64)	23	(10 to 50)
Knee	104	67	(36 to 123)	64	(38 to 107)	124	(86 to 179)	206	(158 to 267)
Limb	5	0	(0 to 26)	14	(5 to 40)	4	(1 to 25)	8	(2 to 28)
Lower back	49	7	(1 to 38)	5	(1 to 26)	66	(40 to 109)	110	(77 to 158)
Lower leg	28	7	(1 to 38)	0	(0 to 17)	66	(40 to 109)	65	(32 to 89)
Lower limb	52	94	(56 to 157)	50	(28 to 89)	35	(18 to 70)	72	(46 to 113)
Neck	45	20	(7 to 59)	32	(15 to 66)	58	(34 to 98)	61	(38 to 99)
Pelvis	36	0	(0 to 26)	32	(15 to 66)	40	(21 to 76)	53	(32 to 89)
Shoulder	13	0	(0 to 26)	5	(1 to 26)	13	(5 to 39)	11	(4 to 34)
Thigh	6	0	(0 to 26)	0	(0 to 17)	18	(7 to 45)	19	(8 to 44)
Upper limb	15	13	(4 to 49)	0	(0 to 17)	18	(7 to 45)	23	(10 to 50)
Wrist	19	0	(0 to 26)	5	(1 to 26)	13	(5 to 39)	42	(23 to 75)
All regions	827	556	(450 to 684)	523	(437 to 624)	1037	(918 to 1169)	1309	(1186 to 1444)

[a]males and females; age-sex standardised based on population figures for England and Wales in 2006
[b]includes consultations coded as upper back, lower back or back

Table 3 Standardised annual consultation prevalence per 10,000 registered persons (aged 3 to 17 years) for each body region - females by age-group

Female (age-group in years) prevalence										
Region	Total [a]	3–5	(95% CI)	6–9	(95% CI)	10–13	(95% CI)	14–17	(95% CI)
Ankle	37	7	(1 to 40)	15	(5 to 43)	45	(24 to 82)	62	(38 to 101)
Back	48	0	(0 to 27)	29	(13 to 63)	54	(31 to 93)	105	(72 to 152)
Back (any [b])	101	0	(0 to 27)	44	(23 to 83)	112	(76 to 164)	205	(157 to 268)
Chest	81	0	(0 to 27)	63	(37 to 107)	49	(27 to 88)	132	(94 to 184)
Elbow	8	0	(0 to 27)	5	(1 to 27)	4	(1 to 25)	4	(1 to 22)
Foot	109	57	(29 to 113)	58	(33 to 101)	170	(124 to 232)	136	(98 to 188)
Hand	49	29	(11 to 73)	5	(1 to 27)	58	(34 to 99)	66	(41 to 105)
Head	72	72	(39 to 131)	58	(33 to 101)	31	(15 to 64)	85	(56 to 129)
Head/neck	12	7	(1 to 40)	10	(3 to 35)	9	(2 to 33)	16	(6 to 40)
Hip	26	7	(1 to 40)	29	(13 to 63)	27	(12 to 58)	47	(27 to 81)
Knee	104	29	(11 to 73)	19	(8 to 50)	94	(61 to 143)	171	(127 to 228)
Limb	5	14	(4 to 52)	5	(1 to 27)	0	(0 to 17)	0	(0 to 15)
Lower back	49	0	(0 to 27)	0	(0 to 19)	54	(31 to 93)	105	(72 to 152)
Lower leg	28	0	(0 to 27)	5	(1 to 27)	40	(21 to 76)	19	(8 to 45)
Lower limb	52	43	(20 to 93)	39	(20 to 76)	22	(10 to 52)	66	(41 to 105)
Neck	45	21	(7 to 63)	24	(10 to 56)	54	(31 to 93)	74	(47 to 115)
Pelvis	36	14	(4 to 52)	5	(1 to 27)	31	(15 to 64)	89	(59 to 133)
Shoulder	13	14	(4 to 52)	0	(0 to 19)	18	(7 to 46)	35	(18 to 66)
Thigh	6	0	(0 to 27)	0	(0 to 19)	0	(0 to 17)	4	(1 to 22)
Upper limb	15	7	(1 to 40)	15	(5 to 43)	13	(5 to 39)	27	(13 to 56)
Wrist	19	7	(1 to 40)	10	(3 to 35)	22	(10 to 52)	43	(24 to 76)
All regions	827	336	(254 to 444)	440	(360 to 537)	818	(711 to 939)	1248	(1126 to 1381)

[a]males and females; age-sex standardised based on population figures for England and Wales in 2006
[b]includes consultations coded as upper back, lower back or back

et al. (1995) demonstrated a higher rate of musculoskeletal consultation in boys in the zero to five year age group. The pattern was reversed in the six to 15 year age group with girls consulting more frequently.

If the higher rate of consultations among boys is confirmed, further research may investigate whether this is due to higher propensity to consult among boys, perhaps driven by different parental concerns, or related to the type of musculoskeletal problems experienced or reported differing among boys and girls. Higher rates of musculoskeletal consultation in boys may be due higher rates of exercise or trauma-related musculoskeletal problems for which parents may be more inclined to bring children to consult for as compared to other musculoskeletal problems. The database used in this study was large with high-quality coding of consultations, and therefore facilitated more in-depth investigation of paediatric patterns by age, sex and body region than many previous studies. However, the database is based within a single region of the UK, which could limit its representativeness. The database has been shown to produce annual consultation prevalence rates for musculoskeletal problems which are comparable to a larger national general practice consultation database [13]. The database has also been used to make international comparisons of consultation prevalence figures, while taking differences in healthcare and recording systems into account [17]. In order to minimise any implications of using a local database, age and sex standardised figures have been presented here. Another potential limitation is that the data analysed was from a single year. There is not enough published data on musculoskeletal consultations to understand the implications of this, but it is possible that changes in both the prevalence and patterns of consultations may change over time.

Conclusions

This study provides new information about primary care patterns of musculoskeletal consultations among children and young people in primary care. The findings reported here improve our understanding of paediatric musculoskeletal problems, provide data on the varied regional paediatric musculoskeletal workload in primary care, and will be useful for planning of healthcare and future research studies.

Abbreviations

CI: Confidence interval; CiPCA: Consultations in primary care archive; GP: General practitioner; STATA v12.0: A statistical software package created by StataCorp; version 12; UK: United Kingdom

Acknowledgements

Acknowledgements are given to the informatics team at the Arthritis Research UK primary care Centre in their contribution to CiPCA.

Funding

This work was supported by Professor Kate Dunn's Wellcome Trust - Career Development Fellowship [083572/Z/07/Z]. CiPCA is funded by the North Staffordshire Primary Care Research Consortium and Keele University Research Institute for Primary Care and Health Sciences. Dr. Albert Tan's work was supported by a grant from the Jean Shanks foundation.

Authors' contributions

All authors (AT, VS, JP, KD) designed the study. AT analysed the data and drafted the manuscript. All authors (AT, VS, JP, KD) contributed to the interpretation of the results and critical revision of the manuscript for important intellectual content and approved the final version of the manuscript.

Ethics approval and consent to participate

Ethics approval for CiPCA was given by the North Staffordshire, Staffordshire, and Black Country Local Research Ethics Committees (REC reference: 03/04). Ethics approval constitutes the use of this anonymised dataset for research and hence individual patient consent is not required. Patients are informed by leaflet that the practice is a research practice and that their anonymised records (with identifiable information removed) may be used for research and that they can opt out if they wish by informing the practice staff. Patients who have asked for their or their children's medical records not to be used for research have a code applied to their records, Type 1 opt out, at their general practice which means their data is excluded during the extraction process. CiPCA operates a research request procedure where all requests are reviewed by the CiPCA Academic Custodianship Committee.

Consent for publication

Not applicable

Competing interests

The authors declare that they have no competing interests.

Author details

[1]Arthritis Research UK Primary Care Centre, Research Institute for Primary Care & Health Sciences, Keele University, Keele, Staffordshire ST5 5BG, UK. [2]Centre for Statistics in Medicine, Oxford Clinical Trial Research Unit , Nuffield Department of Orthopaedics, Rheumatology and Musculoskeletal Sciences, University of Oxford Botnar Research Centre, Windmill Road, Oxford OX3 7LD, UK.

References

1. Jordan KP, Kadam UT, Hayward R, et al. Annual consultation prevalence of regional musculoskeletal problems in primary care: an observational study. BMC Musculoskelet Disord. 2010;11:144.
2. Gunz AC, Canizares M, Mackay C, et al. Magnitude of impact and healthcare use for musculoskeletal disorders in the paediatric: a population-based study. BMC Musculoskelet Disord. 2012;13:98.
3. Roth-Isigkeit A, Thyen U, Stoven H, et al. Pain among children and adolescents: restrictions in daily living and triggering factors. Pediatrics. 2005;115(2):e152–e62.
4. Palermo TM. Impact of recurrent and chronic pain on child and family daily functioning: a critical review of the literature. J Dev Behav Pediatr. 2000; 21(1):58–69.
5. Perquin CW, Hunfeld JA, Hazebroek-Kampschreur AA, et al. The natural course of chronic benign pain in childhood and adolescence: a two-year population-based follow-up study. Eur J Pain. 2003;7(6):551–9. doi: 10.1016/S1090-3801(03)00060-0.
6. Epidemiology d IJ. Of musculoskeletal pain in primary care. Arch Dis Child. 2004;89(5):431–4.
7. King S, Chambers CT, Huguet a, et al. the epidemiology of chronic pain in children and adolescents revisited: a systematic review. Pain. 2011;152(12): 2729–38.
8. de Inocencio J. Musculoskeletal pain in primary pediatric care: analysis of 1000 consecutive general pediatric clinic visits. Pediatrics. 1998;102(6).
9. Kamper SJ, Henschke N, Hestbaek L, et al. Musculoskeletal pain in children and adolescents. Brazilian journal of physical therapy. 2016;20(3):275. https://doi.org/10.1590/bjpt-rbf.2014.0149 [published Online First: 2016/02/18].
10. Bot SD, van der Waal JM, Terwee CB, et al. Predictors of outcome in neck and shoulder symptoms: a cohort study in general practice. Spine 2005; 30(16):E459-EE70.
11. van der Waal JM, Bot SD, Terwee CB, et al. the incidences of and consultation rate for lower extremity complaints in general practice. Ann Rheum Dis. 2006;65(6):809–15. https://doi.org/10.1136/ard.2005.036988 [published Online First: 2005/11/05].
12. Vijlbrief AS, Bruijnzeels MA, van der Wouden JC, et al. Incidence and management of transient synovitis of the hip: a study in Dutch general practice. Br J Gen Pract. 1992;42(363):426–8. [published Online First: 1992/10/01].
13. Jordan K, Clarke AM, Symmons DP, et al. measuring disease prevalence: a comparison of musculoskeletal disease using four general practice consultation databases. Br J Gen Pract. 2007;57(534):7–14.
14. Porcheret M, Hughes R, Evans D, et al. Data quality of general practice electronic health records: the impact of a program of assessments, feedback, and training. J Am Med Inform Assoc. 2004;11(1):78–86.
15. Office for National Statistics: [http://www.statistics.gov.uk/statbase/.
16. Barros AJD, Hirakata VN. Alternatives for logistic regression in cross-sectional studies: an empirical comparison of models that directly estimate the prevalence ratio. BMC Medical Research Methodology. 2003;3:21.
17. Jordan KP, Joud A, Bergknut C, et al. International comparisons of the consultation prevalence of musculoskeletal conditions using population-based healthcare data from England and Sweden. Ann Rheum Dis. 2014; 73(1):212–8. https://doi.org/10.1136/annrheumdis-2012-202634 [published Online First: 2013/01/25].
18. McCormick A, Fleming D, Charlton C. Morbidity statistics from general practice: fourth national study 1991–1992. London; 1995.
19. Bruijnzeels MA, Foets M, van der Wouden JC, et al. Everyday symptoms in childhood: occurrence and general practitioner consultation rates. Br J Gen Pract. 1998;48(426):880–4. [published Online First: 1998/05/30].
20. Hambidge SJ, Davidson AJ, Gonzales R, et al. Epidemiology of pediatric injury-related primary care office visits in the United States. Pediatrics. 2002; 109(4):559–65. [published Online First: 2002/04/03].
21. Fayaz A, Croft P, Langford RM, et al. Prevalence of chronic pain in the UK: a systematic review and meta-analysis of population studies. BMJ Open. 2016;6(6).

6

Hypertrophic osteoarthropathy mimicking a reactive arthritis

Francesco Bozzao[1*], Stella Bernardi[1], Franca Dore[2], Lorenzo Zandonà[2] and Fabio Fischetti[1]

Abstract

Background: Hypertrophic osteoarthropathy (HOA) is a syndrome characterized by abnormal proliferation of skin and periosteal tissues of the extremities. It can be a rare hereditary disease (pachydermoperiostosis) or can be secondary to various diseases, though mostly lung malignancies. Here, we report an unusual clinical presentation of HOA.

Case presentation: A 77-year-old man presented with fever, diarrhea, and an oligoarthritis involving the left knee and the ankles. Since left knee synovial fluid aspiration revealed an aseptic synovitis and *Clostridium Difficile* toxin was detectable in stool samples, a reactive arthritis secondary to a *Clostridium Difficile* induced colitis was initially suspected. However, the presence of a worsened digital clubbing and the lack of a good clinical response to steroid therapy led us to perform a radionuclide bone scanning, which revealed HOA. This turned out to be associated with a lepidic predominant lung adenocarcinoma, which was clinically and radiologically difficult to distinguish from a relapse of pneumonia.

Conclusion: Consistent with the literature, HOA tends to have a variable clinical presentation, mimicking that of various rheumatic diseases. This clinical case shows that HOA can present as a presumptive acute reactive arthritis, and it highlights the importance of patient's follow-up in the differential diagnosis of inflammatory arthritis, especially when a worsened digital clubbing is present.

Keywords: Hypertrophic osteoarthropathy, Reactive arthritis, Lepidic predominant lung adenocarcinoma, Periosteal reaction

Background

Rheumatic paraneoplastic syndromes include musculoskeletal disorders not directly caused by tumor expansion, but related with humoral factors released from deranged cells. These syndromes are rare and challenging to diagnose. Nevertheless, their prompt recognition can be of major clinical importance because they often precede other manifestations of the associated neoplasm [1]. Hypertrophic osteoarthropathy (HOA) can be a primary hereditary disease, but it is most often a rheumatic paraneoplastic syndrome secondary to a lung malignancy [2]. It is characterized by digital clubbing and periostosis of tubular bones [1]. Here, we report the case of a 77-year-old man presenting with an asymmetric oligoarthritis of the lower limbs, which was initially interpreted as a reactive arthritis associated with a *Clostridium Difficile* infection, but later understood to be a HOA associated with a lepidic predominant lung adenocarcinoma. We also performed a review of the literature and a search in Pubmed of other clinical cases of adult patients affected by primary or secondary HOA, in which other rheumatic diseases were initially suspected. For this purpose, we used the combined terms "hypertrophic osteoarthropathy" and "case report" and we selected only English written articles (Table 1).

* Correspondence: francesco.bozzao@gmail.com
[1]Department of Medical Sciences, University of Trieste, Cattinara Teaching Hospital, Strada di Fiume 449, 34149 Trieste, Italy
Full list of author information is available at the end of the article

Case presentation

A 77-year-old man was admitted to our Internal Medicine Department for fever, diarrhea, and a 1-month history of persistent polyarthralgia and prolonged morning stiffness at both ankles and knees. Almost 40 days before, the patient had been hospitalized for an exacerbation of chronic obstructive pulmonary disease (COPD), which was treated

Table 1 Rheumatic disorders mimicking and/or associated with hypertrophic osteoarthropathy

Age/sex	Presentation	Initial diagnosis	Time lapse (months)	Final diagnosis	Ref.
53/M	Diffuse joint effusions; clubbing	Rheumatoid arthritis	Not given	HOA secondary to end-stage cryptogenic cirrhosis, interstitial lung disease	[6]
54/M	Diffuse joint effusions; clubbing; positive RF and anti-CCP	Rheumatoid arthritis	Not given	Primary HOA and rheumatoid arthritis	[12]
30/M	Diffuse joint effusions; positive anti-CCP	Rheumatoid arthritis	12	HOA secondary to primary pulmonary hypertension	[13]
Not given	Diffuse joint effusions; positive RF and anti-CCP	Rheumatoid arthritis	1	HOA secondary to lung tumor and rheumatoid arthritis	[14]
55/M	Left elbow, bilateral wrist and ankle effusions; clubbing	Inflammatory arthritis	3	HOA secondary to small cell carcinoma	[15]
62/M	Bilateral ankle, wrist, right elbow effusions; clubbing	Inflammatory arthritis	4	HOA secondary to non small cell lung carcinoma	[15]
57/F	Clubbing	Inflammatory arthritis	8	HOA secondary to lung adenocarcinoma	[16]
57/M	Right knee effusion; clubbing; positive ANA and anti-Sm	Systemic lupus erythematous	18	HOA secondary to lung adenocarcinoma	[17]
47/F	Bilateral knee effusions; clubbing; positive ANA, anti-ds DNA, anti-SSA e anti-SSB	Systemic lupus erythematous	3	HOA secondary to lung adenocarcinoma	[18]
19/M	Diffuse joint effusions	Juvenile idiopathic arthritis	48	Pachydermoperiostosis	[19]
17/M	Diffuse joint effusions; clubbing	Juvenile idiopathic arthritis	Not given	HOA secondary to hepatopulmonary syndrome	[20]
50/M	Clubbing	Ankylosing spondylitis	36	Primary HOA (incomplete form) and ankylosing spondylitis	[21]
48/F	Diffuse joint effusions	Steroid myopathy	2	HOA secondary to chronic lung transplant rejection	[6]
70/F	Bilateral knee effusions	Infective arthritis	2	HOA secondary to small cell lung cancer	[22]
43/F	Bilateral knee and ankle effusions; clubbing	Lower extremity cellulitis	1	HOA secondary to past lung adenocarcinoma	[23]
66/M	Right knee effusion	Osteoarthritis of the knee	10	HOA secondary to lung adenocarcinoma	[24]

with a fluoroquinolone. Subsequently, he developed a *Clostridium Difficile* induced colitis, treated with oral metronidazole. The patient was a former port worker and had been a heavy smoker for 40 years. Past medical history included ischemic heart disease and arterial hypertension, for which he was taking anti-platelet and anti-hypertensive therapy.

On physical examination, he was febrile (37.9 °C) and had a heart rate of 95 beats/min and a blood pressure of 135/70 mmHg. His oxygen saturation was 96% on room air. His body mass index was 27 Kg/m^2 and he reported a 5 Kg weight loss over the last 3 months. His ankles appeared clearly swollen, with reduced range of motion. There was a tense effusion in the left knee and a moderate joint tenderness in all limbs. Fingers and toes presented with a low grade digital clubbing, whose first appearance could not be precisely dated. Laboratory exams showed C-reactive protein (CRP) of 116.1 mg/L (normal values < 5 mg/L), erythrocyte sedimentation rate (ESR) of 90 mm/hr. (normal values < 35 mm/hr), white blood cells (WBC) of 11.860/mm^3 (normal values between 4.000 and 11.000/mm^3) and a rheumatoid factor of 56 U/mL (normal values < 20 U/ml). Blood and urine cultures were negative. The left knee synovial fluid aspiration showed an aseptic synovitis (8.226 WBC/hpf, with 90% neutrophils, while crystal detection, gram stain and cultures were negative). Moreover, *Clostridium Difficile* toxin in stool samples was still detectable.

Based on this presentation, a reactive arthritis due to a *Clostridium Difficile* induced colitis was suspected and oral vancomycin, oral prednisone, and painkillers were prescribed. Five days later, since fever, diarrhea, and polyarthralgia had apparently resolved, the patient was discharged, and a post-discharge visit was scheduled at the Rheumatology Office 1 month later.

When the patient came to the Rheumatology Office, he reported a relapse of polyarthralgia and joint tenderness while he was gradually reducing oral prednisone. He was slightly febrile (37.5 °C) but had denied relapse of diarrhea. On physical examination, his ankles were still swollen, while the left knee effusion had resolved. The fingers of both hands were also diffusely swollen and digital clubbing had worsened, with an increase of distal phalangeal/interphalangeal depth ratio (greater than 1.05). Lung auscultation revealed fine crackles at the base of the right lung. In laboratory exams, CRP was 101.1 mg/L, ESR was 99 mm/h and WBC was 14.380/mm^3. Chest radiograph was unchanged as compared to that performed when the patient had the COPD exacerbation, revealing a possible patchy infiltrate at the base of the right lung, while radiograph of the ankles was inconclusive (Fig. 1a). At that stage, given the presence of a lung infiltrate and systemic inflammatory features (fever and elevated inflammatory markers), a relapse of right base pneumonia was suspected; thus, an empiric antibiotic therapy with a broad-spectrum penicillin and pain killers were prescribed. In addition, bone scintigraphy and chest computed tomography (CT) were promptly performed. The first revealed increased linear periosteal ^{99}mTc-hydroxymethylene diphosphonate (HMDP) uptake, which is a typical sign of HOA (Fig. 1b). The second revealed a lung infiltrate with a partly ground-glass aspect (Fig. 2).

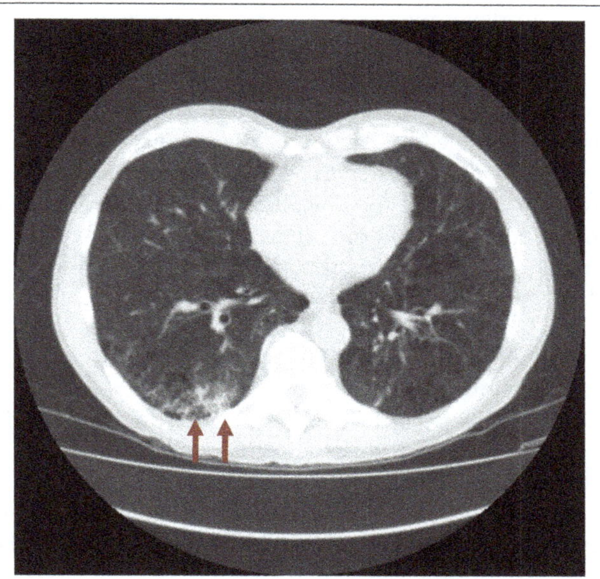

Fig. 2 Chest CT showing lung emphysema with several pulmonary bullae and a lung infiltrate at the right lower lobe (red arrows)

Owing to the high association between HOA and lung malignancies [3], the patient underwent a bronchoscopy with bronchoalveolar lavage (BAL) and transbronchial biopsies of the right lung infiltrate. Unfortunately, biopsies could not be performed because of the complexity in localizing the infiltrate under fluoroscopy. On the other hand, we were unable to schedule a CT-guided percutaneous biopsy or a diagnostic surgery because the patient's general conditions dramatically worsened. He developed high fever (39.4 °C) and severe respiratory failure, which we ascribed to a severe bilateral pneumonia. During the hospitalization in a semi-intensive care unit, bronchoscopy was tried again and, finally, a transbronchial small biopsy could be performed. In the BAL, there were no malignant cells or infectious pathogens; likewise, blood and sputum cultures turned out negative. When the result of the transbronchial biopsy pathology examination (Fig. 3a) became available, showing a lepidic

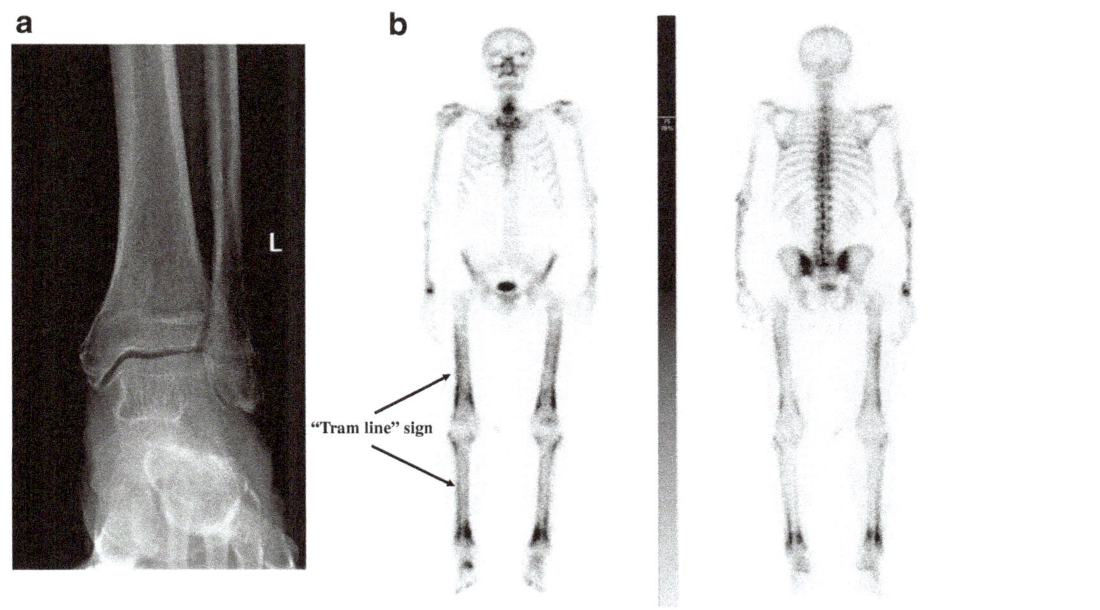

Fig. 1 a Posteroanterior radiograph of the left ankle; (**b**) ^{99m}Tc HMDP bone scintigraphy showing increased linear periosteal tracer uptake ("tram line" sign or "double stripe" sign)

pattern adenocarcinoma, no specific therapy was prescribed due to the extreme gravity of the patient's general conditions. Despite the use of noninvasive ventilation and extended spectrum antibiotic therapy, the patient died 4 days after the biopsy results and roughly 5 months after the initial clinical presentation. Autopsy confirmed the diagnosis of lepidic predominant adenocarcinoma of the right lung, associated with massive bilateral destructive pneumonia and severe emphysema with centrolobular pattern (Fig. 3b).

Discussion

The first interpretation of the patient's complaints was that of a reactive arthritis due to a *Clostridium Difficile* induced colitis. The incidence of *Clostridium Difficile* infections (CDI) is increasing worldwide, and fluoroquinolone use has been implicated in this context [4]. There are several reports of reactive arthritis due to CDI. Based on the literature, this disorder seems to affect young adults, mostly females. It usually develops 10 days after the CDI, and its initial presentation is a monoarthritis or oligoarthritis, most frequently involving the ankles and knees. The criteria for diagnosing a reactive arthritis associated with CDI include: (i) evidence of aseptic synovitis developing during or immediately after colitis; (ii) presence of toxin in stool samples; and (iii) absence of other causes [5]. Based on the initial presentation, which fitted all these criteria, our first hypothesis was that of a reactive arthritis.

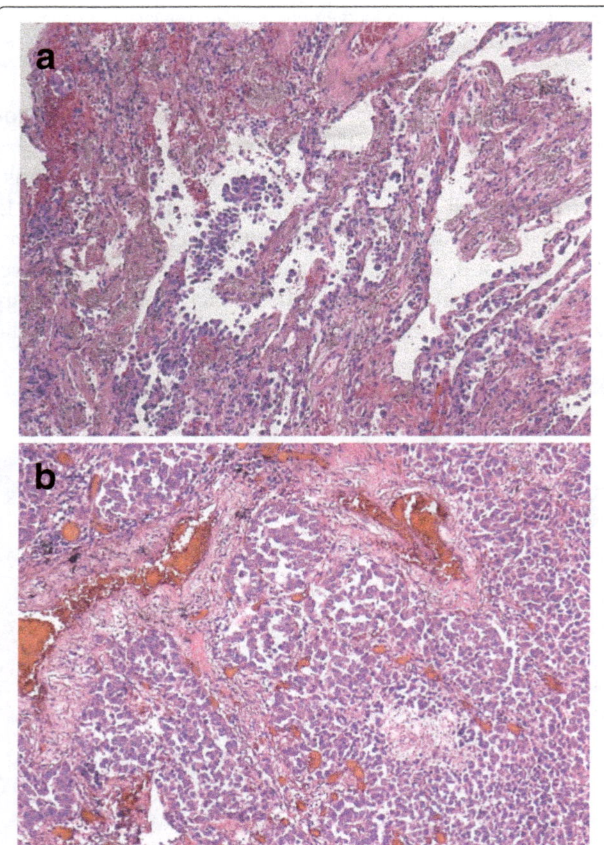

Fig. 3 a Representative Hematoxylin and Eosin (H & E) stained section of transbronchial biopsy specimen, showing thickening of interalveolar septa and atypical pneumocytes proliferating along the surface of alveolar walls, compatible with a lepidic pattern adenocarcinoma of the lung (original magnification 10×); **b** Representative H&E stained section of lung autopsy, showing a lepidic predominant adenocarcinoma of the lung (original magnification 10×)

Nevertheless, the patient's age, his digital clubbing, and the lack of a good clinical response to steroid therapy led us to perform additional exams and finally to the diagnosis of HOA. Hypertrophic osteoartropathy, also known as Pierre Marie-Banberger syndrome, is a condition characterized by the triad of digital clubbing, periosteal reaction of long bones and painful tenderness of the limbs, especially in the lower extremities, sometimes with synovial non-inflammatory effusions of large joints [3]. When all three clinical features are simultaneously present, a complete form of HOA is diagnosed, but most often HOA presents as an incomplete form, with the possibility of digital clubbing being absent [6]. HOA can be a primary hereditary disease (pachydermoperiostosis) or, more commonly, it is secondary to several pathologic conditions, though mostly to lung malignancies (up to 90%) [3]. Digital clubbing, defined as a focal bulbous deformity of the tips of the digits, is one of the oldest clinical signs in medicine and it can be either isolated or associated with HOA. In addition, clubbing can be present in a wide variety of clinical conditions, including both neoplastic and non-neoplastic pulmonary diseases [7]. The quantification of phalangeal depth ratio (distal phalangeal/interphalangeal depth ratio) is one of the methods to measure the degree of digital clubbing and can be helpful to distinguish between patients with pulmonary malignancy and those with COPD. In fact, Baughman and colleagues have demonstrated that a phalangeal depth ratio exceeding 1.05 in a patient with COPD is frequently associated with the presence of bronchogenic carcinoma [7, 8].

Given that in our patient HOA was associated with worsening of digital clubbing and a chest infiltrate, a bronchoscopy was performed, showing a lepidic predominant lung adenocarcinoma, which was then confirmed by the autopsy. It has been shown that diagnosis of lepidic predominant lung adenocarcinoma (formerly known as non-mucinous bronchoalveolar lung cancer) [9] is sometimes quite challenging because it can exhibit radiological features suggestive of interstitial lung disease [10] or it can mimic a recurrent bacterial community acquired pneumonia [11]. In line with these reports, our case highlights that radiological evidence of interstitial lung disease or pneumonia does not rule out a pulmonary malignancy, but warrants further investigations in patients with a high clinical suspicion of lung cancer, such as in the case of HOA.

Diagnosis of HOA tends to be difficult since its clinical presentation can mimic that of other rheumatic diseases [6, 12–24] (Table 1), the first being rheumatoid arthritis [6, 12–14]. Furthermore, the presence of a rheumatic disease does not rule out a diagnosis of HOA, since HOA can also coexist with other rheumatic conditions [12, 14, 21] (Table 1). In addition, periosteal reaction, commonly considered to be the radiological hallmark of HOA [3], can also be present in other disorders [25], including some rheumatic diseases, such as polyarteritis nodosa [26], familial Mediterranean fever [27], Takayasu's arteritis [28], psoriatic arthritis and reactive arthritis [29].

Periosteal reaction is the result of new bone deposition in response to different physical and chemical stimuli, and can develop either as a localized or as a systemic disease. In HOA, periosteal reaction tends to have a symmetric distribution and the earliest lesions are localized at the diaphysis of long bones of lower extremities, typically tibiae and fibulae [3]. Although HOA is most commonly detected with radiography, which can demonstrate periosteal reaction even in asymptomatic patients [3], in our case, this exam turned out to be inconclusive. By contrast, radionuclide bone scan with ^{99}mTc-hydroxymethylene diphosphonate (HMDP), which is considered the most sensitive imaging modality for HOA detection and characterization [3], showed a symmetrically increased linear tracer uptake at the periosteal site (also known as the "tram line" sign), consistent with our clinical suspicion of HOA.

To our knowledge, we are the first to describe a case of HOA mimicking a reactive arthritis, although we cannot exclude the coexistence of both conditions. Some elements, such as the presence of an inflammatory synovial fluid in the left knee and the complete resolution of the effusion in this joint after 1 month of steroid therapy, might suggest that our patient had also suffered from a reactive arthritis secondary to a CDI. Moreover, the inflammatory condition promoted by the reactive arthritis might have contributed to the progression of HOA. In line with this hypothesis, HOA has been found to be associated with several inflammatory conditions such as sarcoidosis [30] and chronic infections [31–34]. Although pathogenesis of HOA is unclear, this condition has been linked to an increased production of prostaglandin E2 (PGE2). For instance, patients with both primary and secondary HOA have much higher urinary levels of PGE2 than healthy individuals [35–37]. PGE2 is a lipid mediator derived from arachidonic acid through the action of enzymes, including the ubiquitous tissue constitutive isoform cyclooxigenase (COX)-1 and the inflammatory or tumor-induced isoform COX-2 [38]. Increased levels of PGE2 might be responsible for secondary overexpression of vascular endothelial growth factor (VEGF), thus inducing neoangiogenesis, new bone formation and edema [36]. Therefore, VEGF inhibitors, such as a monoclonal anti-VEGF antibody and bisphosphonates [30, 39], as well as COX-2 inhibitors [35], have shown to induce relief of bone pain in patients with HOA.

With this in mind, apart from digital clubbing and the chest infiltrate, the other sign that raised our suspicion of an alternative diagnosis was the partial response to initial treatment. Treatment modalities for CDI induced reactive arthritis include NSAIDs, intra-articular corticosteroid injection or systemic corticosteroid therapy [40]. Generally, it is expected that two thirds of patients with reactive arthritis associated with CDI achieve a spontaneous recovery after 60 days from the onset of the colitis [41]. On the other hand, in the case of HOA, only curative treatment of the underlying cause can lead to the complete regression of periostosis and its corresponding symptoms [42].

Conclusion

Our review of the literature confirmed that clinical presentation of HOA can be variable, frequently mimicking that of an inflammatory arthritis. Our case report reminds clinicians to be aware of HOA in elderly patients with a large joint arthritis, even in the presence of features suggestive of an alternative diagnosis, such as a reactive arthritis. For this reason, response to the initial treatment should be closely monitored in order to perform further diagnostic exams when it is only partial. This is particularly true when an occult neoplastic disease is suspected, as in the case of worsened digital clubbing. Furthermore, whenever a HOA is diagnosed, malignancy should be thoroughly searched, even if clinical and radiological exams could be just consistent with infectious or interstitial diseases.

Abbreviations

ANA: Antinuclear antibodies; anti-CCP: Anti-cyclic citrullinated peptide antibodies; Anti-ds DNA: Anti-double stranded DNA antibodies; Anti-Sm: Anti-Smith antibodies; Anti-SSA and Anti-SSB: Anti-Sjogren's syndrome-related antigen A and antigen B; BAL: Broncho-alveolar lavage; CDI: *Clostridium Difficile* infection; COX: Cyclooxigenase; CRP: C-reactive protein; CT: Computed tomography; ESR: Erythrocyte sedimentation rate; HMDP: ^{99}mTc-hydroxymethylene diphosphonate; HOA: Hypertrophic osteoartropathy; hpf: High power field; NSAIDs: Nonsteroidal anti-inflammatory drugs; PGE2: Prostaglandin E2; RF: Rheumatoid factor; VEGF: Vascular endotelial growth factor; WBC: White blood cells

Acknowledgments

Thanks are due to Dr. Georgette Argiris for her precious help in revising this paper.

Authors' contributions

FB examined the patient and contributed to manuscript conception, preparation, and editing. SB contributed to manuscript conception, preparation and editing. FD performed the Nuclear Medicine exams. LZ performed pathological readings. FF examined the patient and contributed to manuscript conception, preparation and editing. All authors read and approved the final manuscript.

Consent for publication
Since the patient was already deceased when this case report was written, patient's next of kin signed a written consent from indicating that he is aware of this case report and the possibility of it being published.

Competing interests
The authors declare that they have no competing interests.

Author details
[1]Department of Medical Sciences, University of Trieste, Cattinara Teaching Hospital, Strada di Fiume 449, 34149 Trieste, Italy. [2]ASUITS, Cattinara Teaching Hospital, Strada di Fiume 449, 34149 Trieste, Italy.

References

1. Manger B, Schett G. Paraneoplastic syndromes in rheumatology. Nat Rev Rheumatol. 2014;10(11):662–70.
2. Coury C. Hippocration fingers and hypertrophic osteoarthropathy. A study of 350 cases. Br J Dis Chest. 1960;54:202–9.
3. Yap FY, Skalski MR, Patel DB, Schein AJ, White EA, Tomasian A, Masih S, Matcuk GR Jr. Hypertrophic Osteoarthropathy: clinical and imaging features. Radiographics. 2017;37(1):157–95.
4. Bartlett JG, Perl TM. The new Clostridium difficile–what does it mean? N Engl J Med. 2005;353(23):2503–5.
5. Legendre P, Lalande V, Eckert C, Barbut F, Fardet L, Meynard JL, Surgers L. Clostridium difficile associated reactive arthritis: case report and literature review. Anaerobe. 2016;38:76–80.
6. Yao Q, Altman RD, Brahn E. Periostitis and hypertrophic pulmonary osteoarthropathy: report of 2 cases and review of the literature. Semin Arthritis Rheum. 2009;38(6):458–66.
7. Myers KA, Farquhar DR. The rational clinical examination. Does this patient have clubbing? JAMA. 2001;286(3):341–7.
8. Baughman RP, Gunther KL, Buchsbaum JA, Lower EE. Prevalence of digital clubbing in bronchogenic carcinoma by a new digital index. Clin Exp Rheumatol. 1998;16(1):21–6.
9. Travis WD, Brambilla E, Nicholson AG, Yatabe Y, Austin JH, Beasley MB, Chirieac LR, Dacic S, Duhig E, Flieder DB, et al. The 2015 World Health Organization classification of lung tumors: impact of genetic, clinical and radiologic advances since the 2004 classification. J Thorac Oncol. 2015;10(9):1243–60.
10. Hammen I. Interstitial lung disease pattern turned out to be a predominantly lepidic lung adenocarcinoma. Respir Med Case Rep. 2017;21:56–8.
11. Cunha BA, Syed U, Mikail N. Bronchoalveolar carcinoma (adenocarcinoma) mimicking recurrent bacterial community-acquired pneumonia (CAP). Heart Lung. 2012;41(1):83–6.
12. Diamond S, Momeni M. Primary hypertrophic osteoarthropathy in a patient with rheumatoid arthritis. J Clin Rheumatol. 2007;13(4):242–3.
13. Sifuentes Giraldo WA, Ahijon Lana M, Gallego Rivera I, Bachiller Corral FJ, Gamir Gamir ML. Hypertrophic osteoarthropathy with acro-osteolysis in a patient with primary pulmonary hypertension. Reumatol Clin. 2012;8(4):208–11.
14. Farhey Y, Luggen M. Seropositive, symmetric polyarthritis in a patient with poorly differentiated lung carcinoma: carcinomatous polyarthritis, hypertrophic osteoarthropathy, or rheumatoid arthritis? Arthritis Care Res. 1998;11(2):146–9.
15. Armstrong DJ, McCausland EM, Wright GD. Hypertrophic pulmonary osteoarthropathy (HPOA) (Pierre Marie-Bamberger syndrome): two cases presenting as acute inflammatory arthritis. Description and review of the literature. Rheumatol Int. 2007;27(4):399–402.
16. Korsten P, Bohnenberger H, Vasko R. Hypertrophic osteoarthropathy presenting as inflammatory arthritis. Arthritis Rheumatol. 2015;67(11):3036.
17. Cruz C, Rocha M, Andrade D, Guimaraes F, Silva V, Souza S, Moura CA, Moura CG. Hypertrophic pulmonary osteoarthropathy with positive antinuclear antibodies: case report. Case Rep Oncol. 2012;5(2):308–12.
18. Aluoch AO, Farbman M, Gladue H. An unusual mimicker of systemic lupus erythematosus: a case report. Open Rheumatol J. 2015;9:27–9.
19. Ibba S, Piga M, Congia M, Cauli A, Mathieu A. Pachidermoperiostosis as a cause of massive joint effusion with polyarticular involvement mimicking juvenile idiopathic arthritis: a case report. Joint Bone Spine. 2016;83(1):113–4.
20. Ede K, McCurdy D, Garcia Lloret M. Hypertrophic osteoarthropathy in the hepatopulmonary syndrome. J Clin Rheumatol. 2008;14(4):230–3.
21. Shinjo SK, Borba EF, Goncalves CR, Levy-Neto M. Ankylosing spondylitis in a patient with primary hypertrophic osteoarthropathy. J Clin Rheumatol. 2007;13(3):175.
22. Meeker J, Lachiewicz PF. An unusual cause of late pain and effusion after total knee arthroplasty: pulmonary hypertrophic osteoarthropathy. A case report. J Bone Joint Surg Am. 2008;90(2):390–2.
23. Mauricio O, Francis L, Athar U, Shah C, Chaudhary M, Gajra A. Hypertrophic osteoarthropathy masquerading as lower extremity cellulitis and response to bisphosphonates. J Thorac Oncol. 2009;4(2):260–2.
24. Swarup I, Mintz DN, Salvati EA. Hypertrophic Osteoarthropathy: an unusual cause of knee pain and recurrent effusion. HSS J. 2016;12(3):284–6.
25. Rana RS, Wu JS, Eisenberg RL. Periosteal reaction. AJR Am J Roentgenol. 2009;193(4):W259–72.
26. Astudillo LM, Rigal F, Couret B, Arlet-Suau E. Localized polyarteritis nodosa with periostitis. J Rheumatol. 2001;28(12):2758–9.
27. Garcia-Gonzalez A, Weisman MH. The arthritis of familial Mediterranean fever. Semin Arthritis Rheum. 1992;22(3):139–50.
28. Kim JE, Kolh EM, Kim DK. Takayasu's arteritis presenting with focal periostitis affecting two limbs. Int J Cardiol. 1998;67(3):267–70.
29. Kettering JM, Towers JD, Rubin DA. The seronegative spondyloarthropathies. Semin Roentgenol. 1996;31(3):220–8.
30. Jayakar BA, Abelson AG, Yao Q. Treatment of hypertrophic osteoarthropathy with zoledronic acid: case report and review of the literature. Semin Arthritis Rheum. 2011;41(2):291–6.
31. Horacio MC, Maria VG, Alonso GL. Hypertrophic osteoarthropathy as a complication of pulmonary tuberculosis. Reumatol Clin. 2015;11(4):255–7.
32. Aziz W, Yates DB. Hypertrophic osteoarthropathy associated with bacterial endocarditis. Rheumatology (Oxford). 1999;38(4):375–7.
33. Chapman SA, Delgadillo D 3rd, MacGuidwin E, Greenberg JI, Jameson AP. Graft infection masquerading as rheumatologic disease: a rare case of Aortobifemoral graft infection presenting as hypertrophic Osteoarthropathy. Ann Vasc Surg. 2017;41:283 e211–8.
34. Puechal X. Whipple's arthritis. Joint Bone Spine. 2016;83(6):631–5.
35. Kozak KR, Milne GL, Morrow JD, Cuiffo BP. Hypertrophic osteoarthropathy pathogenesis: a case highlighting the potential role for cyclo-oxygenase-2-derived prostaglandin E2. Nat Clin Pract Rheumatol. 2006;2(8):452–6. quiz following 456
36. Kozak KR, Milne GL, Bentzen SM, Yock TI. Elevation of prostaglandin E2 in lung cancer patients with digital clubbing. J Thorac Oncol. 2012;7(12):1877–8.
37. Zhang Z, Zhang C, Zhang Z. Primary hypertrophic osteoarthropathy: an update. Front Med. 2013;7(1):60–4.
38. Rotas I, Cito G, Letovanec I, Christodoulou M, Perentes JY. Cyclooxygenase-2 expression in non-small cell lung Cancer correlates with hypertrophic Osteoarthropathy. Ann Thorac Surg. 2016;101(2):e51–3.
39. Kikuchi R, Itoh M, Tamamushi M, Nakamura H, Aoshiba K. Hypertrophic osteoarthropathy secondary to lung cancer: beneficial effect of anti-vascular endothelial growth factor antibody. J Clin Rheumatol. 2017;23(1):47–50.
40. Birnbaum J, Bartlett JG, Gelber AC. *Clostridium difficile*: an under-recognized cause of reactive arthritis? Clin Rheumatol. 2008;27:253–5.
41. Prati C, Bertolini E, Toussirot E, Wendling D. Reactive arthritis due to *Clostridium Difficile*. Joint Bone Spine. 2010;77(2):190–2.
42. Nguyen S, Hojjati M. Review of current therapies for secondary hypertrophic pulmonary osteoarthropathy. Clin Rheumatol. 2011;30(1):7–13.

7

In-vivo study of osseointegration in Prestige LP cervical disc prosthesis

Jigang Lou[1], Beiyu Wang[1], Tingkui Wu[1], Wenjie Wu[2], Huibo Li[3], Ziyang Liu[1] and Hao Liu[1*]

Abstract

Background: A study was designed to quantify the extent of porous osseointegration at the prosthesis-bone interface in the Prestige LP prosthesis containing a plasma-sprayed titanium coating.

Methods: Using an anterior surgical approach, cervical disc arthroplasty was performed in 8 mature male goats at the C3-C4 segment, followed by implantation of the Prestige LP prosthesis. The vertebral specimens were examined using microcomputed tomograph for histomorphometric quantification, and proceeded by routine paraffin processing for histological observation. Hence, the porous osseointegration at the prosthesis-bone interface was evaluated based on histologic and histomorphometric analyses.

Results: At 6 months after surgery, there was no evidence of prosthesis migration, loosening, subsidence, or neurologic or vascular complications. Based on gross histologic analysis, there was excellent porous ingrowth at the prosthesis–bone interface, without significant histopathologic changes. Histomorphometric analysis at the prosthesis-bone interface indicated the mean porous ingrowth of 48.5% ± 10.4% and the total ingrowth range of 36.6 to 59.8%.

Conclusions: As the first comprehensive in vivo investigation into the Prestige LP prosthesis, this project established a successful animal model in the evaluation of cervical disc arthroplasty. Moreover, histomorphometric analysis of porous ingrowth at the prosthesis-bone interface was more favorable for cervical disc arthroplasty with the Prestige LP prosthesis compared to historical reports of appendicular total joint arthroplasty.

Keywords: Cervical disc arthroplasty, Animal model, Porous ingrowth, Osseointegration, Histomorphometry

Background

Cervical disc arthroplasty (CDA) is an exciting new technology to treat symptomatic cervical degenerative disc disease in patients who have failed conservative care. This technology not only allows for the maintenance of normal cervical spinal motion, but also has the potential to prevent or reduce the risk of degeneration at adjacent levels, compared with the conventional fusion techniques [1–3]. However, the complications associated with CDA prostheses have been reported as heterotopic ossification, prosthesis migration and dislocation, prosthesis subsidence, spontaneous fusion, immune tissue reaction and fracture in the adjacent vertebral body [4, 5]. Among these, the most important complication is the prosthesis migration and dislocation, because it often requires reoperation. In previous studies, the incidence of prosthesis dislocation after CDA has been reported as 0.5%–3.06% [6–8]. Hence, it is very essential to improve the initial stability and long-term stability of CDA prostheses in order to lower the risk of prosthesis migration and dislocation.

To date, a variety of commercial and experimental disc prostheses with various design concepts are designed to strive for better initial stability and long-term stability in order to obtain long-term survivorship of CDA prostheses. With regard to the current widely used Prestige LP prosthesis (Medtronic Sofamor Danek, Memphis, TN, USA), with two titanium ceramic composite endplates (Fig. 1), its initial device fixation is mainly attributed to the mechanisms of acute fixation achieved via a series of four rails, two on each prosthesis endplate. Besides, its long-term device fixation is acquired by a porous titanium coating on prosthesis endplate. The primary endplate bearing surface contains two layers of pure titanium, with a pore size of 75–300 μm, which

* Correspondence: liuhao110@126.com
[1]Department of Orthopedics, West China Hospital, Sichuan University, 37 Guoxue Road, Chengdu, Sichuan 610041, China
Full list of author information is available at the end of the article

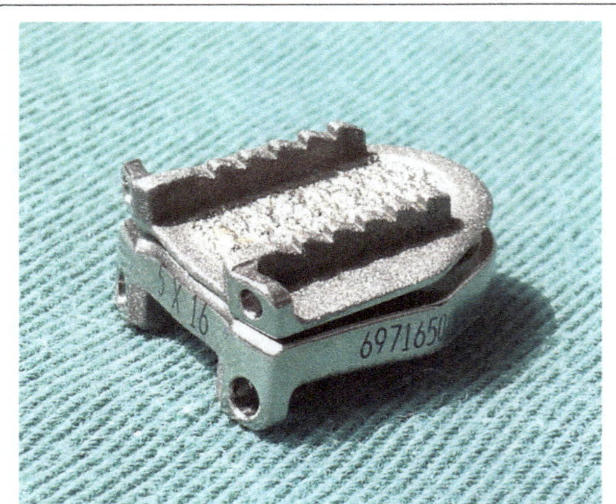

Fig. 1 The Prestige LP prosthesis contains two titanium ceramic composite endplates, with two rails on each endplate and a porous titanium plasma spray coating

serves to increase porosity and surface area and facilitate trabecular ingrowth [9]. The titanium coatings consist of a special adhesive layer (< 90 μm) and a cover layer (< 180 μm). Owing to these features, a porous titanium plasma spray coating on the endplate contacting surfaces facilitates bone ingrowth and promotes the extent of biological osseointegration at the prosthesis-bone interface, ensuring long-term stability. As it is infeasible to quantitatively evaluate the extent of porous osseointegration at the prosthesis-bone interface for patients underwent cervical disc arthroplasty, an animal model is a great alternative.

Serving as the first to demonstrate successful endplate osseointegration in the caprine cervical model, the present study was undertaken to investigate the initial stability and the biologic porous ingrowth characteristics of the Prestige LP artificial cervical disc prosthesis, with success criteria based on radiographic analysis and quantitative histomorphometry.

Methods

Animal research permission

The Institutional Animal Care and Use Committee at the West China Center of Medical Sciences, Sichuan University, Chengdu, Sichuan granted approval for this investigation. Conduct of experimentation on living animals followed the recommendations of the Guide for the Care and Use of Laboratory Animals [10], and under the close supervision of qualified and experienced persons.

Animal model and surgical preparation

Eight mature male goats (2–3 years old, mean weight 30 Kg) from laboratory animal center of Sichuan University were included in this study, and followed for a period of 6 months after surgery. Each animal was sedated with an intravenous injection of anesthetic medications (diazepam 0.2 mg/kg and ketamine HCL 5 mg/kg), followed by endotracheal intubation and general inhalation anesthesia using 1% to 2% isoflurane with continuous intravenous fluids (range 3–6 mL/lb./h) administered for the duration of surgery. In addition, prophylactic intravenous antibiotics (cefazolin sodium, 1 g) and analgesics (butorphanol 0.1 mg/kg) were administered before and after surgery.

Surgical technique and postoperative evaluation

The anterior Smith-Robinson approach to the cervical spine was adapted to the goat model through a right-sided longitudinal incision with length 6- to 8-cm, and a standard anterior cervical discectomy was performed at the C3–C4 intervertebral level. The endplate surfaces were prepared using curettage and a high-speed burr. According to the manufacturer's recommended tools and procedures, the Prestige LP prosthesis was then implanted at the operative disc level (Fig. 2). Blood loss, operating times, and intra- and perioperative complications were quantified.

Observations of ambulatory activities and wound healing were monitored daily, and all animals received analgesics and prophylactic antibiotics for the first 10 days postoperatively. Lateral X-ray films of the cervical spine were taken intra- and post-operatively to confirm the correct position of all disc prostheses (Fig. 3). Euthanasia was performed for each animal using an overdose (150 mg/kg) of concentrated pentobarbital solution (390 mg/mL) at 6 months after surgery. The spinal column then was carefully dissected, immediately placed in double-wrapped

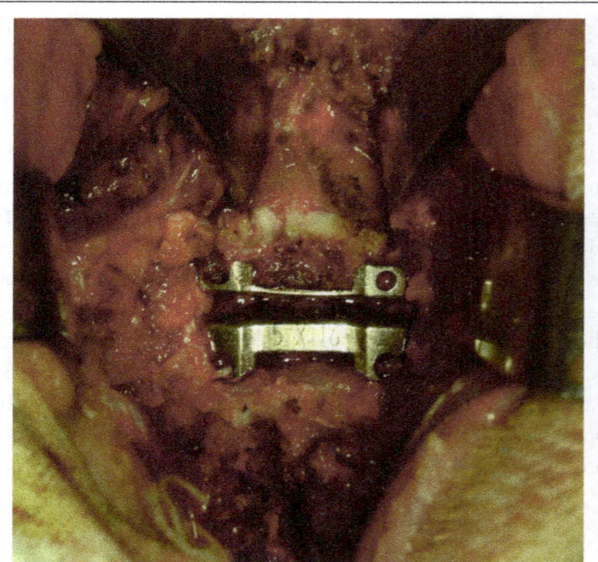

Fig. 2 Anterior intraoperative view. The Prestige LP prosthesis is implanted at the surgical level

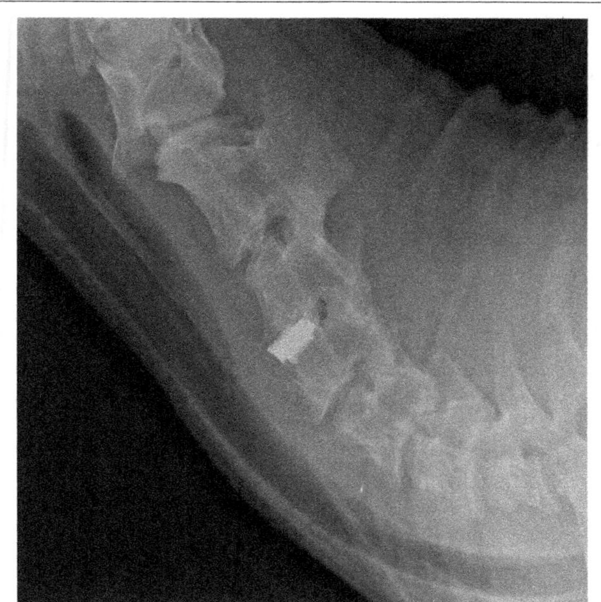

Fig. 3 Lateral X-ray film of the caprine cervical spine demonstrates that the disc prosthesis is in place

plastic specimen bags and frozen at – 20°C for subsequent radiographic and histological examination.

Histology and histomorphometry

The operative motion segments were examined using microcomputed tomograph (Micro-CT) to histomorphometrically quantify the percentage of trabecular ingrowth at the prosthesis-bone interface. The prosthesis surface was traced manually and expressed as a total endplate area pixel count. The regions of trabecular contact were subsequently traced, quantified in pixels, and expressed as a percentage of the total endplate area (% ingrowth = apparent bone contact area/gross total endplate area). The above quantitative evaluation method has been widely used in several previous studies [11–15].

The vertebral specimens were then performed histological evaluation at the Biotechnology Institute Histology Laboratory of Sichuan University. The specimens were fixed in 10% neutral buffered formalin solution, then dehydrated in a series of graded alcohol which was later substituted by dimethylbenzene, and embedded in paraffin. Thereafter, the paraffin embedded sections were cut into 3–5 μm thick using thin-sectioning microtomy, and then treated with two staining techniques: standard Hematoxylin and Eosin and Masson staining.

Statistical analysis

Statistical analysis was performed using SPSS version 19.0 software (SPSS Inc., Chicago, Illinois). Histomorphometric data were presented as the percentage of trabecular bone in contact with the Prestige LP prosthesis (titanium endplates) and statistically compared with historical reports of appendicular total joint arthroplasty using an analysis of variance (ANOVA) with Student–Newman–Keuls test. All data were shown as mean ± standard deviation, and significance was indicated at $P < 0.05$.

Results

All animals survived the procedures and postoperative time period without incidence of vascular, neurologic or infectious complications. The average operating time required was 72.6 ± 17.5 min (range 58–98 min), with an estimated blood loss of less than 50 ml. All animals had a normal recovery by 1 week after surgery, with clinical assessment indicating normal appearance, ambulation, appetite and wound healing. Based on anteroposterior and lateral plain films, there was no evidence of prosthesis migration, loosening, or subsidence at the prosthesis-bone interface.

Histomorphometry

Micro-CT of the operative motion segments showed excellent osseointegration at the prosthesis–bone interface (Fig. 4a and b). Histomorphometric analysis at the prosthesis-bone interface (apparent bone contact area/ gross total endplate area) indicated that the mean porous ingrowth was 48.5% ± 10.4% (total range: 36.6% to 59.8%) at 6 months after surgery, which was higher than that reported for acetabular components, tibial plateaus, and femoral stem components found in the appendicular skeleton (Fig. 5).

Bone histology

As an overall statement, gross histologic analysis of the Prestige LP prosthesis demonstrated excellent ingrowth at the prosthesis–bone interface, without evidence of particulate wear debris or significant histopathologic changes. All the vertebral specimens were fixed and underwent routine paraffin processing and slide preparation. The paraffin embedded sections were cut, slide mounted, and stained using standard Hematoxylin and Eosin and Masson staining. As a result, there were both plenty of proliferated osteoblasts and regenerated osseous tissues in some regions of the prosthesis-bone interface. Moreover, there was a distinct interface between regenerated osseous tissues and mature bone tissues. (Fig. 6a and b).

Discussion

To date, a wide variety of commercial and experimental artificial prosthetic discs are now available on the market or are under clinical trial. Despite with different design concepts, all artificial cervical discs are designed to replace the diseased intervertebral discs to perform their functions. The successful outcome of cervical disc

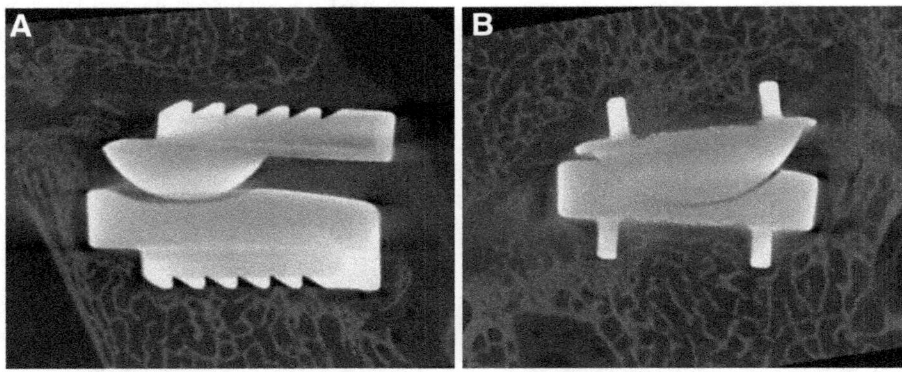

Fig. 4 Microcomputed tomograph of the operative segment. Excellent ingrowth is seen at the prosthesis-bone interface at 6 months after surgery in the mid-sagittal plane (**a**) and specified-coronal plane (**b**)

replacement, on one hand, rests upon the mechanisms of acute fixation, which are accomplished by endplate modifications involving the use of keels, teeth, rails, and serrations providing initial device fixation [16], on the other hand, depends on the extent of biological osseointegration at the prosthesis-bone interface, ensuring long-term device fixation. Therefore, as a current widely used artificial disc, it is very essential to evaluate the initial stability and the biological porous ingrowth characteristics of the Prestige LP prosthesis.

In the current study, radiographic analysis showed no evidence of prosthesis migration, loosening, or subsidence. Most importantly and most challenging is for device to encourage osseointegration at the prosthesis-bone interface in order to minimize the incidence of clinical device loosening or migration after CDA. Based on the histomorphometry data, the mean porous ingrowth was 48.5% ± 10.4%. This demonstrated excellent porous osseointegration at the prosthesis–bone interface for the Prestige LP prosthesis, similar to that reported in several previous studies [13–15]. Moreover, the mean porous ingrowth was much higher than that reported for porous ingrowth found in appendicular total joint arthroplasty (only 20%–30% ingrowth). Harvey et al. [17] found the values of bone ingrowth to be 9.7 ± 5.38% for a composite stem compared with 28.1 ± 5.31% for a titanium alloy stem in a canine total hip arthroplasty model. Jasty et al. [18] retrieved five porous-coated femoral components from patients underwent revision arthroplasty, and found the ingrowth was 4 to 44% (mean 24%). Sumner et al. [19, 20] investigated the uncemented femoral components at 2 years in a canine total hip arthroplasty model, and found the mean ingrowth to be 32.7 ± 4.7% (range 19.7–47.5%) with fiber metal coatings compared with

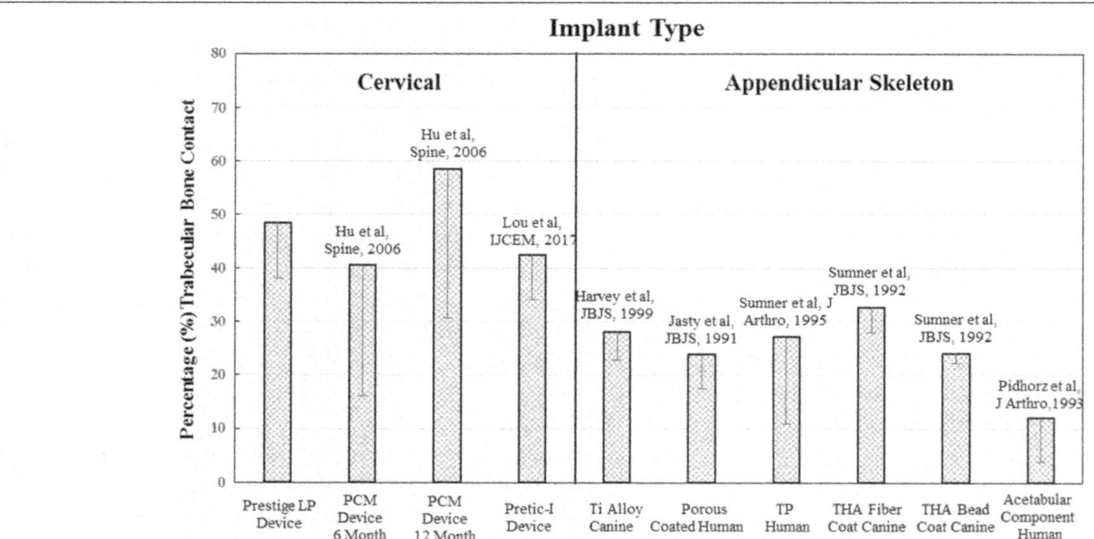

Fig. 5 Porous ingrowth. Percentage of ingrowth–bone contact on the endplate surface. The bar graph compares porous ingrowth in cervical disc arthroplasty and appendicular total joint arthroplasty

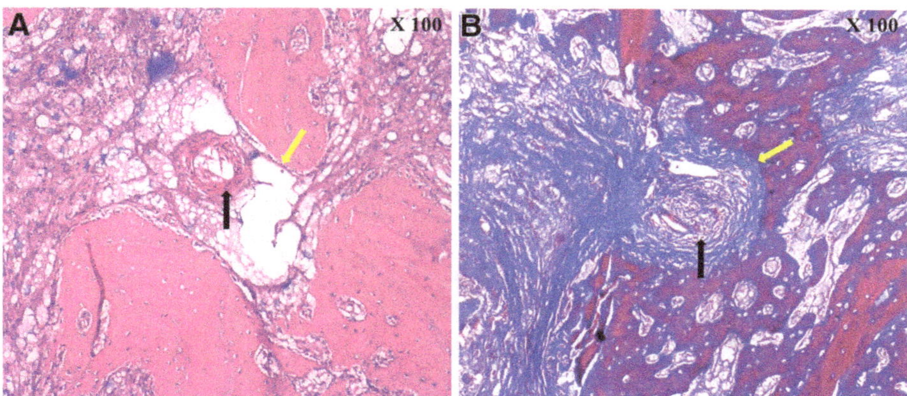

Fig. 6 Sections using standard Hematoxylin and Eosin stain (**a**), Sections using Masson stain (**b**). The proliferated osteoblasts (black arrow). The interface between regenerated osseous tissues and mature bone tissues (yellow arrow)

24.1 ± 1.8% (range 19.0–31.2%) using bead coatings. Pidhorz et al. [21] retrieved 11 cementless acetabular components at autopsy at an average of 41 months (5 weeks to 75 months) after surgery, with mean ingrowth of 12.1 ± 8.2%. As for the improved extent of porous ingrowth in the Prestige LP prosthesis, one reason may be that the rails provide a better primary press-fit fixation, facing toward the bony endplates to resist pull-out, and the porous titanium plasma spray coating facilitates bone ingrowth and significantly encourages osseointegration at the prosthesis-bone interface in the long run. In addition, we postulate that the more favorable porous ingrowth may be the result of acute ligamentotaxis causing long-term and sustained compression across the prosthesis-bone interface.

There is controversy regarding the most accurate method of measuring the porous ingrowth of cementless prostheses [22–24]. The three most widely used methods are microradiography, stained histology, and backscattered electron imaging-scanning electron microscopy (BEI-SEM). In this study, we adopted microradiography and stained histology to evaluate the porous ingrowth at the prosthesis-bone interface. It turned out that there was evidence of excellent osseointegration at the prosthesis–bone interface. Sumner et al. [25] compared the porous ingrowth of acetabular cups using the three methods, finding that BEI-SEM and histologic sections possessed comparable results, whereas microradiography underestimated the porosity of the porous coating by a mean of 17% and simultaneously overestimated the amount of bony ingrowth by a mean of 0.8%.

There are still some aspects need to be improved in the current study. First, the caprine model used only a 6-month follow-up period and a small sample size. It is expected that longer follow-up evaluation with greater numbers of subjects would be required to obtain a more reliable measure of the biological osseointegration of CDA with the Prestige LP prosthesis. In addition, it is a relatively simplified design for the Prestige LP prosthesis with a porous titanium plasma spray coating. A unique bioactive TiCaPHA (titanium/calcium phosphate/hydroxyapatite) coating is more favorable to encourage osseointegration at the prosthesis-bone interface [13, 14]. Moreover, the prosthesis may possess stronger surface and more favorable porous osseointegration through the procedure for an electrochemically bonded coating than a plasma-sprayed coating [12].

Conclusions

In summary, as the first comprehensive in vivo investigation into the Prestige LP prosthesis, the present project established a successful animal model for CDA. Moreover, histomorphometric analysis of porous ingrowth at the prosthesis-bone interface was more favorable for CDA with the Prestige LP prosthesis, compared to historical reports of appendicular total joint arthroplasty.

Abbreviations

BEI-SEM: Backscattered electron imaging-scanning electron microscopy; CDA: Cervical disc arthroplasty; Micro-CT: Microcomputed tomograph; TiCaPHA: Titanium/calcium phosphate/hydroxyapatite

Acknowledgements

We would like to thank Dr. Li Tian for her highly valuable participation in animal care and operations.

Funding

This study was supported by the foundation of Science & Technology Department of Sichuan Province (grant No. 0040205301C35), PR China.

Authors' contributions

HL, JL, BW, WW, and HL conceived and designed the experiments. TW and ZL analyzed the data. HL and JL wrote the paper. All authors read and approved the final manuscript.

Consent for publication

Not applicable.

Competing interests

The authors declare that they have no competing interests.

Author details

[1]Department of Orthopedics, West China Hospital, Sichuan University, 37 Guoxue Road, Chengdu, Sichuan 610041, China. [2]Department of Orthopedics, Southwest Hospital, the Third Military Medical University, Chongqing, China. [3]Department of Orthopedics, Qianfoshan Hospital, Shandong University, Jinan, Shandong, China.

References

1. Sasso RC, Smucker JD, Hacker RJ, Heller JG. Artificial disc versus fusion: a prospective, randomized study with 2-year follow-up on 99 patients. Spine (Phila Pa 1976). 2007;32:2933–40.
2. Phillips FM, Allen TR, Regan JJ, Albert TJ, Cappuccino A, Devine JG, et al. Cervical disc replacement in patients with and without previous adjacent level fusion surgery: a prospective study. Spine (Phila Pa 1976). 2009;34:556–65.
3. Maldonado CV, Paz RD, Martin CB. Adjacent-level degeneration after cervical disc arthroplasty versus fusion. Eur Spine J. 2011;20(Suppl 3):403–7.
4. Cavanaugh DA, Nunley PD, Kerr EJ 3rd, Werner DJ, Jawahar A. Delayed hyper-reactivity to metal ions after cervical disc arthroplasty: a case report and literature review. Spine (Phila Pa 1976). 2009;34:E262-5.
5. Thaler M, Hartmann S, Gstöttner M, Lechner R, Gabl M, Bach C. Footprint mismatch in total cervical disc arthroplasty. Eur Spine J. 2013;22:759–65.
6. Goffin J, Van Calenbergh F, van Loon J, Casey A, Kehr P, Liebig K, et al. Intermediate follow-up after treatment of degenerative disc disease with the Bryan cervical disc prosthesis: single-level and bi-level. Spine (Phila Pa 1976). 2003;28:2673–8.
7. Anderson PA, Sasso RC, Riew KD. Comparison of adverse events between the Bryan artificial cervical disc and anterior cervical arthrodesis. Spine (Phila Pa 1976). 2008;33:1305–12.
8. Ozbek Z, Ozkara E, Arslantas A. Implant migration in cervical disk Arthroplasty. World Neurosurg. 2017;97:390–7.
9. Rahbek O, Overgaard S, Jensen TB, Bendix K, Søballe K. Sealing effect of hydroxyapatite coating: a 12-month study in canines. Acta Orthop Scand. 2000;71:563–73.
10. Mason TJ, Matthews M. Aquatic environment, housing, and management in the eighth edition of the guide for the care and use of laboratory animals: additional considerations and recommendations. J Am Assoc Lab Anim Sci. 2012;51:329–32.
11. Cunningham BW, Lowery GL, Serhan HA, Dmitriev AE, Orbegoso CM, McAfee PC, et al. Total disc replacement arthroplasty using the AcroFlex lumbar disc: a non-human primate model. Eur Spine J. 2002; 11(Suppl 2):S115–23.
12. McAfee PC, Cunningham BW, Orbegoso CM, Sefter JC, Dmitriev AE, Fedder IL. Analysis of porous ingrowth in intervertebral disc prostheses: a nonhuman primate model. Spine (Phila Pa 1976). 2003;28:332–40.
13. Hu N, Cunningham BW, McAfee PC, Kim SW, Sefter JC, Cappuccino A, et al. Porous coated motion cervical disc replacement: a biomechanical, histomorphometric, and biologic wear analysis in a caprine model. Spine (Phila Pa 1976). 2006;31:1666–73.
14. Cunningham BW, Hu N, Zorn CM, McAfee PC. Bioactive titanium calcium phosphate coating for disc arthroplasty: analysis of 58 vertebral end plates after 6- to 12-month implantation. Spine J. 2009;9:836–45.
15. Lou J, Wu W, Li H, Wang B, Liu H. Analysis of bony ingrowth in novel cervical disc prosthesis. Int J Clin Exp Med. 2017;10:10196–201.
16. Cunningham BW, Hu N, Zorn CM, McAfee PC. Comparative fixation methods of cervical disc arthroplasty versus conventional methods of anterior cervical arthrodesis: serration, teeth, keels, or screws? J Neurosurg Spine. 2010;12:214–20.
17. Harvey EJ, Bobyn JD, Tanzer M, Stackpool GJ, Krygier JJ, Hacking SA. Effect of flexibility of the femoral stem on bone-remodeling and fixation of the stem in a canine total hip arthroplasty model without cement. J Bone Joint Surg Am. 1999;81:93–107.
18. Jasty M, Bragdon CR, Maloney WJ, Haire T, Harris WH. Ingrowth of bone in failed fixation of porous-coated femoral components. J Bone Joint Surg Am. 1991;73:1331–7.
19. Sumner DR, Turner TM, Urban RM, Galante JO. Remodeling and ingrowth of bone at two years in a canine cementless total hip-arthroplasty model. J Bone Joint Surg Am. 1992;74:239–50.
20. Sumner DR, Kienapfel H, Jacobs JJ, Urban RM, Turner TM, Galante JO. Bone ingrowth and wear debris in well-fixed cementless porous-coated tibial components removed from patients. J Arthroplast. 1995;10:157–67.
21. Pidhorz LE, Urban RM, Jacobs JJ, Sumner DR, Galante JO. A quantitative study of bone and soft tissues in cementless porous-coated acetabular components retrieved at autopsy. J Arthroplast. 1993;8:213–25.
22. Engh CA, Zettl-Schaffer KF, Kukita Y, Sweet D, Jasty M, Bragdon C. Histological and radiographic assessment of well functioning porous-coated acetabular components. A human postmortem retrieval study. J Bone Joint Surg Am. 1993;75:814–24.
23. Urban RM, Jacobs JJ, Sumner DR, Peters CL, Voss FR, Galante JO. The bone-implant interface of femoral stems with non-circumferential porous coating. J Bone Joint Surg Am. 1996;78:1068–81.
24. Bloebaum RD, Rhodes DM, Rubman MH, Hofmann AA. Bilateral tibial components of different cementless designs and materials. Microradiographic, backscattered imaging, and histologic analysis. Clin Orthop Relat Res. 1991;268:179–87.
25. Sumner DR, Bryan JM, Urban RM, Kuszak JR. Measuring the volume fraction of bone ingrowth: a comparison of three techniques. J Orthop Res. 1990;8:448–52.

Musculoskeletal pain and associated factors among Ethiopian elementary school children

Manayesh Delele[1], Balamurugan Janakiraman[1], Abey Bekele Abebe[1*], Ararso Tafese[2] and Alexander T. M. van de Water[1,3]

Abstract

Background: Ethiopian school children often carry school supplies in heavy school bags and encounter limited school facilities. This stresses their vulnerable musculoskeletal system and may result in experiencing musculoskeletal pain. High prevalence of musculoskeletal pain has been documented, but data on musculoskeletal pain among elementary school children in Ethiopia is lacking. To determine the prevalence of musculoskeletal pain and associated factors among elementary school children in Gondar, Ethiopia.

Methods: Cross-sectional study was conducted among children from six randomly selected elementary schools. Sample size was determined proportionally across school grades and governmental and private schools to ensure variety within the sample. Data collection consisted of physical measurements including height, weight and schoolbag weight, and a structured questionnaire on musculoskeletal pain, mode of transport, walking time and school facilities. Data were analysed descriptively and through uni- and multivariate logistic regression model.

Results: In total 723 children participated. The overall prevalence of self-reported musculoskeletal pain was 62%, with a significant difference between school types (governmental 68% versus private 51%). Shoulder, neck and lower leg/knee were most commonly reported. Walking to and from school for ≥20 min (OR = 2.94, 95% CI 2.05 to 4.21) and relative school bag weight (OR = 2.57, 95% CI 1.48 to 4.47) were found significantly associated with self-report musculoskeletal pain. Children with carrying heavy school supplies and also walking long duration have a 3.5 (95% CI = 1.80–6.95) times greater chance of reporting pain as compared to those who carry lesser weighed bags and reported shorter walking duration at the same time.

Conclusions: Prevalence of self-reported musculoskeletal pain was high among children attending public schools and also those who walked a long way to and from school. Long walking duration and relative school bag weight were significantly associated with musculoskeletal pain. These findings can inform policymakers to provide transportation services and other facilities at elementary schools. The findings of this study should be interpreted with caution due to possible social desirability bias with higher prevalence of self-reported pain and more so in children population.

Keywords: Musculoskeletal pain, School children, School bag, Walking distance, Ethiopia

* Correspondence: abeybekele@gmail.com
[1]Department of Physiotherapy, School of Medicine and Health Sciences, University of Gondar and Gondar University specialized comprehensive hospital, Gondar, Ethiopia
Full list of author information is available at the end of the article

Background

Musculoskeletal pain among school-aged children is a well-known concern as acknowledged by WHO interdisciplinary experts studying school environments [1]. The overall lifetime prevalence of musculoskeletal symptoms among school children in developed countries ranges from 16 to 86% [2–4] and in developing countries these figures are higher, ranging from 46.3 to 88.8% [5–9].

Ethiopia is one of the fastest developing countries in Africa. There is a sustained increase in the number of both public and private schools and the educational system is evolving. The expanding school syllabus has resulted in children having to carry more school supplies, while many Ethiopian schools still have low resource facilities lacking to offer student lockers in schools and transport coverage to and from schools [10, 11]. Although some researchers debate that there is still lack of evidence on the short and long-term effects of determinants of musculoskeletal pain among school children [12], others report that children's developing musculoskeletal system is negatively influenced by factors such as heavy school bags, lack of locker facilities, walking to and from school, sitting postures, method of carrying school supplies, body mass index and furniture facilities [13–15]. For example, excessive school bag weight could in the long term result in deteriorating biomechanical effects on the rapidly growing musculoskeletal system of young aged children. These findings formed the basis for recommended school bag weight limits. Professional associations advise that school children should carry no more than 15 to 20% of their bodyweight [16–18].

Although implied, literature searching revealed that the burden of musculoskeletal pain among school children and its associations have not been established or explored in Ethiopia. Considering the additional burden of child health issues and potential long-term effects of musculoskeletal pain in children on communities and society in a developing country like Ethiopia, it is important to gain an understanding of the extent of this problem. Therefore, this study aimed to investigate the prevalence and to determine the associated factors of musculoskeletal pain among private and public elementary school children in Gondar city, Ethiopia.

Methods

Study setting

An institution-based cross-sectional descriptive study was carried out from February 2016 to June 2016. The study was done at 43 public and 21 private elementary schools in Gondar city (300,000 inhabitants, estimated), which is located 741 km North West of Addis Ababa, Ethiopia. Informed consent was obtained from parents/caregivers and school teachers, and assent was obtained from participating children. Ethical approval was obtained from the Gondar University School of Medicine research and ethical review committee (SOM/047/7/08).

Study participants

The population of interest comprised of all elementary school children's of both sexes, aged 18 or less and living in Gondar city. Inclusion criteria were parental consent, children assent, ability to ambulate independently and ability to wear school bag while standing. Children with known congenital or structural deformities or recent surgery (within 3 months) were excluded.

Sample size determination

In total 47,286 elementary school children were registered as student in private and government schools in Gondar city by the local government school authority bureau. The required sample size was calculated using Epi Info software version 7.0 (Centres for Disease Control and prevention, USA) and was based on this registered population. The following assumptions were used to determine the sample size based on single population proportion: prevalence of 50% since no past regional data exist, confidence level of 95%, design effect of 2. The derived sample size was $n = 768$. Accounting for an estimated non-response or refusal rate of 10%, the required sample size was $n = 845$.

Sampling procedure

A multistage sampling was implemented. The schools were stratified into governmental and private elementary schools. In each strata, schools were proportionally selected based on random selection. Within the selected school, the samples were proportionally allocated based on the total number of children in that school and from each grade, randomly from grade 1 to 8 using their alphabetically ordered list. Children were sampled based on the proportion of gender in the selected grade of the randomly selected six schools.

Data collection procedure and materials

Prior to data collection, a one-day intensive training was given to data collectors (community-based rehabilitation workers). A pre-test of data collection was carried out with 42 elementary school children from one Gondar city school, prior to actual data collection. Those children were excluded from participation in the main study. Modifications and corrections of the measurement procedures were made based on analyses of pre-test data.

The data collection process was supervised by the principal investigator (MD) on a daily basis to ensure accuracy, completeness and consistency. Consequently, amendments and corrections were made before the start of the next working day.

Elementary school children, who had informed consent from their teacher and a parent/caregiver and assented, were enrolled in the study. First, height of the children was measured to the nearest 1 cm using a stadiometer, and weight was measured using a digital weighing scale (Electrolux, Korea) to the nearest 1 kg. The children, dressed in school uniforms, were instructed to remove their shoes before measuring weight. Weight was initially measured with children standing on the weighing scale with their school bag and then without their school bag. The difference between the two recorded weights was recorded as weight of the school bag. Recalibration of the weighing scale was done after each measurement. Since children carry a lunch box and water bottle, the data were collected only in morning sessions. Body Mass Index (BMI) was calculated, adjusted for children and categorised (https://www.cdc.gov/healthyweight/assessing/bmi/childrens_bmi/about_childrens_bmi.html, [19]).

We used a structured questionnaire to record demographic data such as age, gender and grade level, and associated factors of musculoskeletal pain such as type of school bag, mode of transport, walking time to school, locker facilities, type of furniture at school, time spent sitting, time of physical education. Musculoskeletal symptoms in different body regions were assessed using an Amharic translation of a modified version of the Standardised Nordic questionnaires for musculoskeletal symptoms [20]. The questionnaire includes a body map to allow children to report musculoskeletal pain by labelling the body location and a happy-face sad-face visual pain scale for pain intensity was used. Four rating categories (never, occasionally, frequently and every day) were used to record presence of musculoskeletal pain/symptoms. Care was taken by the data collectors to simplify the questions as much as possible, accompany parents or class teacher during pain reporting and explanations were given whenever questions arose.

Data analysis

Data were coded and entered into Epi Info software version 7.0 and IBM Statistical Package for Social Sciences (SPSS) version 24 for Windows for statistical analyses. Data entry with the original data was done by the data collector and the main investigator (MD) supervising each other to enhance correctness. In addition, the data was checked by two other researchers (AB and AvdW) for completeness, accuracy and clarity. Descriptive statistics (frequencies, percentages, means and standard deviations (SD)) were used for all participant characteristics and associated factors of musculoskeletal pain.

With musculoskeletal pain (categories: none versus present) as dependent variable, bivariate and multivariate binary logistic regression analyses were executed to examine the association with different independent variables. Independent variables included in the regression models were, age (categorised 5–10, 11–15 and > 15), BMI (categorised underweight, normal weight, overweight and obese), type of school (governmental and private), mode of transport (walking and motorised transport), walking duration (categorised no walking, < 20 min and ≥ 20 min), way of carrying school supplies, percentage of school bag's weight of body weight (categorised 0–10%, 10–20, > 20%). Multiple regression and interaction terms were used to examine the potential association between school bag weight and musculoskeletal pain differed by hypothesized variables, including gender, type of school, and walking duration. Variables were inputted into the model using forced entry and categories were used as covariates for detailed analyses. Results were considered statistically significant when 95% confidence intervals not containing unity (equal to p-value < 0.05) for both main effects and interaction terms. Initially, bivariate analyses were conducted and independent variables that were found statistically significant were included in multivariate analysis. When clear subgroups seemed present in the data, significance testing (Pearson χ^2) and, if appropriately sized subgroups per category remained, logistic regression were performed.

Results

Sample characteristics

Out of 845 consent forms dispatched to six elementary schools in Gondar city, 723 parents (85.6%) consented for their children to participate. This is 94.1% of the power calculated sample size ($n = 768$). The 723 elementary school children were from four governmental schools ($n = 497$; 68.9%) and two private schools ($n = 226$; 31.1%). The mean age of the participants was 11.5 years (SD 2.7 years) and 58.5% ($n = 423$) was female. A normal weight children adjusted BMI was recorded in 524 (72.5%) children, whereas 148 (20.5%) were found being underweight. More sample characteristics are presented in Table 1.

Musculoskeletal pain

Four hundred and fifty one ($n = 451$, 62.4%) students reported to have experienced musculoskeletal pain in the previous 12 months. Reported prevalence of musculoskeletal pain was nearly equal for female (63.6%, $n = 269$) as for male (60.7%, $n = 182$) participants. A significant difference was observed in musculoskeletal pain prevalence between type of schools (private 50.9% versus governmental 67.6%; χ^2 (1, $n = 723$) =17.8, $p < 0.001$, $phi = -0.16$). Most participating children who reported musculoskeletal pain felt this in one (66.2%, $n = 294$) or two body regions (25.7%, $n = 114$). The most frequently recorded regions of

Table 1 Sample characteristics and distribution of musculoskeletal pain among school children, Ethiopia

Variables	Sample totals		Musculoskeletal pain			
			Yes		No	
	n	(%)	n	(%)	n	(%)
All participants	723	(100%)	451	(62.4%)	272	(37.6)
Age (in years)						
5–10	272	(37.6%)	173	(23.9%)	99	(13.7%)
11–15	397	(54.9%)	238	(32.9%)	159	(22.0%)
> 15	54	(7.5%)	40	(5.5%)	14	(1.9%)
Sex						
Male	300	(41.5%)	182	(25.2%)	118	(16.3%)
Female	423	(58.5%)	269	(37.2%)	154	(21.3%)
Height (in cm) as mean (SD)	133.1	(13.7)	131.9	(13.2)	135.1	(14.4)
Weight (in kg) as mean (SD)	30.4	(8.7)	29.7	(8.5)	31.5	(8.9)
BMI children adjusted percentiles						
Underweight < 5%	148	(20.5%)	98	(13.6%)	50	(6.9%)
Healthy weight 5–85%	524	(72.5%)	324	(44.8%)	200	(27.7%)
Overweight 85–95%	41	(5.7%)	24	(3.3%)	17	(2.4%)
Obese 95%	10	(1.4%)	5	(0.7%)	5	(0.7%)
Type of school						
Governmental	497	(68.9%)	336	(46.5%)	161	(22.3%)
Private	226	(31.3%)	115	(15.9%)	111	(15.4%)
School grade						
Grade 1–4	380	(52.6%)	240	(33.2%)	140	(19.4%)
Grade 5–8	343	(47.4%)	211	(29.2%)	132	(18.3%)
Mode of Transport						
Walking	546	(75.5%)	368	(50.9%)	178	(24.6%)
School bus	115	(15.9%)	49	(6.8%)	66	(9.1%)
Public transport	14	(1.9%)	6	(0.8%)	8	(1.1%)
Private transport	48	(6.6%)	28	(3.8%)	20	(2.8%)
Method of carrying school supplies						
Backpack	587	(81.2%)	363	(50.2%)	224	(31.0%)
Single strap	93	(12.9%)	58	(8.0%)	35	(4.8%)
Handbag	6	(0.8%)	2	(0.3%)	4	(0.6%)
Without bag in hand	37	(5.1%)	28	(3.9%)	9	(1.2%)
Preference of backpack carrying	(*n* = 587)					
Right side	10	(1.7%)	9	(1.5%)	1	(0.2%)
Left side	2	(0.3%)	2	(0.3%)	0	(0%)
Both shoulder together	575	(98.0%)	352	(48.7%)	223	(30.8%)
Preference of single strap carrying	(*n* = 93)					
Right shoulder	64	(68.8%)	41	(44.1%)	23	(24.7%)
Left shoulder	18	(19.4%)	10	(10.8%)	8	(8.6%)
Alternatively(Left/Right)	11	(11.8%)	7	(7.5%)	4	(4.3%)

Table 1 Sample characteristics and distribution of musculoskeletal pain among school children, Ethiopia *(Continued)*

Variables	Sample totals		Musculoskeletal pain			
			Yes		No	
	n	(%)	n	(%)	n	(%)
Walking duration						
No walking	177	(24.5%)	83	(11.5%)	94	(13.0%)
< 20 min	50	(6.9%)	16	(2.2%)	34	(4.7%)
≥ 20 min	496	(68.6%)	352	(48.7%)	144	(19.9%)
Bag weight in % of bodyweight						
0–10%	250	(34.6%)	142	(19.6%)	108	(14.9%)
11–20%	380	(52.6%)	240	(33.2%)	140	(19.4%)
> 20%	93	(12.9%)	69	(9.5%)	24	(3.3%)

experienced musculoskeletal pain was the shoulder (24.9%, $n = 180$) and the least reported musculoskeletal pain region was wrist (5.8%, $n = 42$). An overview of the prevalence of all regions is presented in Fig. 1.

The pain intensity of the majority of participating children who reported musculoskeletal pain was moderate ($n = 352$, 78.1% of 451). Forty-one participants (9.1%) reported severe intensity pain and 58 (12.9%) had mild intensity pain.

Associated factors of musculoskeletal pain

Walking was the main mode of transport to and from school (75.5%, $n = 546$) followed by a school bus (15.9%, $n = 115$). Mode of transport between type of schools was vastly different (χ^2 (3, $n = 723$) = 490.4, $p < 0.001$, phi = 0.82), with most children from private schools going by school bus ($n = 113$, 50%) or other motorised transport (total $n = 172$, 77.0% versus 23.0%) and nearly all children from governmental schools going by foot ($n = 494$, 99.4% versus 0.6%).

Of those who walked, 68.6% ($n = 496$) walked to school for 20 min or more, which constitutes a subgroup in which a greater prevalence of musculoskeletal pain was found (48.7%, $n = 352$). The school supplies carried by children in both governmental and private schools weighted a mean of 3.84 kg (SD 1.57, range 0-14 kg) and were most commonly carried in a backpack was (81.5%, $n = 589$). Considerable weight (11–20%) was carried by 380 children (52.6%) and 93 children (12.9%) carried supplies weighing > 20% of body weight.

Other relevant factors potentially related to musculoskeletal pain showed no variance between grades or schools. All participants sat more than 330 min per day at school and had less than 100 min of physical education per week. Schools provided no locker facilities for their students' school supplies.

Regression analysis

Prior to analysis, eleven variables potentially related to musculoskeletal pain were identified for regression

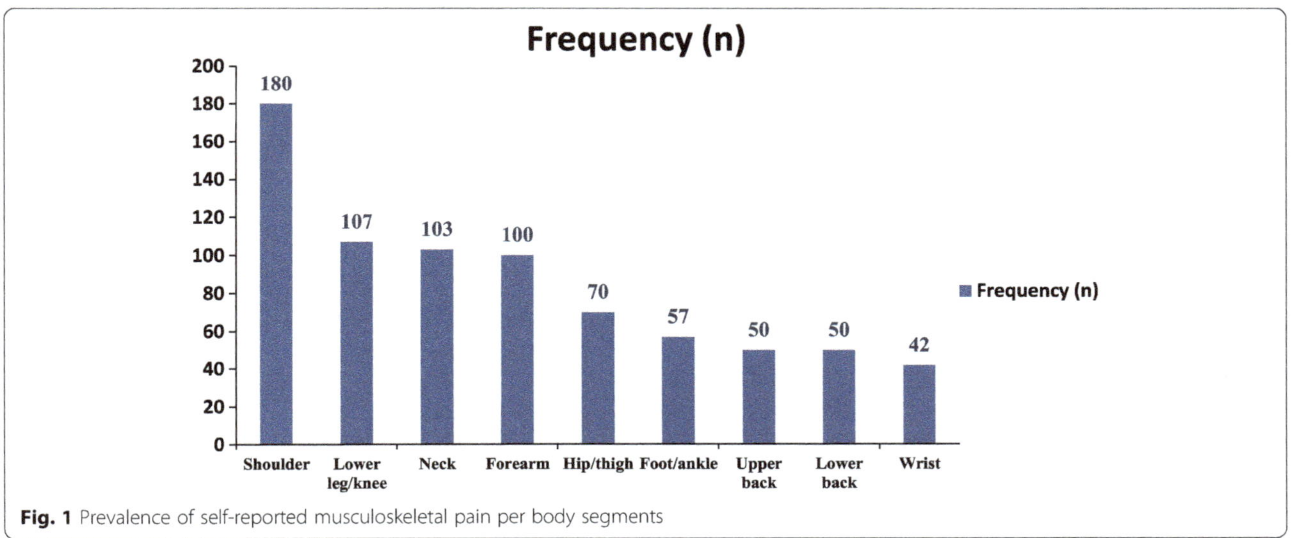

Fig. 1 Prevalence of self-reported musculoskeletal pain per body segments

analysis: age, BMI, type of school, type of school by school bag weight, school bag weight by gender, type of school by duration of walking, mode of transport, duration of walking, duration of walking by school bag weight, method of carrying of school supplies, and relative school bag weight. Of those, age, BMI method of carrying school supplies and type of school by school bag weight in % of body weight were found not significantly associated in univariate analyses (Table 2). The remaining six variables were significant (Table 2) and were evaluated prior to multivariate analysis. Type of school (private or governmental) was significantly related to mode of transport (motorised or walking) and, therefore, both related to walking duration (no walking, < 20 min, ≥ 20 min) violating the assumption of collinearity. Also, multivariate testing revealed that type of school and mode of transport were not significant when adjusting for other included variables and were subsequently removed from the analysis.

The final multivariate regression model (Table 3) included the categorised variables walking duration and relative school bag weight for main effects, type of school by walking duration and school bag weight by walking duration for interaction effects. It was statistically significant (Model χ^2 (4, $n = 723$) = 65.21, $p < 0.001$), explained 9.1 to 12.5% of variance and classified 66.8% of cases correctly. A non-significant finding was that walking for < 20 min may be protective of musculoskeletal pain as explained by the coefficient below 1 in the logistic regression model, but that walking for ≥20 min significantly increases the odds of musculoskeletal pain by almost 3 (OR = 2.94, 95%CI 2.05 to 4.21). The model also showed that the heavier the schoolbag the more likely it is to have musculoskeletal pain. Compared to 0–10%, the odds increase by 1.5 if the bag weights 10–20% of body weight, and 2.6 if the bag weights > 20% of body weight (Table 3). The interaction effect between heavier school bag weight expressed in percentage of body weight and longer walking duration was also significant (AOR = 3.53, 95% CI: 1.80–6.95, $p < 0.001$).

Given the significant difference between school types on transportation, subgroup regression analysis (splitting data on private and government schools) was considered. Although, the same variables (walking ≥20 min, relative school bag weight) remained significant in both subgroup models, group sizes in certain categories were too small for adequate analysis.

Table 2 Results of univariate logistic regression of factors associated with musculoskeletal pain among school children, Ethiopia

Variable	Crude Odds ratio	95% CI interval		P
		Lower	Upper	
Age (5–10 years)				
10–15 years	0.86	0.62	1.18	0.34
> 15 years	1.64	0.85	3.15	0.14
Bag/body weight (0–10%)				
10–20%	1.30	0.94	1.81	0.11
> 20%	2.19	1.29	3.71	0.00
BMI (underweight)				
Normal	0.83	0.56	1.21	0.33
Overweight	0.72	0.36	1.46	0.36
Obese	0.51	0.14	1.85	0.31
Carrying supplies (back pack)				
Single strap	1.02	0.65	1.61	0.92
Hand bag	0.31	0.06	1.70	0.18
In hand (no bag)	1.92	0.89	4.14	0.10
Mode of transport (walking)				
Motorized	0.43	0.30	0.60	0.00
Type of school (private)				
Governmental	2.01	1.46	2.78	0.00
Walking duration (no walking)				
< 20 min	0.53	0.27	1.04	0.06
≥ 20 min	2.77	1.95	3.94	0.00
Bag/body weight X Gender	1.138	0.83	1.56	0.42
Bag/body weight X Type of school	1.061	0.71	2.45	0.89
Bag/body weight X Walking duration	5.761	2.67	9.41	0.00
Type of school X walking duration	4.27	1.93	9.44	0.00

Discussion

This is the first study that investigated prevalence of musculoskeletal pain and associated factors among elementary school children in Ethiopia. The overall prevalence of musculoskeletal pain in this sample was 62.4% and the two main significantly associated factors were walking time to

Table 3 Multivariate logistic regression predicting likelihood of musculoskeletal pain among school children, Ethiopia

Variable	Adjusted Odds ratio	95% CI interval		P
		Lower	Upper	
Walking duration < 20 min	0.53	0.27	1.04	0.07
Walking duration ≥20 min	2.94	2.05	4.21	0.00
Bag/body weight 10–20%	1.46	1.04	2.06	0.03
Bag/body weight > 20%	2.57	1.48	4.47	0.00
Bag/body weight X Walking duration	3.534	1.80	6.95	0.00
Type of school X walking duration	0.64	0.29	1.37	0.24
Constant	0.62			0.17

Note: R^2 = 0.091 (Cox & Snell), 0.125 (Nagelkerke). Model χ^2 (4, n = 723) =65.21, $p < 0.001$. Correctly predicted 66.8%

school and relative weight of the school bag. A clear difference in mode of transport was observed between private (school bus) and governmental schools (walking), but the same factors remained significantly associated. These findings can aid formulating organisational recommendations for elementary schools in Ethiopia.

The prevalence of musculoskeletal pain found in the current study is similar to the results of studies done in Greece (64.2%) and India (63.2%) [6, 21]. Other studies, however, have found higher or lower prevalence rates. For example, a cross-sectional study done in Uganda [9] reported a prevalence of musculoskeletal pain of 88.8% in 532 students of 10–21 years old. A Brazilian cross-sectional study with a convenience sample of 262 children aged 6–12 years reported musculoskeletal pain to be present in 51.1% [22]. Possible reasons for different prevalence rates in these studies might be the sample size, age variation, environmental factors and facilities.

Walking to school with supplies for a longer period of time (heavy school bags and walking for 20 min) was found to be significantly associated with musculoskeletal pain. These findings are consistent with other studies which reported that long time walking with a school bag is significantly associated with back pain [6, 9, 12, 22, 23]. For example, a survey conducted in Australia reported that adolescents with long time walking with school supplies reported more musculoskeletal complaints than those who utilized transport facilities [24]. A study conducted in Uganda found that methods of carrying school supplies and long duration of walking were significantly associated with low back pain [9]. They found an Adjusted OR = 0.073 (95%CI 0.007 to 0.731) for those who carried school supplies in the hand compared to those carrying a hand bag with supplies, which can be explained (when converted as 1/0.073) as those who carried school supplies in the hand being 13.7 times more likely to experience musculoskeletal pain. Possible reason could be the position of upper extremities while holding the materials in the hand. As found in this study, heavy bags of more than 20% of body weight can also influence musculoskeletal pain. The interaction between heavier school bag weight in % of body weight and longer walking duration suggest that the children carrying heavier school supplies and at the same time walking longer have 3.5 times higher chances of developing musculoskeletal pain than those carrying lighter school supplies and/or walking lesser duration to or from school.

Other clear findings from this study with potential for organisational adjustments, is the difference between private and governmental schools with regards to the prevalence of musculoskeletal pain and mode of transport, and the facilities and physical (in)activity at schools. Walking to school appeared a significant associated factor for students of both governmental and private schools. The majority of private school children (77%) had motorised transport to school which could be a reason for the significantly lower prevalence of musculoskeletal pain in this group (50% versus 67%). A likely reason is the socio-economic status of families of school children attending governmental and private schools. Schools are recommended to provide transport services for school children living farther away from school.

Similarly, schools are recommended to provide locker facilities to store school supplies, such as books, to facilitate reducing school bag weight. Other factors such as poor ergonomic furniture, long sitting times and lack of varied physical activity through physical education should be taken into consideration by school authorities aiming to decrease musculoskeletal pain in their students.

Study limitations

This study has provided well-powered insight into the prevalence, type of musculoskeletal pain and associated factors in school children in North-West Ethiopia. Although 94% of the calculated sample size was reached, post-hoc power analysis show 100% power was reached with the higher than anticipated prevalence. A few limitations can be mentioned to benefit future research. Schoolbag weight was recorded only once. Consequently, the recorded data did not account for the variance of school bag weight during a typical week. In addition, this study reported current pain and pain history rather than pain while carrying their school bag, which could lead to possible differences in estimation of the association between school bag weight and pain. Also, psychological factors, postural assessment and personal (home) factors were not considered. Personal factors could include help with household duties or farming. However, the results should be interpreted with caution because the findings are based on self-reported pain among children. The potential for social desirability bias due social attention seeking by children during pain reporting may occur. At same time it is difficult to attempt objective verification of pain among children. Nevertheless, the present findings indicate that transport specific interventions and school bag weight monitoring programs by schools is needed to reduce musculoskeletal pain.

Conclusion

In conclusion, more than 60% of school children experienced musculoskeletal pain partly explained by the associated factors walking long distance to school and carrying heavy school bags. Other factors that may help explain musculoskeletal pain in children and should be explored in future studies. In the meantime, school authorities are recommended to provide transportation services to reduce the impact of long walking duration and provide locker facilities in schools for students to keep their school supplies in order to decrease weight, frequency and duration of carriage.

Abbreviations

BMI: Body Mass Index; WHO: World Health Organization

Acknowledgments

The authors are grateful to the University of Gondar for funding. The author's gratitude and appreciation goes to the school children, parents, teachers and data collectors. We are also grateful to Dr. Solomon Mekonen for providing the measurement tools.

Funding

This work was fully funded by University of Gondar. The funder has no role in the design of the study and collection, analysis, and interpretation of data and in writing the manuscript.

Authors' contributions

MD brought the original idea, was involved in the proposal writing, designed the study, and participated in all the implementation stages of the project. MD also analyzed data and wrote the initial version of the manuscript. BJ, AB, and AT participated in the conception of the original idea and were involved in proposal writing. BJ, AB, AT and AvdW were involved with data analysis. AvdW checked and reran data analyses and extensively rewrote the the manuscript prior to submission. BJ, AB and AvdW critically revised the manuscript for important intellectual content. All the authors read and approved the final version of the manuscript.

Consent for publication

Not applicable.

Competing interests

The authors declare that they have no competing interests.

Author details

[1]Department of Physiotherapy, School of Medicine and Health Sciences, University of Gondar and Gondar University specialized comprehensive hospital, Gondar, Ethiopia. [2]Department of Public Health, School of Medicine and Health Sciences, University of Gondar, Gondar, Ethiopia. [3]School of Physiotherapy, Academy of Health, Saxion University of Applied Sciences, Enschede, The Netherlands.

References

1. WHO IRIS: The burden of musculoskeletal conditions at the start of the new millenium : report of a WHO scientific group. 2017 [cited 2017 Apr 10]. Available from: http://apps.who.int/iris/handle/10665/42721
2. Pant K, Kaur H, Sidhu M. Assessment of problems faced by school children while carrying school bags. Int J Sci Res. 2016;5(2):210–15.
3. Azuan M, Zailina H, Shamsul BMT, Asyiqin N, Azhar MN, Aizat IS. Neck, upper back and lower back pain and associated risk factors among primary school children. J Appl Sci. 2010;10(5):431–5.
4. AAslund C, Starrin B, Nilsson KW. Social capital in relation to depression, musculoskeletal pain, and psychosomatic symptoms: a cross-sectional study of a large population-based cohort of Swedish adolescents. BMC Public Health. 2010;10(1):715.
5. Janakiraman B, Ravichandran H, Demeke S, Fasika S. Reported influences of backpack loads on postural deviation among school children: a systematic review. J Educ Health Promot. 2017;6
6. Balamurugan J. School bags and musculoskeletal pain among elementary school children in Chennai city. Int J Med Sci Clin Invent. 2014;1(6):302–9.
7. Woolf AD, \AAkesson K. Understanding the burden of musculoskeletal conditions. BMJ 2001;322(7294):1079–1080.
8. Dianat I, Javadivala Z, Allahverdipour H. School bag weight and the occurrence of shoulder, hand/wrist and low back symptoms among Iranian elementary schoolchildren. Health Promot Perspect. 2011;1(1):76–85.
9. Mwaka ES, Munabi IG, Buwembo W, Kukkiriza J, Ochieng J. Musculoskeletal pain and school bag use: a cross-sectional study among Ugandan pupils. BMC Res Notes. 2014;7:222.
10. Brief YLP. Educational choices in Ethiopia: what determines whether poor children go to school? 2006;
11. Education for All 2015 National Review Report: Ethiopia. efa2015review@unesco.org.
12. Jafri Mohd. Rohani. A multifactorial model based on self-reported back pain among Nigerian schoolchildren and the associated risk factors. World Appl Sci J 2013;21(6):812–818.
13. Negrini S, Carabalona R. Backpacks on! Schoolchildren's perceptions of load, associations with back pain and factors determining the load. Spine. 2002; 27(2):187–95.
14. Ren L, Jones RK, Howard D. Dynamic analysis of load carriage biomechanics during level walking. J Biomech. 2005;38(4):853–63.
15. Siambanes D, Martinez JW, Butler EW, Haider T. Influence of school backpacks on adolescent back pain. J Pediatr Orthop. 2004;24(2):211–7.
16. Communications Group of the American Occupational Therapy Association. (2002). Summary of the literature from 1999–2002.
17. American Academy of Orthopaedic Surgeons. Kids and backpacks [on-line]. 2001. Available: http://orthoinfo.aaos.org/fact/thr_report.cfm.
18. Dianat I, Javadivala Z, Asghari-Jafarabadi M, Asl Hashemi A, Haslegrave CM. The use of schoolbags and musculoskeletal symptoms among primary school children: are the recommended weight limits adequate? Ergonomics. 2013;56(1):79–89.
19. Bekele A, Janakiraman B. Physical therapy guideline for children with malnutrition in low income countries : clinical commentary. J Exerc Rehabil. 2016;12(4):266–75.
20. Kuorinka I, Jonsson B, Kilbom A, Vinterberg H, Biering-Sørensen F, Andersson G, et al. Standardised Nordic questionnaires for the analysis of musculoskeletal symptoms. Appl Ergon. 1987;18(3):233–7.
21. Hulsegge G, van Oostrom SH, Picavet HSJ, Twisk JWR, Postma DS, Kerkhof M, et al. Musculoskeletal complaints among 11-year-old children and associated factors: the PIAMA birth cohort study. Am J Epidemiol. 2011 Oct;174(8):877–84.
22. Pereira DS, Castro SS, Bertoncello D, Damião R, Walsh IA. Relationship of musculoskeletal pain with physical and functional variables and with postural changes in school children from 6 to 12 years of age. Braz J Phys Ther. 2013;17(4):392–400.
23. Papadopoulou D, Malliou P, Kofotolis N, Emmanouilidou MI, Kellis E. The association between grade, gender, physical activity, and back pain among children carrying schoolbags. Arch Exerc Health Dis. 2013;4(1):234–42.
24. Haselgrove C, Straker L, Smith A, O'Sullivan P, Perry M, Sloan N. Perceived school bag load, duration of carriage, and method of transport to school are associated with spinal pain in adolescents: an observational study. Aust J Physiother. 2008;54(3):193–200.

9

"Revision of subtrochanteric femoral nonunions after intramedullary nailing with dynamic condylar screw"

Sebastian Lotzien[1,2*], Valentin Rausch[1], Thomas Armin Schildhauer[1] and Jan Gessmann[1]

Abstract

Background: Nonunions of the subtrochanteric region of the femur after previous intramedullary nailing can be difficult to address. Implant failure and bone defects around the implant significantly complicate the therapy, and complex surgical procedures with implant removal, extensive debridement of the nonunion site, bone grafting and reosteosynthesis usually become necessary. The purpose of this study was to evaluate the records of a series of patients with subtrochanteric femoral nonunions who were treated with dynamic condylar screws (DCS) regarding their healing rate, subsequent revision surgeries and implant-related complications.

Methods: We conducted a retrospective chart review of patients with aseptic femoral subtrochanteric nonunions after failed intramedullary nailing. Nonunion treatment consisted of nail removal, debridement of the nonunion, and restoration of the neck shaft angle (CCD), followed by DCS plating. Supplemental bone grafting was performed in all atrophic nonunions. All patients were followed for at least six months after DCS plating.

Results: Between 2002 and 2017, we identified 40 patients with a mean age of 65.4 years (range 34–91 years) who met the inclusion criteria. At a mean follow-up period of 26.3 months (range 6–173), 37 of the 40 (92.5%) nonunions healed successfully (secondary procedures included). The mean healing time of the 37 patients was 11.63 months (± 12.4 months). A total of 13 of the 40 (32.5%) patients needed a secondary revision surgery; one patient had a persistent nonunion, nine patients had persistent nonunions leading to hardware failure, two patients had deep infections requiring revision surgery, and one patient had a peri-implant fracture due to low-energy trauma four days after the index surgery.

Conclusions: The results indicate that revision surgery of subtrochanteric femoral nonunions after intramedullary nailing with dynamic condylar screws is a reliable treatment option overall. However, secondary revision surgery may be indicated before final healing of the nonunion.

Keywords: Subtrochanteric nonunion, Pseudarthrosis, DCS, Dynamic condylar screw, Intramedullary nailing, Hardware failure

Background

Subtrochanteric femoral fractures account for approximately 25% of all hip fractures and have a bimodal age and sex distribution [1]. The subtrochanteric region is defined as the area between the lesser trochanter and the femoral isthmus, which is five centimeters below the trochanter [2, 3]. The femur is exposed to biomechanical forces due to the osseous anatomic conditions in the region, as well as the skeletal muscles surrounding the hip joint. Shear forces specifically affect the cancellous bone of the proximal femur, whereas bending forces especially affect the cortical bones of the subtrochanteric area and the shaft [4–6]. Nonoperative treatment of subtrochanteric femur fractures is associated with a high rate of complications [7]. Although the most recent literature does not emphasise the superiority of intramedullary fixation with nail systems (IMN), it should be however considered as a primary treatment option more particular in

* Correspondence: SebastianLotzien@hotmail.com
[1]BG University Hospital Bergmannsheil, Bochum, Germany
[2]Department of General and Trauma Surgery, Ruhr University Bochum, Bürkle-de-la-Camp-Platz 1, 44789 Bochum, Germany

elderly patients [8, 9]. Nevertheless, extramedullary fixation with a 95° angled blade plate and plate-sliding screw systems also has significant value in current surgical therapy [1]. IMN seems to have biomechanical advantages due to a shorter lever arm compared to the extramedullary components. However, these advantages are partially outweighed by a difficult closed reduction [10]; screw cut outs, screw migration peri-implantary femoral fractures, malunion and nonunion are not uncommon [11–13]. General risk factors [14], as well as local risk factors due to the magnitude of trauma, can lead to delayed bone healing or nonunion in as many as 20% of subtrochanteric femur fractures [15–18]. A significant increase in nonunions of the proximal femur is expected in the future, especially in patients older than 80 years. This is due to demographic changes and the consequently greater number of proximal fractures of the femur in the population [19–21]. Nonunions of the subtrochanteric region of the femur after prior IMN can be difficult to address. Implant failure and bone defects around the implant significantly complicate the therapy, and complex surgical procedures with implant removal, extensive debridement of the nonunion site, bone grafting and reosteosynthesis usually become necessary [22]. The Dynamic Condylar Screw (DCS; Synthes, Bettlach, Switzerland) has been designed for the internal fixation of fractures of the distal and subtrochanteric regions of the femur and has superior biomechanical properties compared to the blade plate [23–25]. The purpose of this study was to evaluate a series of DCS treatments of patients with subtrochanteric femoral nonunions following IMN regarding healing rate, secondary surgeries and implant-related complications.

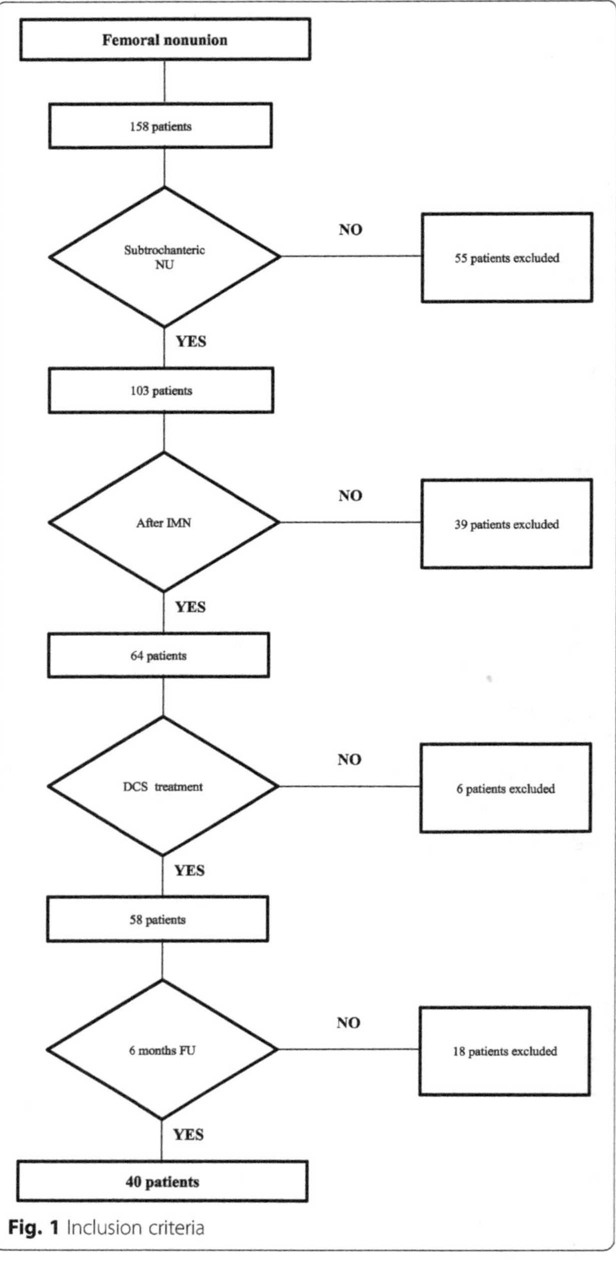

Fig. 1 Inclusion criteria

Methods

The electronic medical database at the authors' institution was searched for patients 18 years of age or older with aseptic subtrochanteric femoral nonunions after failed IMN and DCS treatment at our institution (Fig. 1). Nonunion was defined as a lack of union six months after trauma, including predictable nonunion with a lack of callus formation, gap distraction and implant breakage or progressive loosening of the nail/locking screws (Fig. 2) [26]. All patients treated with a DCS subsequent to IM nail removal (index procedure) in this time period were included in the study if an adequate follow-up period of at least six months was available. The nonunions were radiologically classified according to the pattern of callus formation. Atrophic nonunions showed little callus formation, and hypertrophic nonunions showed an extuberant callus formation with a horse-shoe or elephant-foot configuration [27]. Patients were followed through regular visits at our outpatient clinic six weeks, twelve weeks and six months after the index procedure. After the initial visits, additional visits were scheduled at different intervals until bone union was radiologically confirmed. Clinical and radiological results were analyzed at the latest follow-up examination. The primary outcome measure was time to healing calculated in months. The secondary outcome measures included complications after the index operation and hip function at the last follow-up visit. Complications were recorded regarding persistent nonunion with or without hardware failure, infection and revision surgery. Radiological results were assessed using antero-posterior and lateral radiographs. Whenever in doubt, a computerized tomography (CT)

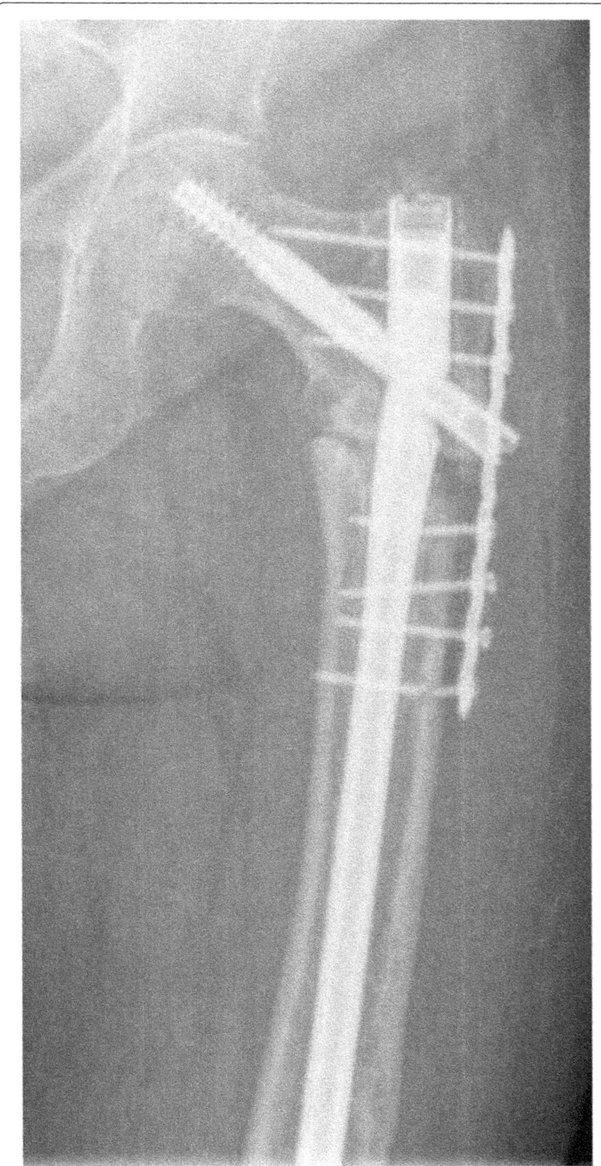

Fig. 2 An 86-year-old female patient with a persistent femoral nonunion after nailing and having already undergone revision with augmentation plating. There is a lack of callus formation and radiographic breakage of the nail and two screws with varus deformation of the femur with a CCD of 104

was used to confirm bony union. Union was defined as a radiologically detectable callus bridge or at least three healed cortices on the radiographs. Deep infection was defined as an infection with microbial detection leading to revision surgery [28]. Infection leading to nonunion was listed as a complication and was also counted as nonunion.

The 40 included patients had been referred to our hospital for nonunion treatment. Additional information about each patient was gathered, including demographics, comorbidities and trauma mechanism. The fractures were classified according to the Seinsheimer classification and the Orthopaedic Trauma Association (OTA) classification system as well [29]. To conduct subgroup comparisons, the patients were sorted into two different groups (Table 1). Patients without further revision surgery after the index procedure were sorted into group 1. Patients who needed secondary revision surgery were sorted into group 2.

Surgical technique

Eighteen different surgeons performed the index procedures. Cefazolin (two grams intravenously) was administered for perioperative antibiotic prophylaxis 30 min before the skin incision. The patient was placed in a supine position on a radiolucent table. Radiographic examinations were used to guide the osteotomy and the positioning of the implant. The initial approach was incorporated and extended distally into the lateral approach, with the fracture site fully exposed. The nail was removed and extensive debridement of the fracture site and nonunion site, including removing fibrotic tissue and necrotic bone, was performed until the bleeding bone was exposed. A collection of tissue samples was collected for microbiological analysis. After the screw insertion into the femoral neck, the DCS plate was then inserted over the lag screw. The plate length was selected according to the surgeon's preference (9–22 holes). The CCD angle was restored by reduction of the shaft to the plate and was maintained with a reduction clamp. The degree of valgus correction depended on the preoperative measured neck shaft angle. To allow proper valgus correction, the plate may have been precontoured using plate benders before plate application (Figs. 3 and 4). An articulated tension device was used to produce compression on the nonunion zone before the additional screws were inserted. If available, cancellous bone graft harvested from the ipsilateral iliac crest was used as graft material in case of an atrophic nonunion. If not available, allograft (Tutogen Medical GmbH, Germany) was utilized. The use of an additional 4.5-mm limited contact dynamic compression plate (LCDCP) placed orthogonally onto the anterior proximal face of the femur was used at the surgeon's discretion (Figs. 5, 6 and 7). Physical therapy was initiated one day after the index procedure. During the first six weeks, weight bearing was delayed, with toe-touch bearing allowed.

Patient characteristics were described by their mean and standard deviation, as well as their minimum and maximum values. Normality of variables was tested with the Shapiro-Wilk test. Significance was calculated using a t-test, Wilcoxon-Mann-Whitney test, contingency tables and Fischer's exact test. A p-value of 0.05 or less was considered statistically significant. In the

Table 1 Group comparison

	Group 1 ($n = 27$)	Group 2 ($n = 13$)	p-value
Sex			0.58
Female	16 (59.26%)	8 (61.54%)	
Male	11 (40.74%)	5 (38.46%)	
Fracture-type[a]			0.32
Seinsheimer Type IIA	3	2	
Seinsheimer Type IIB	1	2	
Seinsheimer Type IIIA	10	3	
Seinsheimer Type IIIB	–	1	
Seinsheimer Type IV	2	–	
Seinsheimer Type V	1	–	
OTA-type[a]			0.54
32A1	1	2	
32A2	–	–	
32A3	3	2	
32B2	10	4	
32B3	2	–	
32C2	–	–	
32C3	1	–	
Trauma mechanism[b]			0.61
Low energy	16	9	
High energy	6	3	
Nonunion-type			0.53
hypertrophic	3/27 (11.1%)	2/13 (15.4%)	
atrophic	24/27 (88.9%)	11/13 (84.6%)	
Age	64.96 ± 15.87	66.31 ± 12.66	0.35
BMI[c]	26.9 ± 5.41	29.91 ± 5.6	0.57
Time to index procedure (months)	10.37 ± 7.2	8.85 ± 5.77	0.67
Prior surgeries per particpant	0.22 ± 0.42	0.69 ± 1.18	0.21
Mean operation time (minutes)	156.74 ± 42.63	149.08 ± 41.36	0.59
Number of red blood cell units tranfused	2.96 ± 3.57	3.15 ± 3.46	0.87
Lenght of hospital stay (days)	14.74 ± 5.45	15.77 ± 8.64	0.89
Diabetes mellitus	3/27 (11.1%)	0/13 (0%)	0.54
Steroid use	3/27 (11.1%)	0/13 (0%)	0.54
Smoking	3/27 (11.1%)	3/13 (23.1%)	0.37
Osteoporosis	2/27(7.4%)	3/13(23.1%)	0.31
Bony healing	27/27(100%)	10/13(76.92%)	0.03
Healing time (months)	7.96 ± 6.53	23.11 ± 26.57	0.01
Follow-up (months)	21.48 ± 17.52	36.15 ± 50.7	0.54

[a]incomplete dataset; in 15 participants Information could not be gathered due to incomplete medical records at admission to our clinic
[b]incomplete dataset; in six participants Information could not be gathered due to incomplete medical records at admission to our clinic
[c]incomplete dataset; in one participant Information could not be gathered due to incomplete medical records at admission to our clinic

case of missing data due to the retrospective design of the study, the specific missing information was marked and explained. If further calculation was performed with an incomplete dataset, listwise deletion was used. Data were analyzed using SPSS Statistics version 23 and Microsoft Excel version 14.5.9.

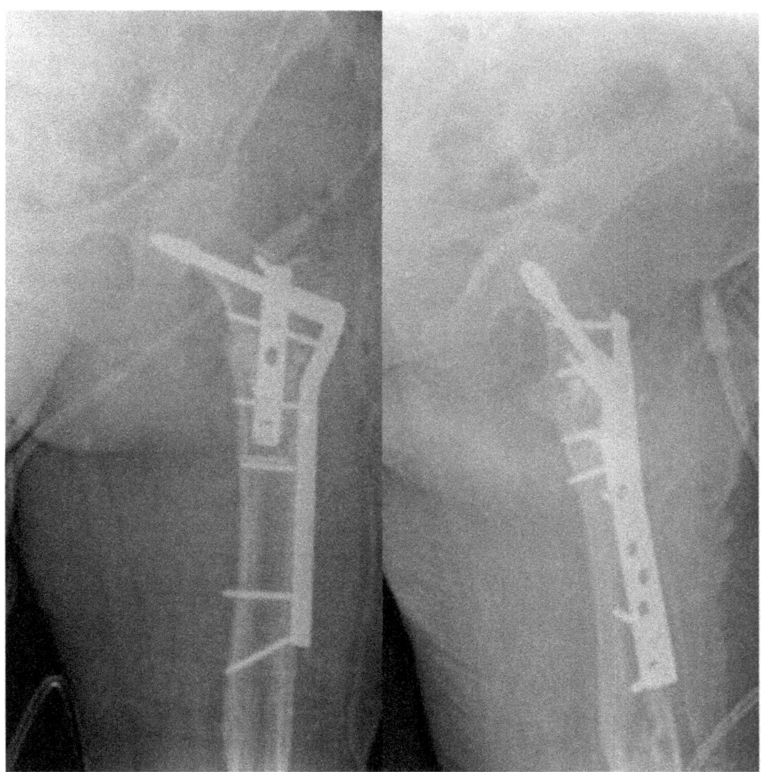

Fig. 3 Postoperative X-rays after nail removal, restoration of the CCD (126°) and DCS treatment with a precontoured plate by leaving the augmentation plate in situ

Results

Between January 2002 and July 2017, 40 patients fulfilled the inclusion criteria and were included in the study. The average length of the follow-up period was 26.3 months (range 6–173 months), with a median of twelve months. The mean age of the 24 women and 16 men upon admittance to our clinic was 65.4 years (range 34–91 years). Regarding clinical constellations, initial fractures were treated with a gamma nail (fa. Stryker) in 17 patients, and a proximal femoral nail (PFN; fa. Zimmer) was used in eight patients. Fifteen fractures were treated by Targon-, Sirius-, Trigen-, Vero-, Friedel or Orthofix intramedullary nails. Among these cases, ten of the 40 patients (23.3%) had already undergone revision surgery after nailing, including for dynamization of the nail, bone grafting, additional augmentation plate insertion or exchange nailing (Fig. 2). A total of three patients had undergone more than one revision surgery. Of the 40 total nonunions, nine (22.5%) were associated with implant failure at admission to our hospital (Fig. 5). The 40 aseptic nonunions were classified as atrophic in 35 (87.5%) cases and as hypertrophic in five (12.5%) patients.

The index surgery was performed at an average of 9.88 months (± 6.7 months) and a median of nine months after the initial nailing. The mean operation time was 154.25 min (range 70–265 min). In 18 patients (45%), an additional LCDCP was used. With the exception of ten patients, an autologous cancellous bone graft taken from the anterior iliac crest was used. In five patients, a demineralized bone matrix was applied instead of an autologous bone graft. The remaining five patients without additional bone grafting had hypertrophic nonunions. The preoperative CCD of the 40 patients prior to the index procedure was 118° (range 101° – 131°). The mean postoperative CCD was calculated to be 128° (range 114° – 142°) with a mean valgus correction of ten degrees. The mean length of the hospital stay was 15.08 days (range 6–40 days). On average, three units of red blood cells were transfused during the hospital stays (range 0–12 units).

Bony union was achieved in 27 of the 40 nonunions (67.5%) after the index procedure. A total of 13 of the 40 (32.5%) patients needed secondary revision surgery, including one persistent nonunion (2.5%), nine persistent nonunions leading to hardware failure (22.5%), two deep infections requiring revision (5%) and one peri-implantary fracture (2.5%) due to low-energy trauma four days after index surgery (Table 2). Within the study group, neither sex nor initial fracture type, trauma mechanism, nonunion type, age, BMI, time to index procedure, number of

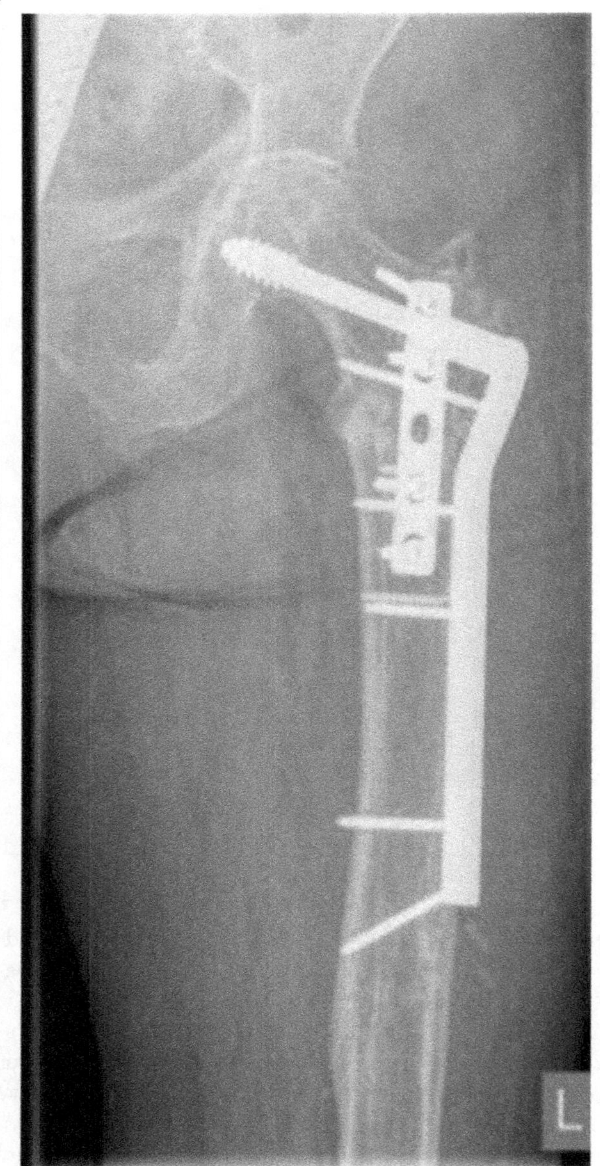

Fig. 4 Final follow-up visit six months after index procedure showing bony union

revisions prior to index procedure, operation time, number of transfused red blood cell units, diabetes mellitus, steroid use, smoking or osteoporosis was a significant factor for revision surgery after the index procedure (Table 1). Ultimately, 37 of the 40 (92.5%) nonunions healed (subsequent surgical procedures included). The mean healing time of the 37 patients was 11.63 months (± 12.4 months). In one case, the patient did not reach union and was treated with a total hip replacement (THR) seven months after the index procedure. Another 90-year-old female patient underwent a resection arthroplasty due to persistent hip infection. Additionally, a 72-year-old female did not reach union, with radiographs showing implant failure with varus deformity and screw loosening; nevertheless, she was fully mobilized without pain using forearm crutches and did not agree to further revision. Revision surgery was a significant factor in unsuccessful bony healing and prolonged healing time within the study period (bony healing $p = 0.03$; healing time $p = 0.01$).

Revision surgery was performed at a mean of 4.9 months after the index procedure (range 4 days – 12 months). In cases of a persistent nonunion with hardware failure ($n = 9$), removal of the plate and a revision procedure using the same implant again or a double plate construct (DCS + anterior LCDCP; $n = 4$) and iliac bone crafting was performed after a mean of 5.9 months (range 1–15 months). In one case, a patient developed a femoral head necrosis with screw cut-out and was treated with THR. In the case of a persistent nonunion without implant failure ($n = 1$), further revision with additional anterior plating using LCDCP and iliac bone crafting was performed. Due to infections ($n = 2$), local surgical debridement was performed leaving the plate in situ with subsequent antibiotic therapy. Implant removal was performed in seven patients after a mean follow-up period of 14 months (range 6–24 months) due to a planned foreign body removal or local pain sensation. Of the 13 patients, a subcategory of eight patients (20%) needed a second additional surgery. Second revisions were performed a mean of two months (range 6 days – 8 months) after the first revision. Second revision surgeries were necessary due to implant failure ($n = 4$), persisting nonunion without implant failure ($n = 1$) and a deep infection requiring surgical debridement ($n = 3$). In the case of a hardware failure, the same revision procedure with double plating was repeated. In the three patients with infections, debridement was repeated in two patients. In one case, resection arthroplasty resulting in a Girdlestone situation was performed. The nonunion without implant failure was treated with an iliac bone graft and demineralized bone matrix. A total of three of the 13 patients (7.5%) patients needed one or more additional surgeries, leading to two cases of osseous consolidation and one case of persisting nonunion.

At the final follow-up visit, a full range of motion of the hip was seen in ten of the 40 (25%) hips. The other 30 hips (75%) had a limited range of motion, with a minimum of 90° of hip flexion. A total of 15 patients (37.5%) could walk without any walking aids, nine patients (22.5%) walked with forearm crutches and eight patients (20%) walked with a walking frame. Two patients used a wheelchair (5%). One patient was bedridden (2.5%). In five patients, postoperative mobility could not be evaluated due to a lack of data.

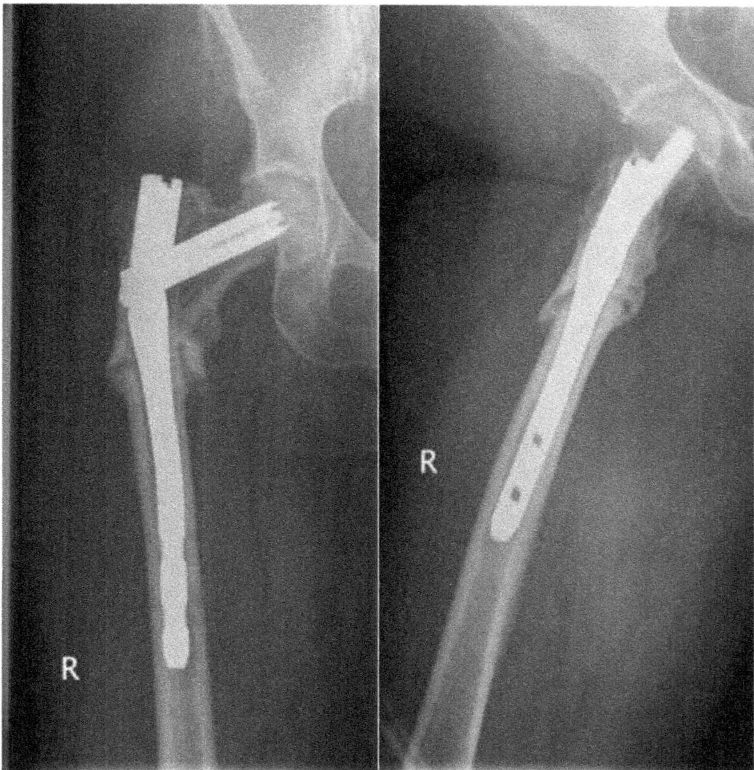

Fig. 5 AP and lateral radiographs of a 56-year-old female patient with a hypertrophic nonunion after nailing with an implant failure and varus nonunion of the femur with a CCD of 109

Discussion

The purpose of this study was to evaluate a series of DCS treatments of subtrochanteric femoral nonunions following IMN regarding the healing rate and implant-related complications. To the best of our knowledge, our patient series of 40 subtrochanteric femoral nonunions represents the largest study reporting on a standardized salvage DCS procedure after failed intramedullary nailing.

Nonunions of the subtrochanteric region of the femur are uncommon; however, they are difficult to treat. In addition to general risk factors [14], mechanobiological properties such as the stability of fracture fixation influence the cellular processes in the healing tissue [30]. Cephalomedullary interlocking nails have improved the results of subtrochanteric fractures with high union rates and have decreased the incidence of fixation failure [1, 31–33]. However, use of IMN remains technically demanding and requires proper reduction and correct positioning of the implant [34]. Malreduction in either the coronal (comminution of the medial cortex) or sagittal plane leads to prolonged time to union for subtrochanteric fractures [10, 35, 36]. Percutaneous reduction maneuvers and minimally invasive techniques can be useful in obtaining proper reduction [3]. Immediate unrestricted weight bearing appears to be a safe postoperative regime for subtrochanteric femoral fractures treated by IMN [1]. Early mobilization can not only lower mortality and morbidity rates but also impel functional recovery in patients with proximal femur fracture [37, 38]. If nonunion occurs after intramedullary nailing, options for reconstruction include dynamization of the nail, exchange nailing, bone grafting, augmentative plating, nail removal and plating or prosthetic replacement. The length of the proximal fragment, femoral deformities and defects in the femoral bone stock guide decision-making. The presence of hardware and poor bone stock from prior fixation attempts can compromise stable fixation [39]. In the treatment of subtrochanteric femoral nonunion, a variety of implants have been used with variable success. The treatment of subtrochanteric aseptic nonunions is rarely reported, and sample sizes in published studies have been small [39]. Barquet et al. [40] presented a study of 29 patients with subtrochanteric nonunions managed by the removal of previous implants ($n = 9$ after nailing; $n = 20$ after open reduction and internal fixation (ORIF) with blade plate, dynamic compression plate or DCS), open correction osteotomy if needed ($n = 3$), secondary osteosynthesis with a gamma nail (overreaming to provide biologic augmentation) and bone grafting in case of loss of bone

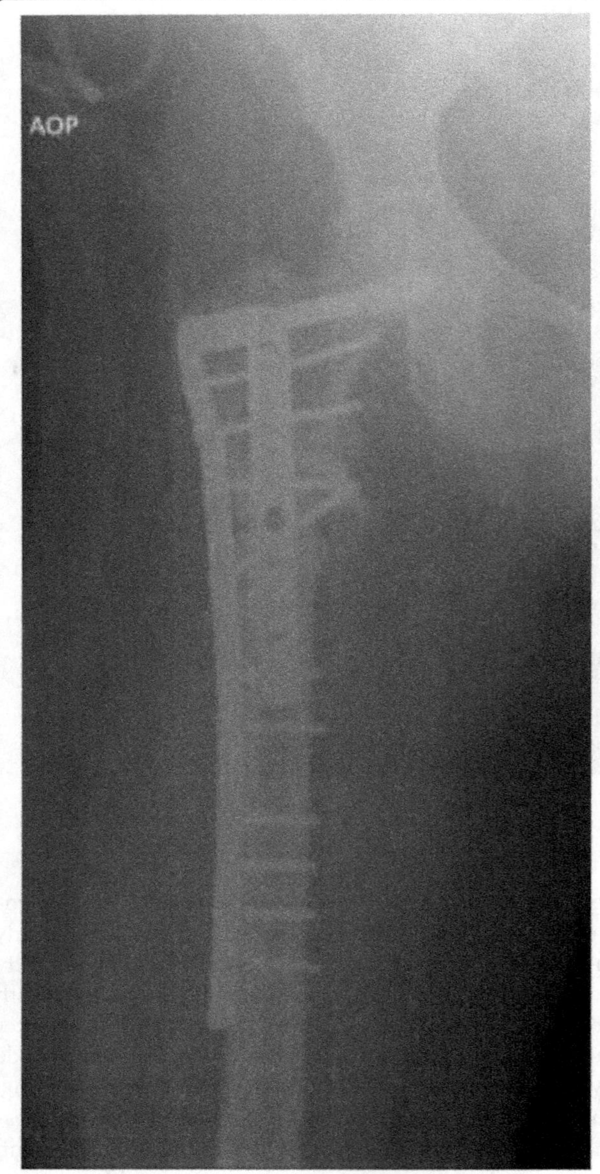

Fig. 6 X-ray after implant removal, nonunion debridement, restoration of the CCD (131°) and ORIF utilizing a DCS with an additional LCDCP

substance ($n = 5$) [40]. Of these nonunions, 23 (88%) healed after the index procedure. Except for one case (96%), all nonunions healed in a mean of seven months. In total, three implant failures (11.5%) were detected. Severe comminution and fragment diastasis or varus alignment were mentioned as influencing factors for persisting nonunion [41]. Wu treated 21 patients with subtrochanteric nonunions after ORIF or IMN (all described patients remained unhealed after one to six previous surgical treatments) with locked nail stabilization [42]. The patient age ranged from 19 to 56, with a median of 36 years. No patients required additional surgery with a healing rate of 100% after one year. Nail dynamization alone offers a minimally invasive treatment option for patients without unacceptable bony deformity or limb shortening. Dynamization has been shown to be effective [43, 44], but its effectiveness according to subtrochanteric nonunions has not been proven yet. In a study including 19 patients, Kang et al. [22] showed that the union rate with the exchange of previous implants, in addition to the complete removal of fibrous tissue and bone grafting, was better than in those with retained hardware in the treatment of subtrochanteric nonunion (ten vs. nine) [22]. In contrast to the abovementioned techniques that rely on renailing or nail dynamization, plate revision of the subtrochanteric femoral nonunions has also been reported. Focusing on the enhancement of mechanical and biological preconditions (subsumed as the diamond concept [45]), Giannoudis et al. [46] presented a study of 14 subtrochanteric nonunions after initial IMN revised with ORIF (95 degree angle blade, $n = 11$) or IMN (Affixus® Hip Fracture nail, $n = 3$) [46]. In total, one revision surgery due to a blade plate failure was necessary. Finally, all 14 nonunions healed after an average of 6.8 months. De Vries used blade plating in 33 subtrochanteric nonunions (mean age of 53 years) and reported a healing rate of 96.9% ($n = 32$) [47]. The average time to healing was five months. According to the functional outcome of the united nonunions measured by the Merle d'Aubigne score [48], ten patients scored as excellent, 15 scored as good and seven as fair outcomes. In total, nine postoperative complications (27.3%) after the index surgery were mentioned. These complications required six revisions, including three "minor" revisions such as one postoperative hematoma that required drainage, one protruding tip of the plate for partial removal of the implant and one superficial wound infection requiring debridement. In total, three "major" complications led to revision surgery including one collapse of the femoral head, one implant failure leading to THR and one refracture after implant removal leading to a revision with IMN and ultimately leading to union.

According to the current literature, there is no strong evidence to support the use of either IMN or extramedullary devices in the revision of subtrochanteric nonunions. Despite the development of new implants and increasing knowledge of nonunion, the treatment of postoperative complications and persisting nonunion still presents a challenge. To date, no prospective randomized study has been published; therefore, level IV studies are currently the best available evidence [49]. We presented a large series of late plate fixations of subtrochanteric femoral nonunions following IMN. In our current study, the final healing rate was 92.5% (37/40). A

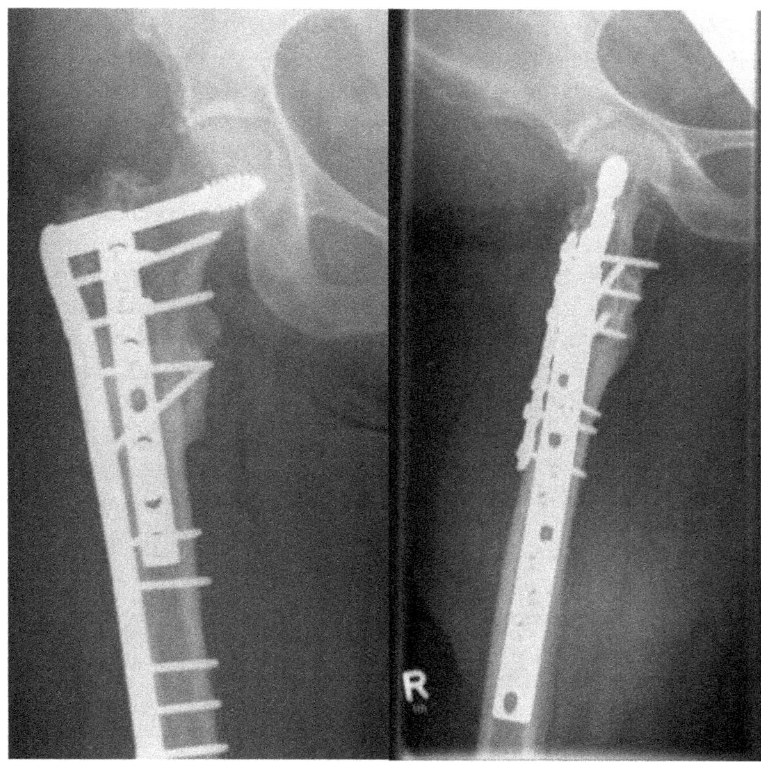

Fig. 7 X-rays of the same patient showing a healed nonunion six months after index treatment

Table 2 Additional information about the patients with implant failure after index procedure

Case number	Age	DCS Construction (holes)	Additional plate	Complication	Therapie
3	58	14	No	Infection	Surgical debridement leaving the plate in situ in addition to antibiotic therapy
4	67	16	No	Periimplant fracture four days after index procedure	Add. Plate
5	52	8	No	Persisting nonuinon without implant failure	Add. Plate + bone grafting
10	72	14	Yes	Implant failure; prox. Plate broken between hole 1/2	Re-ORIF with double plate construction + bone grafting
11	87	14	Yes	Implant failure; prox. Plate broken between hole 2/3	Re-ORIF+ bone grafting
14	69	16	Yes	Implant failure; prox. Plate broken between hole 3/4	Re-ORIF+ bone grafting
21	59	16	No	Implant failure; Plate broken between hole 7/8	Re-ORIF+ bone grafting
24	56	[a]	No	Implant failure; prox. Plate broken between hole 8/9	Re-ORIF with double plate construction + bone grafting
26	50	12	Yes	Implant failure; prox. Plate broken between hole 3/4	Re-ORIF with double plate construction + bone grafting
31	68	14	Yes	Implant failure; Screws broken distal 4 screws with implant loosenig	Re-ORIF+ bone grafting
40	75	16	No	Implant failure; Screw cut out	THR
53	91	12	No	Infection	Surgical debridement leaving the plate in situ in addition to antibiotic therapy
54	58	14	Yes	Implant failure; prox. Plate broken between hole 3/4	Re-ORIF with double plate construction

[a]Plate type remained unknown do to lacking data

significant number of the initial nonunions (87.5%) were classified as atrophic nonunions. Therefore, fracture healing seemed to be disturbed more by biology than by biomechanics. Internal fixation causes significant additional damage to soft tissues in settings where bone healing is already compromised by prior procedures and implants [50]. Positive results have been reported for closed reduction and biologic plating by DCS for treating subtrochanteric fractures [51, 52]. In contrast, extensive debridement of the atrophic nonunion sites with bone grafting [53, 54] is one of the key factors in treatment of a nonunion. Therefore, complete exposure and opening of the nonunion site is necessary for successful surgical nonunion treatment. Additionally, in cases where significant deformities require proper anatomic reduction (for patients with very short proximal fragments with complex deformities or large bone defects), the theoretical advantages of biological plating or exchange nailing are refuted.

Our data series has a relatively high number of postoperative complications leading to revision surgery (13/40). Rosso et al. [55] and Kulkarni et al. [52] reported a high implant failure rate (26%) in elderly patients (> 50 years) using DCS for unstable subtrochanteric and intertrochanteric femoral fracture treatment. Most of the abovementioned studies included younger patients [42, 47]. The mean age in Giannoudis's study was 68.4 years. Except for one 63-year-old patient, all of the mentioned complications ($n = 6$) occurred in patients older than 74 years [46]. Our study includes a large number of elderly patients. The average age of patients upon admittance to our clinic was 65.6 years. In total, 85% patients were 50 years old or older. Most of the patients were older than 60 years (64.6%) or 70 years (41.7%) at admittance. Thus, age was not a significant factor for revision surgery in our study because both groups (Groups 1 and 2) seemed to belong to a high-risk group suffering from implant failure or complications. For these patients, less favorable results and high implant failure rates have been reported previously [56]. Cement-augmented techniques have been described and might be possible alternatives in fracture and implant fixation; however, no study has explored subtrochanteric femoral nonunion treatment [57, 58]. Hip arthroplasty after failed fixation of trochanteric and subtrochanteric fractures might be another alternative; however, several studies highlighted the challenge of the procedure with comparable or even higher complication rates [59, 60]. The strengths of the present study are the relatively large population compared to other studies focusing on nonunions after IMN and the use of one type of implant as the revision procedure.

We acknowledge the limitations of the study. First, only retrospective data gathered from a local electronic database without a defined follow-up protocol is presented. Second, there is a heterogeneity of the study cohort. We included all participants with subtrochanteric nonunions following IMN regardless of the type of initial trauma, type of nonunion and the number of prior revisions. Although there was no significant impact on bony healing in any of these categories, in our cohort group that might be a result of subgroup analysis with small group samples. Third, the index procedure was performed over the course of 15 years observational time by 18 different surgeons with varying levels of experience. Fourth, the 40 included patients had been referred to our hospital for nonunion treatment. Additional information about inital fracture treatment was limited and the rate of nonunion after fracture treatment was not available.

Conclusions

This study shows that treatment of subtrochanteric nonunions is still a challenge. Despite high overall healing rates, a significant number of patients needed secondary surgical revisions, especially among elderly patients.

Abbreviations

BMI: Body mass index; CCD: Neck shaft angle; CT: Computerized tomography; DCS: Dynamic condylar screw; IMN: Intramedullary nail; LCDCP: Limited contact dynamic compression plate; ORIF: Open reduction internal fixation; OTA: Orthopaedic Trauma Association; PFN: Proximal femoral nail; PRS: Prospective and randomized

Acknowledgements

Not Applicable.

Funding

We acknowledge support by the DFG Open Access Publication Funds of the Ruhr-Universität Bochum.

Authors' contributions

SL, VR, TS and JG have contributed to the conception and design of the study, acquisition of data, analysis and interpretation of the data. SL, VR, TS and JG have approved the final version of this manuscript.

Consent for publication

All patients gave written consent for publication of their anonymized data.

Competing interests

On behalf of all authors, the corresponding author states that there is no conflict of interest.

References

1. Joglekar SB, Lindvall EM, Martirosian A. Contemporary management of subtrochanteric fractures. Orthop Clin North Am. 2015;46:21–35.
2. Bedi A, Le TT. Subtrochanteric femur fractures. Orthop Clin North Am. 2004; 35:473–83.
3. Tomas J, Teixidor J, Batalla L, Pacha D, Cortina J. Subtrochanteric fractures: treatment with cerclage wire and long intramedullary nail. J Orthop Trauma. 2013;27:e157–60.
4. Gdoutos EE, Raftopoulos DD, Baril JD. A critical review of the biomechanical stress analysis of the human femur. Biomaterials. 1982;3:2–8.
5. Williams JF, Svensson NL. An experimental stress analysis of the neck of the femur. Med Biol Eng. 1971;9:479–93.
6. Koch JC. The laws of bone architecture. Am J Anat. 1917;21:177–298.
7. Velasco RU, Comfort TH. Analysis of treatment problems in subtrochanteric fractures of the femur. J Trauma Acute Care Surg. 1978;18:513–23.

8. Parker MJ, Handoll HH. Gamma and other cephalocondylic intramedullary nails versus extramedullary implants for extracapsular hip fractures in adults. Cochrane Database Syst Rev. 2010;9:CD000093.
9. Liu P, Wu X, Shi H, Liu R, Shu H, Gong J, Yang Y, Sun Q, Wu J, Nie X, Cai M. Intramedullary versus extramedullary fixation in the management of subtrochanteric femur fractures: a meta-analysis. Clin Interv Aging. 2015;10: 803–11.
10. Park SH, Kong GM, Ha BH, Park JH, Kim KH. Nonunion of subtrochanteric fractures. Comminution or Malreduction. Pak J Med Sci. 2016;32:591–4.
11. Boldin C, Seibert FJ, Fankhauser F, Peicha G, Grechenig W, Szyszkowitz R. The proximal femoral nail (PFN)--a minimal invasive treatment of unstable proximal femoral fractures: a prospective study of 55 patients with a follow-up of 15 months. Acta Orthop Scand. 2003;74:53–8.
12. Pires RE, Santana EO Jr, Santos LE, Giordano V, Balbachevsky D, Dos Reis FB. Failure of fixation of trochanteric femur fractures: clinical recommendations for avoiding Z-effect and reverse Z-effect type complications. Patient Saf Surg. 2011;5:17.
13. Menezes DF, Gamulin A, Noesberger B. Is the proximal femoral nail a suitable implant for treatment of all trochanteric fractures? Clin Orthop Relat Res. 2005;439:221–7.
14. Calori GM, Albisetti W, Agus A, Iori S, Tagliabue L. Risk factors contributing to fracture non-unions. Injury. 2007;38(Suppl 2):S11–8.
15. Craig NJ, Sivaji C, Maffulli N. Subtrochanteric fractures. A review of treatment options. Bull Hosp Jt Dis. 2001;60:35–46.
16. Sims SH. Subtrochanteric femur fractures. Orthop Clin North Am. 2002;33: 113–26.
17. Maquet P, Pelzer-Bawin G. Mechanical analysis of inter- and subtrochanteric fractures of the femur. Acta Orthop Belg. 1980;46:823–8.
18. Parker MJ, Dutta BK, Sivaji C, Pryor GA. Subtrochanteric fractures of the femur. Injury. 1997;28:91–5.
19. Iorio R, Robb WJ, Healy WL, Berry DJ, Hozack WJ, Kyle RF, Lewallen DG, Trousdale RT, Jiranek WA, Stamos VP, Parsley BS. Orthopaedic surgeon workforce and volume assessment for total hip and knee replacement in the United States: preparing for an epidemic. J Bone Joint Surg Am. 2008; 90:1598–605.
20. Lohmann R, Frerichmann U, Stockle U, Riegel T, Raschke MJ. Proximal femoral fractures in the elderly. Analysis of data from health insurance providers on more than 23 million insured persons--part 1. Unfallchirurg. 2007;110:603–9.
21. Frerichmann U, Raschke MJ, Stockle U, Wohrmann S, Lohmann R. Proximal femoral fractures in the elderly. Data from health insurance providers on more than 23 million insured persons--part 2. Unfallchirurg. 2007;110:610–6.
22. Kang SH, Han SK, Kim YS, Kim MJ. Treatment of subtrochanteric nonunion of the femur: whether to leave or to exchange the previous hardware. Acta Orthop Traumatol Turc. 2013;47:91–5.
23. Floyd JC, O'Toole RV, Stall A, Forward DP, Nabili M, Shillingburg D, Hsieh A, Nascone JW. Biomechanical comparison of proximal locking plates and blade plates for the treatment of comminuted subtrochanteric femoral fractures. J Orthop Trauma. 2009;23:628–33.
24. Lundy DW, Acevedo JI, Ganey TM, Ogden JA, Hutton WC. Mechanical comparison of plates used in the treatment of unstable subtrochanteric femur fractures. J Orthop Trauma. 1999;13:534–8.
25. Radford PJ, Howell CJ. The AO dynamic condylar screw for fractures of the femur. Injury. 1992;23:89–93.
26. Yang JS, Otero J, McAndrew CM, Ricci WM, Gardner MJ. Can tibial nonunion be predicted at 3 months after intramedullary nailing? J Orthop Trauma. 2013;27:599–603.
27. Megas P. Classification of non-union. Injury. 2005;36(Suppl 4):S30–7.
28. Trampuz A, Zimmerli W. Diagnosis and treatment of infections associated with fracture-fixation devices. Injury. 2006;37(Suppl 2):S59–66.
29. Seinsheimer F. Subtrochanteric fractures of the femur. J Bone Joint Surg Am. 1978;60:300–6.
30. Claes L. Mechanobiologie der frakturheilung teil 2. Unfallchirurg. 2017; 120:23–31.
31. Bergman GD, Winquist RA, Mayo KA, Hansen ST Jr. Subtrochanteric fracture of the femur. Fixation using the Zickel nail. J Bone Joint Surg Am. 1987;69: 1032–40.
32. Barquet A, Francescoli L, Rienzi D, Lopez L. Intertrochanteric-subtrochanteric fractures: treatment with the long gamma nail. J Orthop Trauma. 2000;14: 324–8.
33. Roberts CS, Nawab A, Wang M, Voor MJ, Seligson D. Second generation intramedullary nailing of subtrochanteric femur fractures: a biomechanical study of fracture site motion. J Orthop Trauma. 2002;16:231–8.
34. Jahangir AA, Perez EA, Russell TA. Intramedullary nailing of subtrochanteric fractures: relevant anatomy and entry portals, supine, or lateral positioning. Tech Orthop. 2008;23:113–7.
35. Riehl JT, Koval KJ, Langford JR, Munro MW, Kupiszewski SJ, Haidukewych GJ. Intramedullary nailing of subtrochanteric fractures--does malreduction matter? Bull Hosp Jt Dis. 2014;72:159–63.
36. Choi JY, Sung YB, Yoo JH, Chung SJ. Factors affecting time to bony union of femoral subtrochanteric fractures treated with intramedullary devices. Hip Pelvis. 2014;26:107–14.
37. Kubiak EN, Beebe MJ, North K, Hitchcock R, Potter MQ. Early weight bearing after lower extremity fractures in adults. J Am Acad Orthop Surg. 2013;21:727–38.
38. Kim JW, Byun SE, Chang JS. The clinical outcomes of early internal fixation for undisplaced femoral neck fractures and early full weight-bearing in elderly patients. Arch Orthop Trauma Surg. 2014;134:941–6.
39. Haidukewych GJ, Berry DJ. Nonunion of fractures of the subtrochanteric region of the femur. Clin Orthop Relat Res. 2004;419:185–8.
40. Barquet A, Mayora G, Fregeiro J, Lopez L, Rienzi D, Francescoli L. The treatment of subtrochanteric nonunions with the long gamma nail: twenty-six patients with a minimum 2-year follow-up. J Orthop Trauma. 2004;18:346–53.
41. Barquet A. The treatment of subtrochanteric nonunions with the long gamma nail: twenty-six patients with a minimum 2-year follow-up. J Orthop Trauma. 2005;19:294 author reply 294.
42. Wu CC. Locked nailing for shortened subtrochanteric nonunions: a one-stage treatment. Clin Orthop Relat Res. 2009;467:254–9.
43. Brumback RJ, Uwagie-Ero S, Lakatos RP, Poka A, Bathon GH, Burgess AR. Intramedullary nailing of femoral shaft fractures. Part II: fracture-healing with static interlocking fixation. J Bone Joint Surg Am. 1988;70:1453–62.
44. Wu CC. The effect of dynamization on slowing the healing of femur shaft fractures after interlocking nailing. J Trauma. 1997;43:263–7.
45. Giannoudis PV, Einhorn TA, Marsh D. Fracture healing: the diamond concept. Injury. 2007;38(Suppl 4):S3–6.
46. Giannoudis PV, Ahmad MA, Mineo GV, Tosounidis TI, Calori GM, Kanakaris NK. Subtrochanteric fracture non-unions with implant failure managed with the "diamond" concept. Injury. 2013;44(Suppl 1):S76–81.
47. de Vries JS, Kloen P, Borens O, Marti RK, Helfet DL. Treatment of subtrochanteric nonunions. Injury. 2006;37:203–11.
48. D'Aubigne RM, Postel M. Functional results of hip arthroplasty with acrylic prosthesis. J Bone Joint Surg Am. 1954;36-A:451–75.
49. Brighton B, Bhandari M, Tornetta P 3rd, Felson DT. Hierarchy of evidence: from case reports to randomized controlled trials. Clin Orthop Relat Res. 2003;413:19–24.
50. Gautier E, Ganz R. The biological plate osteosynthesis. Zentralbl Chir. 1994; 119:564–72.
51. Celebi L, Can M, Muratli HH, Yagmurlu MF, Yuksel HY, Bicimoğlu A. Indirect reduction and biological internal fixation of comminuted subtrochanteric fractures of the femur. Injury. 2006;37:740–50.
52. Kulkarni SS, Moran CG. Results of dynamic condylar screw for subtrochanteric fractures. Injury. 2003;34:117–22.
53. Egol KA, Nauth A, Lee M, Pape HC, Watson JT, Borrelli J Jr. Bone grafting: sourcing, timing, strategies, and alternatives. J Orthop Trauma. 2015; 29(Suppl 12):S10–4.
54. Kulachote N, Sa-ngasoongsong P, Sirisreetreerux N, Chanplakorn P, Fuangfa P, Suphachatwong C, Wajanavisit W. Demineralized bone matrix add-on for acceleration of bone healing in atypical subtrochanteric femoral fracture: a consecutive case-control study. Biomed Res Int. 2016;2016:4061539.
55. Rosso R, Babst R, Marx A, Hess P, Heberer M, Regazzoni P. Proximal femoral fractures. Is there an indication for the condylar screw (DCS)? Helv Chir Acta. 1992;58:679–82.
56. Garnavos C, Peterman A, Howard PW. The treatment of difficult proximal femoral fractures with the Russell-Taylor reconstruction nail. Injury. 1999; 30:407–15.
57. Lee PC, Hsieh PH, Yu SW, Shiao CW, Kao HK, Wu CC. Biologic plating versus intramedullary nailing for comminuted subtrochanteric fractures in young adults: a prospective, randomized study of 66 cases. J Trauma. 2007;63: 1283–91.

58. Tzioupis C, Panteliadis P, Gamie Z, Tsiridis E. Revision of a nonunited subtrochanteric femoral fracture around a failed intramedullary nail with the use of RIA products, BMP-7 and hydroxyapatite: a case report. J Med Case Rep. 2011;5:87.
59. Enocson A, Mattisson L, Ottosson C, Lapidus LJ. Hip arthroplasty after failed fixation of trochanteric and subtrochanteric fractures: a cohort study with 5–11 year follow-up of 88 consecutive patients. Acta Orthop. 2012;83:493–8.
60. Exaltacion JJ, Incavo SJ, Mathews V, Parsley B, Noble P. Hip arthroplasty after intramedullary hip screw fixation: a perioperative evaluation. J Orthop Trauma. 2012;26:141–7.

10

Evaluation of mitochondrial function in chronic myofascial trigger points - a prospective cohort pilot study using high-resolution respirometry

Michael J. Fischer[1,2,3], Gergo Horvath[4], Martin Krismer[3], Erich Gnaiger[5], Georg Goebel[6] and Dominik H. Pesta[7,8,9*]

Abstract

Background: Myofascial trigger points (MTrPs) are hyperirritable areas in the fascia of the affected muscle, possibly related to mitochondrial impairment. They can result in pain and hypoxic areas within the muscle. This pilot study established a minimally invasive biopsy technique to obtain high-quality MTrP tissue samples to evaluate mitochondrial function via high-resolution respirometry. Secondary objectives included the feasibility and safety of the biopsy procedure.

Methods: Twenty healthy males participated in this study, 10 with a diagnosis of myofascial pain in the musculus (m.) trapezius MTrP (TTP group) and 10 with a diagnosis of myofascial pain in the m. gluteus medius (GTP group). Each participant had 2 muscle biopsies taken in one session. The affected muscle was biopsied followed by a biopsy from the m. vastus lateralis to be used as a control. Measurements of oxygen consumption were carried out using high-resolution respirometry.

Results: Mitochondrial respiration was highest in the GTP group compared to the TTP group and the control muscle whereas no differences were observed between the GTP and the control muscle. When normalizing respiration to an internal reference state, there were no differences between muscle groups. None of the participants had hematomas or reported surgical complications. Patient-reported pain was minimal for all 3 groups. All participants reported a low procedural burden.

Conclusions: This pilot study used a safe and minimally invasive technique for obtaining biopsies from MTrPs suitable for high-resolution respirometry analysis of mitochondrial function. The results suggest that there are no qualitative differences in mitochondrial function of MTrPs of the trapezius and gluteus medius muscles compared to the vastus lateralis control muscle, implying that alterations of mitochondrial function do not appear to have a role in the development of MTrPs.

Keywords: Mitochondria, Myofascial trigger points, High-resolution respirometry, Mitochondrial function, Muscle biopsy

* Correspondence: dominik.pesta@ddz.uni-duesseldorf.de
[7]Institute for Clinical Diabetology, German Diabetes Center, Leibniz Institute for Diabetes Research, Heinrich-Heine-University, Düsseldorf, Germany
[8]German Center for Diabetes Research (DZD), München-Neuherberg, Germany
Full list of author information is available at the end of the article

Background

Myofascial pain syndrome is a leading cause of chronic musculoskeletal pain [1] with a lifetime incidence estimated to be up to 85% [2, 3]. It is characterized by local and referred pain, weakness, and restricted mobility [2]. Almost half of sick leave in the European Union is due to musculoskeletal disorders, which imposes a tremendous burden to healthcare resources [4].

Myofascial trigger points (MTrPs), a common and ubiquitous condition with (and cause of) myofascial pain [2, 5], were first identified by American researchers Travell and Simons, who described them as the dominant factor responsible for pain and functional limitations in the neuromusculoskeletal system [1]. MTrPs are palpable, taut bands found in stiff muscle that cause spontaneous pain (active MTrPs) or pain provoked by compression of the nodule (latent MTrPs) [2, 6]. This pain is often referred to other parts of the body, even in the absence of persisting nerve damage. Paresthesia, muscle weakness without primary atrophy, restricted mobility, proprioceptive disorders with impaired coordination, and autonomic reactions can also be caused by MTrPs [2, 6].

MTrPs are possibly caused by chronic overload, overstretching, or by direct trauma of the affected muscles [2, 5–7]. This can result in acute or chronic musculoskeletal pain, experienced by almost everyone during their lifetime. MTrPs have been found in 20–85% of the general population [8–11]. They can be treated holistically with stretching techniques, massage, pain medication, trigger point infiltration, dry needling, electrical stimulation, ultrasound, and cold laser treatment [2, 6, 12]. Myofascial pain syndrome can be initiated by the following events: damage to the sarcoplasmic reticulum, malfunction of the motor end plate, activation and sensitization of nociceptors [by adenosine triphosphate (ATP)], or the release of vasoneuroactive substances [5, 6, 13, 14]. The direct lesion of muscle fibers or persistently increased muscle tone are common factors related to the initial development of MTrPs [2, 5, 15].

The etiology of MTrPs is poorly understood. One of the earliest theories of trigger point formation states a continued shortening of the sarcomeres [6]. This is caused by extended calcium release from the sarcolemma due to abnormal endplate activity. ATP demand increases upon reuptake of calcium into the sarcoplasmic reticulum and induces relaxation of the muscle [13, 16]. Impairment of mitochondrial function due to a reduced cytochrome oxidase system stemming from a deficiency of freely accessible iron leads to an energy crisis within the muscle [17, 18]. Mitochondrial content determines the aerobic capacity of a muscle and is impaired in chronic musculoskeletal pain [18–22]. Lack of ATP propagates contracture and the resulting compressed capillary circulation can cause a hypoxic environment [1]. Data from respirometric studies on athletes, obese individuals, patients with diabetes or heart failure, and sedentary people indicate that hypoxia and ischemia can significantly affect and potentially impair mitochondrial function [23–35]. Inflammatory processes may also play a role as an increased concentration of inflammatory mediators including bradykinin, substance P, calcitonin gene-related peptides, tumor necrosis factor-alpha, and interleukins (ILs), such as IL-6, IL-1β, and IL-8 have been reported to be detected by in vivo microdialysis in MTrPs in humans [14].

In order to improve therapies and therapeutic tools for the treatment of MTrPs, understanding the mechanisms involved in their etiology is necessary. Elucidation of cell communication and signal transduction [15] or mitochondrial function from muscle biopsy samples to explore mechanisms at the level of the muscle cell are promising approaches. Based on the 'energy crisis theory' and disrupted mitochondrial energy metabolism in MTrPs, we assessed mitochondrial function in MTrPs in the present study.

The primary aim of this pilot study was to establish the clinical use of a minimally invasive biopsy technique to obtain high-quality muscle tissue from MTrPs in sufficient amount in order to evaluate their mitochondrial function via high-resolution respirometry. Secondary objectives included evaluation of the feasibility of the procedure in terms of patient acceptance and safety of the biopsy technique.

Methods

Study design and participants

In this prospective cohort pilot study using high-resolution respirometry to evaluate mitochondrial function in MTrPs, the primary endpoints were mitochondrial function expressed as oxygen flux (JO_2; pmol $O_2.s^{-1}.mg^{-1}$) and flux control ratios (FCR). Secondary endpoints to access the feasibility of the biopsy procedure in terms of patient acceptance were patient-reported pain, based on a Numeric Rating Scale (NRS) of 0–10, and patient-reported burden of procedure, based on a scale of 0–4, with 0 = extreme and 4 = none. Secondary endpoints to assess the safety of the procedure included: clinical wound assessment, consisting of assessing signs for local infection and inflammation (increased local temperature, swelling, redness and increased wound exudate), hematoma volume (assessed by ultrasound examination), and surgical complications.

This study took place at the Department for Rehabilitation Medicine of the General Hospital Hall in Tirol, Austria lasting from October 2013 through February 2014. The local television station for the province of Tyrol with approximately 50,000 viewers daily, ran a news documentary on myofascial pain and announced the study. Interested patients were advised to contact the principal investigator (PI), who determined their eligibility, obtained their informed consent, and enrolled them into the study. The study sample comprised 20 patients. Male patients aged 18–45 years with a clinical diagnosis of myofascial pain syndrome within the shoulder-neck muscles or the lumbogluteal region and the presence of an MTrP, defined as a firm palpation of a hard, tender nodule resulting in a spontaneous pain complaint [1], with symptoms present for 1 to 12 months were included. Exclusion criteria were:

- Signs that the participant's prescriptive compliance was not expected (e.g., lack of cooperation)
- Disorders of the respiratory tract
- Neurological disorders, in particular neurodegenerative and neuromuscular diseases
- Disorders of the cardiovascular system or the musculoskeletal system
- Civil servants and military service personnel.

Those who met the inclusion criteria and additionally provided written informed consent were enrolled into the study. According to their specific pathology, participants were allocated to either a gluteus medius myofascial trigger point (GTP) or a descending trapezius myofascial trigger point (TTP) group with 10 participants in each group.

During the baseline visit, the participants' demographic and anthropometric data were recorded, including weight, height, body mass index (BMI), type of sports practice, number of hours per week each sport was practiced, and smoking status. Each MTrP was assessed in terms of location, to determine if it was latent or active, and for pain. A MTrP was defined as being "active" if it caused spontaneous pain and referred pain pattern as described by Simons and Travell and as "latent", if pain was provoked only by compression of the nodule [2, 6]. Patients reported pain following the compression of their trigger points [1]. Laboratory examinations were performed to analyze levels of C-reactive protein, creatine-kinase, and lactate dehydrogenase, as well as prothrombin time. Biopsies were obtained at baseline from GTP, TTP and the musculus (m.) vastus lateralis as control muscle, respectively, and analyzed as described below using high-resolution respirometry. Participants were asked to return to the study site for a follow-up visit 1 week after the biopsy.

During the follow-up visit, clinical wound assessment and an ultrasound examination was performed to determine hematoma volume. Surgical complications were reported and treated. Patient acceptance was assessed based on patient-reported pain (spontaneous pain at the trigger point without compression) and the burden of the biopsy procedure.

Muscle biopsy sampling

Prior to performing the study procedures, the PI, an experienced surgeon who previously performed over 100 muscle biopsies on patients with neuromuscular disorders, was trained on the study biopsy procedure, which involved performing 10 biopsies (as described below) on a freshly slaughtered pig.

Local anesthesia was applied to the superficial skin covering the MTrP of each participant. Percutaneous biopsy sampling [36] optimized with a suction-enhancement technique was used to obtain muscle biopsies of the m. trapezius MTrP or the m. gluteus medius MTrP from each participant, using a small Bergstrom muscle biopsy needle, 8 swg (4.0 mm) × 100 mm (Dixons Surgical Instruments, Essex, United Kingdom). Biopsies were also obtained from the m. vastus lateralis of each participant to serve as a control sample.

Each muscle specimen was immediately placed in ice-cold biopsy preservation solution (BIOPS) containing 2.77 mM CaK_2EGTA (ethylene glycol traacetic acid) buffer, 7.23 mM K_2EGTA buffer, 0.1 μM free calcium, 20 mM imidazole, 20 mM taurine, 50 mM 2-(*N*-morpholino) ethanesulfonic acid hydrate (MES), 0.5 mM dithiothreitol, 6.56 mM $MgCl_2{\cdot}6H_2O$, 5.77 mM ATP, and 15 mM phosphocreatine (pH 7.1).

A blinded assessor, who did not know the origin of the muscle specimens or the participants' diagnoses, evaluated the muscle specimens. After careful dissection of each muscle sample using forceps, fibers were chemically permeabilized via incubation in 2 ml of BIOPS containing saponin (50 μg/ ml) for 30 min [37]. Muscle fibers were subsequently incubated for 10 min at 4 °C in ice-cold mitochondrial respiration medium (MiR06; 0.5 mM EGTA, 3 mM $MgCl_2$, 60 mM K-lactobionate, 20 mM taurine, 10 mM KH_2PO_4, 20 mM HEPES, 110 mM sucrose, and 1 g/l bovine serum albumin essentially fatty acid free, adjusted to pH 7.1, 2800 units/mg solid catalase lypophilized powder). The fibers' wet weight was measured on a microbalance (Mettler Toledo, Greifensee, Switzerland).

Each biopsy specimen was evaluated for visual quality (based on a scale of 1–5, with 1 = poor and 5 = excellent) and for quantity (based on wet weight in mg).

High-resolution respirometry

A blinded assessor performed high-resolution respirometry on the muscle specimens and the related data collection and analysis. Measurements of oxygen consumption were carried out at 37 °C using the 2-chamber titration-injection respirometer Oxygraph-2 k (Oroboros Instruments, Innsbruck, Austria). All experiments were carried out in a hyperoxygenated chamber to prevent any potential oxygen diffusion limitation [37]. Oxygen concentration (μM = nmol/ml) and oxygen flux ($pmol.s^{-1}.mg^{-1}$; negative time derivative of oxygen concentration, divided by muscle wet weight) were recorded using DatLab software (Oroboros Instruments). For the substrate-uncoupler-inhibitor titration protocol, the following substrates were added (as final concentrations):

- Malate (2 mM) and glutamate (10 mM) to support leak respiration without adenylates (LEAK, L_N).
- Active respiration was stimulated by addition of adenosine diphosphate (2.5 mM) and pyruvate (5 mM) yielding complex I (CI)-supported oxidative phosphorylation (OXPHOS) capacity (CI_P).
- After titration of carbonyl cyanide p-(trifluoromethoxy) phenylhydrazone (FCCP; a total of 1.5 μM in steps of 0.5 μM) electron transfer capacity (ETC) of CI (CI_E) was recorded.
- Subsequently, succinate (10 mM) was added to stimulate maximal ETC of CI and CII ($CI + II_E$).
- Finally, rotenone (0.5 μM) was added to inhibit CI, yielding ETC of CII (CII_E) and antimycin A (2.5 μM) and malonic acid (5 mM) to yield residual oxygen consumption (ROX).

Statistical analysis

Data were extracted from the DatLab-program and compiled into a spreadsheet. SPSS for Windows (SPSS, 2009, Chicago, IL) was used for subsequent statistical analysis. Data were checked for normal distribution by Kolmogorov-Smirnov test, depending on the distribution. Baseline and endpoint data were analyzed using descriptive statistics. The difference between the mean values of the different muscle groups was assessed by a one-way analysis of variance. The significance level was set at $p \leq 0.01$; $p \leq 0.05$ and of $p \leq 0.1$ were considered as trends. Data are presented as mean ± standard deviation (SD). Because this is an explorative study, no correction for multiple testing was applied. There were no previous data available from the literature to perform a sample size calculation for this pilot study. Analysis was performed on a per-protocol basis.

Results

The baseline demographic, anthropometric and clinical characteristics of the participants were similar for both groups and are summarized in Table 1.

A representative mitochondrial trace of one participant for evaluating mitochondrial function is shown in Fig. 1.

Quantitative differences in mitochondrial function

With the exception of L_N, mass-specific CI_P (53.5 ± 19.3 vs 37.9 ± 6.3 $pmol.s^{-1}.mg^{-1}$), CI_E (79.8 ± 37.6 vs 56.0 ± 20.7 $pmol.s^{-1}.mg^{-1}$), $CI + II_E$ (131.5 ± 55.5 vs 85.9 ± 29.2 $pmol.s^{-1}.mg^{-1}$) and CII_E (76.9 ± 27.6 vs 47.9 ± 11.4 $pmol.s^{-1}.mg^{-1}$) were all lower (all $p < 0.05$) in the TTP than in the GTP (Fig. 2). $CI + II_E$ of the TTP was lower compared to the control m. vastus lateralis (131.5 ± 55.5 vs 100.5 ± 30.8 $pmol.s^{-1}.mg^{-1}$, $p < 0.05$). No differences were observed in any respiratory state between the GTP and the control m. vastus lateralis.

Qualitative differences in mitochondrial function

When normalizing respiratory states for the internal reference state of maximal ETC of CI + II, the resulting FCRs reflect important qualitative alterations in mitochondrial function (Fig. 3). Surprisingly, there were no differences across all groups for FCR, indicating no qualitative differences with regard to mitochondrial function between GTP, TTP, and m. vastus lateralis.

Biopsy assessment, safety and acceptance of the biopsy procedure for all 3 muscle groups are summarized in Table 2. Muscle samples of very good quality and similar

Table 1 Comparison of baseline characteristics of gluteus medius and descending trapezius myofascial trigger point (MTrP) groups

Parameter	Gluteus Medius MTrP (n = 10)	Descending Trapezius MTrP (n = 10)
Age (y)	38.7 ± 5.1 (21–42)	37.6 ± 6.2 (31–45)
Pain intensity NRS	6.8 ± 1.2	6.2 ± 1.5
Weight (kg)	81.2 ± 17.5	86.2 ± 12.8
Height (m)	1.8 ± 0.08	1.8 ± 0.06
Smoker, n (%)	7 (70%)	6 (60%)
Body Mass Index (kg/m^2)	26.1 ± 3.6	24.9 ± 4.2
Physical activities/sports (minutes/week)	216 ± 154.8	185 ± 90.6
Laboratory tests		
C-reactive protein ($mg.dl^{-1}$)	0.11 ± 0.12	0.15 ± 0.25
Creatine kinase ($U.l^{-1}$)	222.5 ± 161.3	204.6 ± 128.5
Lactate dehydrogenase ($U.l^{-1}$)	182.1 ± 26.9	186.3 ± 38.0
Prothrombin time (%)	101.9% ± 11.7	107.1 ± 11.9

Values are mean ± SD; *NRS* Numeric Rating Scale

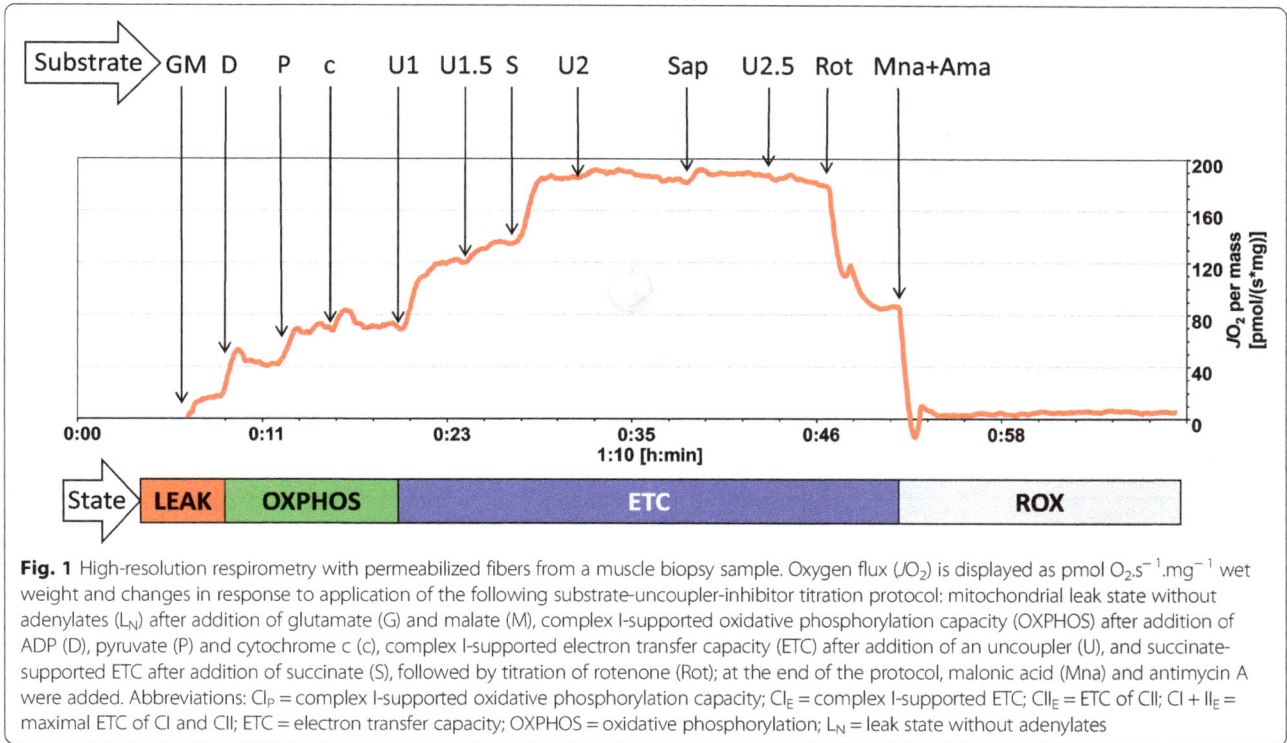

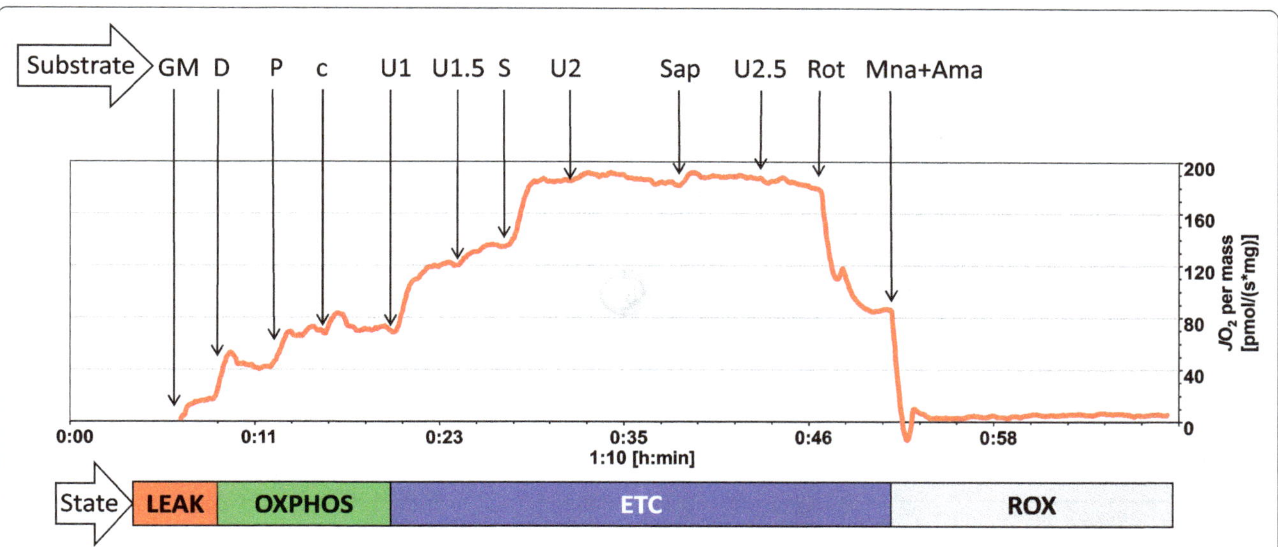

Fig. 1 High-resolution respirometry with permeabilized fibers from a muscle biopsy sample. Oxygen flux (JO_2) is displayed as pmol $O_2.s^{-1}.mg^{-1}$ wet weight and changes in response to application of the following substrate-uncoupler-inhibitor titration protocol: mitochondrial leak state without adenylates (L_N) after addition of glutamate (G) and malate (M), complex I-supported oxidative phosphorylation capacity (OXPHOS) after addition of ADP (D), pyruvate (P) and cytochrome c (c), complex I-supported electron transfer capacity (ETC) after addition of an uncoupler (U), and succinate-supported ETC after addition of succinate (S), followed by titration of rotenone (Rot); at the end of the protocol, malonic acid (Mna) and antimycin A were added. Abbreviations: CI_P = complex I-supported oxidative phosphorylation capacity; CI_E = complex I-supported ETC; CII_E = ETC of CII; $CI + II_E$ = maximal ETC of CI and CII; ETC = electron transfer capacity; OXPHOS = oxidative phosphorylation; L_N = leak state without adenylates

yield were obtained from all 3 muscle groups. None of the groups had hematomas or surgical complications. The mean pain reported for the biopsy procedure was higher for the TTP group (1.1 ± 2.3) than for the GTP (0.25 ± 0.35) and control (0.2 ± 0.4), although pain was generally minimal for all 3 groups. For all 3 muscle groups, participants reported a low procedural burden.

Discussion

This pilot study demonstrates the feasibility of a minimally invasive biopsy technique to obtain muscle tissue from an MTrP in sufficient amount and quality for high-resolution respirometry analysis of mitochondrial function. The use of fresh muscle biopsy samples for high-resolution respirometry allows for the direct measurement of oxygen consumption and provides detailed information about mitochondrial functional integrity and energetic capacity (Figs. 2 and 3). Previous histological examination of MTrP biopsies revealed mitochondrial swelling, resulting in reduced ATP concentrations and blood flow and increased metabolic stress that contributed to persistent MTrPs [2]. In the

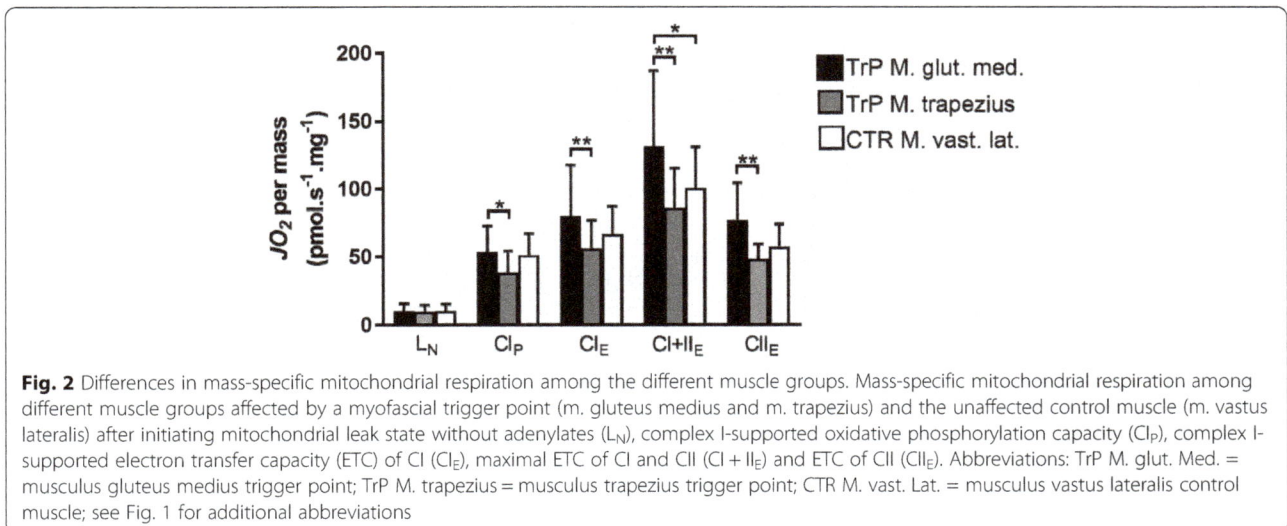

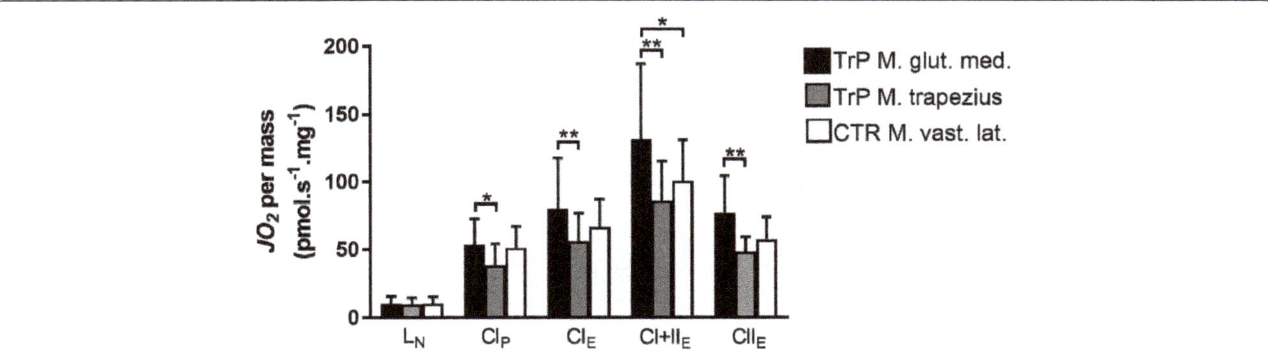

Fig. 2 Differences in mass-specific mitochondrial respiration among the different muscle groups. Mass-specific mitochondrial respiration among different muscle groups affected by a myofascial trigger point (m. gluteus medius and m. trapezius) and the unaffected control muscle (m. vastus lateralis) after initiating mitochondrial leak state without adenylates (L_N), complex I-supported oxidative phosphorylation capacity (CI_P), complex I-supported electron transfer capacity (ETC) of CI (CI_E), maximal ETC of CI and CII ($CI + II_E$) and ETC of CII (CII_E). Abbreviations: TrP M. glut. Med. = musculus gluteus medius trigger point; TrP M. trapezius = musculus trapezius trigger point; CTR M. vast. Lat. = musculus vastus lateralis control muscle; see Fig. 1 for additional abbreviations

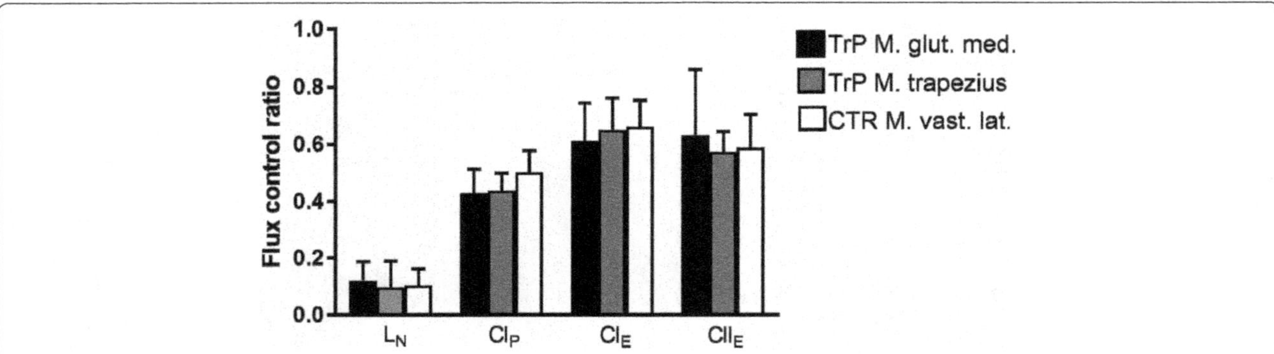

Fig. 3 Respiratory states normalized for the internal reference state of electron transfer capacity (ETC). Normalizing respiration for ETC of CI and CII (CI + II_E) results in flux control ratios, which reflect important mitochondrial qualitative alterations in mitochondrial function. The leak state without adenylates (L_N), complex I-supported oxidative phosphorylation capacity (CI_P), complex I-supported ETC (CI_E), and ETC of CII (CII_E) are displayed, and all states are normalized to maximal ETC of CI and CII (CI + II_E). Abbreviations: TrP M. glut. Med. = musculus gluteus medius trigger point; TrP M. trapezius = musculus trapezius trigger point; CTR M. vast. Lat. = musculus vastus lateralis control muscle; see Fig. 1 for additional abbreviations

current study, high-resolution respirometry provides evidence that the presence of an MTrP for up to 12 months does not influence mitochondrial function in the corresponding muscle. There were no qualitative differences in mitochondrial function among the MTrP samples and the control samples. Our results suggest that mitochondria do not have role in the development of MTrPs.

The presence of quantitative differences in respiratory capacity, enzymatic equipment, and fiber type distribution between different muscles of the human body is well established [38–40]. It has been shown that mitochondrial density in the arm is half of that in the leg in a cohort of healthy males [40]. It is therefore not surprising that, in the current study, quantitative differences exist with regard to mitochondrial function among the m. gluteus medius, the m. vastus lateralis, and the m. trapezius. In humans, the 2 former muscles are energetically challenged and extensively involved in locomotion, while the trapezius muscle has mainly postural functions with low level sustained muscle activity above resting level. [41]. Mass-specific mitochondrial respiration (expressed per mg of muscle tissue) was highest in m. gluteus medius, followed by m. trapezius and m. vastus lateralis (Fig. 2), whereas mitochondrial respiration normalized to maximal ETC of CI + CII was not different between the different muscles (Fig. 3). Normalization for maximal respiration yields lower and upper limits of 0.0 and 1.0 (0% and 100%). Internal normalization has the advantage of expressing respiratory control independent of mitochondrial content and will hence indicate any qualitative changes within the respiratory system. Our results suggest that changes in mass-specific mitochondrial respiration are mainly the result of changes in mitochondrial content as naturally present between different muscles of the human body.

Until now, it was not known if mitochondria also play a role in the development and manifestation of MTrPs. Our results indicate that qualitative skeletal muscle bioenergetics are not impaired in muscles affected by a trigger point. As our study only involved in vitro analysis,

Table 2 Biopsy yield, quality, safety, and acceptance of biopsy procedure for gluteus medius myofascial trigger point (GTP) and descending trapezius myofascial trigger point (TTP) samples and control (vastus lateralis) samples

	GTP ($n = 10$)	TTP ($n = 10$)	Vastus Lateralis ($n = 20$)
Mean biopsy yield (mg)	3.7 ± 1.6	3.4 ± 2.2	3.8 ± 2.1
Mean microscopic biopsy quality (1–5)[a]	4.9 ± 0.32	4.7 ± 0.48	4.7 ± 0.47
Clinical wound assessment (number of patients without signs for local infection and inflammation), n	10	10	20
Mean ultrasonic volume of hematoma (cm^3)	0	0	0
Surgical complications, n	0	0	0
Mean pain (NRS) at biopsy location after 7 days	0.25 ± 0.35	1.1 ± 2.3	0.2 ± 0.4
Procedure burden at biopsy location (1–4)[b]	3.2 ± 0.8	3.1 ± 0.99	3.1 ± 0.91

Values are mean ± SD
[a]Microscopic biopsy quality scale of 1–5: 1 = poor, 2 = fair, 3 = good, 4 = very good, and 5 = excellent
[b]Procedure burden scale of 1–4: 1 = very high, 2 = high, 3 = low, and 4 = none
NRS Numeric Rating Scale

we cannot exclude, however, possible in vivo impairments of mitochondrial function. Based on our results, we assume that alterations in mitochondrial function do not play a major role in the development of trigger points, at least up to 12 months after diagnosis.

It will be challenging to identify the point at which mitochondrial function is possibly impaired in the affected muscle. However, this is clinically important, as interventions at the point where impaired mitochondrial function is still reversible will prevent disease progression to a level where mitochondrial function is irreversibly damaged. It therefore remains highly relevant to study mitochondrial function and its relation to trigger point development and progression.

Although not intended as therapeutic intervention, the diagnostic biopsy procedure resolved the reported pain intensity in almost all patients. This response is similar to dry needling interventions for myofascial trigger points [6]. There is a significant bias in the assessment of pain levels at baseline and 1 week after the biopsy procedure in our study. Pain intensity was assessed pre biopsy by palpation and pressure applied to the trigger point. One week post biopsy, only spontaneous reported pain intensity was documented. The authors wanted to reduce patient discomfort and possible surgical wound-related complications. By choosing a later time point in future studies, this bias can be eliminated. In the current study, pain reduction was not an intended outcome measure, therefor pain assessment was not identical at both time points. This pilot study, being exploratory in nature, was limited by its sample size comprising a homogeneous, younger, male population. MTrPs are more prevalent in women and elderly individuals [2, 12], and impaired mitochondrial function is also more prevalent in older populations [42–45]. A large-scale clinical trial including women and older adults is necessary to confirm our findings.

A further limitation of our study is the lack of a clear presentation of clinical data. One inclusion criteria was the documentation of duration of trigger point-related pain complaint. Patients were included into the study if pain existed more than one and less than twelve months, without documenting the exact duration.

This study did assess pain related to the biopsy procedure, but these data were not collected during/immediately after the procedure. Therefore, the findings related to the acceptability of the procedure are limited in terms of pain.

Conclusions

This pilot study used a minimally invasive and safe technique for obtaining biopsies from MTrPs suitable for high-resolution respirometry analysis of mitochondrial function in MTrPs. The results suggest that there are no qualitative differences with regard to mitochondrial function in biopsies of MTrPs of the m. trapezius and m. gluteus medius muscles compared to control biopsies of the vastus lateralis muscle, therefore implying that alterations of mitochondrial function do not appear to have a role in the development of MTrPs, at least up to 12 months after diagnosis.

Abbreviations

31P-MRS: Phosphorus-31 magnetic resonance spectroscopy; ATP: adenosine triphosphate; BIOPS: biopsy preservation solution; BMI: Body-Mass Index; CI + II_E: maximal ETC of CI and CII; CI: Complex I; CII: Complex II; CII_E: ETC of CII; CI_P: Complex I-supported oxidative phosphorylation capacity; ETC: electron transfer capacity; FCR: flux control ratio; GTP: gluteus medius myofascial trigger point; IL: interleukin; L_N: leak state without adenylates; m.: musculus; mtDNA: mitochondrial DNA, the mitochondrial genome; MTrP: myofascial trigger point; NRS: Numeric Rating Scale; OXPHOS: oxidative phosphorylation; PCr: phosphocreatine; PI: principal investigator; ROS: reactive oxygen species; TTP: descending trapezius myofascial trigger point

Acknowledgments

The authors would like to thank Kristen Eckert and Dr. Marissa Carter of Strategic Solutions, Inc. (Cody, WY, USA) for their assistance in writing and editing this manuscript.

Funding

MJF received a personal grant from the German Society for Manual Medicine (DGMM) and from the Poullain Foundation for the position of a senior postdoc for 2 years. This work was supported by the Austrian Science Fund (FWF), project no. J3267. The funding body did not have a role in the design of the study, collection, analysis, and interpretation of data; and in writing the manuscript.

Authors' contributions

MJF: managed the entire project, designed the study, analyzed and interpreted data, and provided major contributions to writing the manuscript, tables and figures; GH: performed high-resolution respirometry and managed the respirometry data; MK: analyzed and interpreted data and revised the manuscript; EG: helped design the study, analyzed and interpreted data and supervised high-resolution respirometry and revised the manuscript; GG: wrote the statistical analysis plan and supervised statistical analysis; DP: helped design the study, analyzed and interpreted data, and provided major contributions to writing the manuscript. All authors read and approved the final manuscript.

Consent for publication

Not applicable.

Competing interests

The authors declare that there are no competing interests.

Author details

[1]Vamed Rehabilitation Center Kitzbuehel, Kitzbuehel, Austria. [2]Department of Rehabilitation Medicine, Hanover Medical School, Hanover, Germany. [3]Department of Orthopedics, Medical University Innsbruck, Innsbruck, Austria. [4]Department of Medical Biochemistry, Semmelweis University, Budapest, Hungary. [5]D. Swarovski Research Laboratory, Department of Visceral, Transplant and Thoracic Surgery, Medical University Innsbruck, Innsbruck, Austria. [6]Department of Medical Statistics, Informatics and Health Economics, Medical University Innsbruck, Innsbruck, Austria. [7]Institute for Clinical Diabetology, German Diabetes Center, Leibniz Institute for Diabetes Research, Heinrich-Heine-University, Düsseldorf, Germany. [8]German Center for Diabetes Research (DZD), München-Neuherberg, Germany. [9]Department of Sport Science, University of Innsbruck, Innsbruck, Austria.

References

1. Simons D, Travell J, Simons L. Travell, Simons & Simons' myofascial pain and dysfunction: the trigger point manual. 3rd ed. Baltimore: Williams & Wilkins; 2019.
2. Jafri MS. Mechanisms of myofascial pain. Int Sch Res Notices. 2014;2014.
3. Simons DG. Clinical and etiological update of myofascial pain from trigger points. J Musculoskelet Pain. 1996;4(1–2):93–121.
4. Bevan S, Quadrello T, McGee R, Madhon M, Vavrosky A, Barham L. Fit for work? Musculoskeletal disorders in the European workforce. London: The Work Foundation; 2009.
5. Bron C, Dommerholt JD. Etiology of myofascial trigger points. Curr Pain Headache Rep. 2012;16(5):439–44.
6. Shah JP, Thaker N, Heimur J, Aredo JV, Sikdar S, Gerber L. Myofascial trigger points then and now: a historical and scientific perspective. PM R. 2015;7(7):746–61.
7. Alijevic O, Kellenberger S. Subtype-specific modulation of acid-sensing ion channel (ASIC) function by 2-guanidine-4-methylquinazoline. J Biol Chem. 2012;287(43):36059–70.
8. Zuil-Escobar JC, Martínez-Cepa CB, Martín-Urrialde JA, Gómez-Conesa A. Prevalence of myofascial trigger points and diagnostic criteria of different muscles in function of the medial longitudinal arch. Arch Phys Med Rehabil. 2015;96(6):1123–30.
9. Chiarotto A, Clijsen R, Fernández-de-las-Peñas C, Barbero M. The prevalence of myofascial trigger points in spinal disorders: a systematic review and meta-analysis. Arch Phys Med Rehabil. 2016;97(2):316–37.
10. Fernández-de-las Peñas C, Dommertholt J. Myofascial trigger points: A peripheral or central phenomenon? Current Rheum Rep. 2014;16(1):395.
11. Grieve R, Barnett S, Coghill N, Cramp F. The prevalence of latent myofascial trigger points and diagnostic criteria of the triceps surae and upper trapezius: a cross sectional study. Physiotherapy. 2013;99(4):278–84.
12. Pal US, Kumar L, Mehta G, Singh N, Singh G, Singh M, et al. Trends in management of myofacial pain. Natl J Maxillofac Surg. 2014;5(2):109–16.
13. Gerwin R. The taut band and other mysteries of the trigger point: an examination of the mechanisms relevant to the development and maintenance of the trigger point. J Musculoskelet Pain. 2008;16(1–2):115–21.
14. Shah JP, Gilliams EA. Uncovering the biochemical milieu of myofascial trigger points using in vivo microdialysis: an application of muscle pain concepts to myofascial pain syndrome. J Bodyw Mov Ther. 2008; 12(4):371–84.
15. Fischer MJ, Strasser E, Scheibe RJ. Going in deeper and deeper: signal transduction pathways in myofascial trigger points: a narrative review. Int Musculoskelet Med. 2011;33(2):64–74.
16. Hagberg H. Intracellular pH during ischemia in skeletal muscle: relationship to membrane potential, extracellular pH, tissue lactic acid and ATP. Pflugers Arch. 1985;404(4):342–7.
17. Gerdle B, Ghafouri B, Ernberg M, Larsson B. Chronic musculoskeletal pain: review of mechanisms and biochemical biomarkers as assessed by the microdialysis technique. J Pain Res. 2014;7:313–26.
18. Larsson B, Björk J, Henriksson KG, Gerdle B, Lindman R. The prevalences of cytochrome c oxidase negative and superpositive fibres and ragged-red fibres in the trapezius muscle of female cleaners with and without myalgia and of female healthy controls. Pain. 2000;84(2–3):379–87.
19. Weibel ER, Hoppeler H. Exercise-induced maximal metabolic rate scales with muscle aerobic capacity. J Exp Biol. 2005;208(Pt 9):1635–44.
20. Bengtsson A. The muscle in fibromyalgia. Rheumatology (Oxford). 2002; 41(7):721–4.
21. Larsson B, Björk J, Kadi F, Lindman R, Gerdle B. Blood supply and oxidative metabolism in muscle biopsies of female cleaners with and without myalgia. Clin J Pain. 2004;20(6):440–6.
22. Bengtsson A, Henriksson KG, Larsson J. Muscle biopsy in primary fibromyalgia. Light-microscopical and histochemical findings. Scand J Rheumatol. 1986;15(1):1–6.
23. Brandão ML, Roselino JE, Piccinato CE, Cherri J. Mitochondrial alterations in skeletal muscle submitted to total ischemia. J Surg Res. 2003;110(1):235–40.
24. Gnaiger E. Capacity of oxidative phosphorylation in human skeletal muscle: new perspectives of mitochondrial physiology. Int J Biochem Cell Biol. 2009; 41(10):1837–45.
25. Zoll J, Sanchez H, N'Guessan B, Ribera F, Lampert E, Bigard X, et al. Physical activity changes the regulation of mitochondrial respiration in human skeletal muscle. J Physiol. 2002;543(Pt 1):191–200.
26. Mogensen M, Bagger M, Pedersen PK, Fernström M, Sahlin K. Cycling efficiency in humans is related to low UCP3 content and to type I fibres but not to mitochondrial efficiency. J Physiol. 2006;571(Pt 3):669–81.
27. Mettauer B, Zoll J, Sanchez H, Lampert E, Ribera F, Veksler V, et al. Oxidative capacity of skeletal muscle in heart failure patients versus sedentary or active control subjects. J Am Coll Cardiol. 2001;38(4):947–54.
28. Rasmussen UF, Rasmussen HN. Human quadriceps muscle mitochondria: a functional characterization. Mol Cell Biochem. 2000;208(1–2):37–44.
29. Rasmussen UF, Krustrup P, Bangsbo J, Rasmussen HN. The effect of high-intensity exhaustive exercise studied in isolated mitochondria from human skeletal muscle. Pflugers Arch. 2001;443(2):180–7.
30. Rasmussen UF, Rasmussen HN, Krustrup P, Quistorff B, Saltin B, Bangsbo J. Aerobic metabolism of human quadriceps muscle: in vivo data parallel measurements on isolated mitochondria. Am J Physiol Endocrinol Metab. 2001;280(2):E301–7.
31. Bakkman L, Sahlin K, Holmberg HC, Tonkonogi M. Quantitative and qualitative adaptation of human skeletal muscle mitochondria to hypoxic compared with normoxic training at the same relative work rate. Acta Physiol (Oxf). 2007;190(3):243–51.
32. Walsh B, Tonkonogi M, Sahlin K. Effect of endurance training on oxidative and antioxidative function in human permeabilized muscle fibres. Pflugers Arch. 2001;442(3):420–5.
33. Anderson EJ, Lustig ME, Boyle KE, Woodlief TL, Kane DA, Lin CT, et al. Mitochondrial H_2O_2 emission and cellular redox state link excess fat intake to insulin resistance in both rodents and humans. J Clin Invest. 2009;119(3):573–81.
34. Phielix E, Schrauwen-Hinderling VB, Mensink M, Lenaers E, Meex R, Hoeks J, et al. Lower intrinsic ADP-stimulated mitochondrial respiration underlies in vivo mitochondrial dysfunction in muscle of male type 2 diabetic patients. Diabetes. 2008;57(11):2943–9.
35. Pesta D, Hoppel F, Macek C, Messner H, Faulhaber M, Kobel C, et al. Similar qualitative and quantitative changes of mitochondrial respiration following strengths and endurance training in normoxia and hypoxia in sedentary humans. Am J Physiol Regul Integr Comp Physiol. 2011;301(4):R1078–87.
36. Bergstrom J. (1975) Percutaneous needle biopsy of skeletal muscle in physiological and clinical research. Scand J Clin Lab Invest. 1975;35(7):609–16.
37. Pesta D, Gnaiger E. High-resolution respirometry: OXPHOS protocols for human cells and permeabilized fibers from small biopsies of human muscle. Methods Mol Biol. 2012;810:25–58.
38. Edgerton VR, Smith JL, Simpson DR. Muscle fibre type populations of human leg muscles. Histochem J. 1975;7(3):259–66.
39. Jacobs RA, Díaz V, Meinild AK, Gassmann M, Lundby C. The C57Bl/6 mouse serves as a suitable model of human skeletal muscle mitochondrial function. Exp Physiol. 2013;98(4):908–21.
40. Gnaiger E, Boushel R, Søndergaard H, Munch-Andersen T, Damsgaard R, Hagen C, et al. Mitochondrial coupling and capacity of oxidative phosphorylation in skeletal muscle of Inuit and Caucasians in the arctic winter. Scand J Med Sci Sports. 2015;25(Suppl 4):126–34.
41. Wall-Scheffler CM, Chumanov E, Steudel-Numbers K, Heiderscheit B. Electromyography activity across gait and incline: The impact of muscular activity on human morphology. Am J Phys Anthropol. 2010;143(4):601–11.
42. Seo DY, Lee SR, Kim N, Ko KS, Rhee BD, Han J. Age-related changes in skeletal muscle mitochondria: the role of exercise. Integr Med Res. 2016;5(3):182–6.

11

Reattachment of the flexor and extensor tendons at the epicondyle in elbow instability: a biomechanical comparison of techniques

Andreas Lenich[2†], Christian Pfeifer[4†], Philipp Proier[1], Roman Fleer[1], Coen Wijdicks[5], Martina Roth[5], Frank Martetschläger[3] and Jonas Pogorzelski[1*]

Abstract

Background: Elbow dislocation represents a common injury, especially in the younger population. If treated surgically, the reattached tendons require a high amount of primary stability to allow for an early rehabilitation to avoid postoperative stiffness. The purpose of this study was to assess the biomechanical properties of a single and a double row technique for reattachment of the common extensor and common flexor muscles origin. We hypothesized that the double row technique would provide greater stability in terms of pullout forces than the single row technique.

Methods: Twelve cadaveric specimens were randomized into two groups of fixation methods for the common extensor tendon or the common flexor tendon at the elbow (1): a single row technique using two knotted 3.0 mm suture anchors, and (2) a double row technique using an additional knotless 3.5 mm anchor. The repairs were cyclically loaded over 500 cycles at 1 Hz from 10 N to a maximum of 100 N (extensors) or 150 N (flexors), and then pulled to failure. Stiffness and maximum load at failure and mode of failure were recorded and calculated.

Results: No significant differences in stiffness were observed between the two techniques for both the extensor and flexor reattachment ($P = 0.701$ and $P = 0.306$, respectively). The mean maximum load at failure indicated that the double row construct was significantly stronger than the single row construct. This was found to be true for both the extensor and flexor reattachment (213.6; SD 78.7 N versus 384.1; SD 105.6 N, $P = 0.010$ and 203.7; SD 65.8 N versus 318.0; SD 64.6 N, $P = 0.013$, respectively).

Conclusions: The double row technique provides significant greater stability to the reattached common flexor or extensor origin to the medial or lateral epicondyle. Thus, it should be considered in the development of improved repair techniques for stabilizers of the elbow.

Study design: Controlled laboratory study.

Keywords: Elbow, Dislocation, Reattachment, Common extensor muscle origin, Common flexor muscle origin

* Correspondence: jonas.pogorzelski@tum.de
[†]Andreas Lenich and Christian Pfeifer contributed equally to this work.
[1]Department of Orthopedic Sports Medicine, Technical University of Munich, Klinikum rechts der Isar, Ismaninger Str. 22, 81675 Munich, Germany
Full list of author information is available at the end of the article

Background

The elbow is the most commonly dislocated joint in children and the second most dislocated joint in adults with an estimated incidence of elbow dislocations in the general United States population of about 5.21 per 100,000 person-years [1, 2]. The stabilizing structures of the elbow joint are typically classified as primary, secondary, and dynamic stabilizers [3, 4]. More precisely, primary stabilizers include the bony ulno-humeral articulation, the lateral collateral ligament (LCL) complex as well as the medial collateral ligament (MCL) complex. Secondary stabilizers include the radial head, the anterior and posterior joint capsule, and the common flexor and extensor muscle origins. Finally, the biceps muscle, the brachialis muscle, the anconeus muscle, and the triceps muscle are classified as dynamic stabilizers [3, 4].

While simple elbow dislocations – defined as acute dislocations without concomitant significant fractures - may be accessible through non-operative treatment, complex dislocations involving fractures of the radial head or neck, olecranon, coronoid, humeral condyles or epicondyles typically require surgical intervention [5, 6]. Even though the majority of dislocations can be considered "simple", "complex" cases still occur in up to 20% of patients suffering from a traumatic elbow dislocation [7]. As the postoperative results have been historically hampered by frequent stiffness with or without recurrent instability, discussions have been raised, whether to augment to the reduction with some type of external fixation or whether the length of postoperative immobilization should be prolonged [8, 9]. However, there is actual consensus in the literature that early rehabilitation following simple elbow dislocation is the best way to prevent range of motion deficits [10]. Whether an early postoperative rehabilitation is safe for the reconstructed certainly depends on the stability of the refixated structures.

Therefore, the objective of this study was to assess the biomechanical properties of a single and a double row technique for re-fixation of the common extensor muscles and common flexor muscles origin. We hypothesized that the double row technique would provide greater stability in terms of pullout strengths than the single row technique.

Methods

Specimen preparation

As a cadaveric study, our institution does not require Institutional Review Board (IRB) approval. The study was performed using 12 fresh-frozen, human cadaveric humeri of male donors only, which were donated to our research laboratory. Radial head compression tests were performed to exclude specimens with osteoporosis. More precisely, as mechanical stability of the radial head is known to correlate with bone quality, static axial compression load was applied on the cartilage surface until breakage with a speed of 10 mm/min and subsequently a load-over-displacement analysis performed [11, 12]. To ensure equal bone quality before testing, all specimen with significant deviations in the mean load-over-displacement curve were discarded. All specimens were less than 65 years of age (mean, 55.6 years; standard deviation (SD) 12.0 years), with no history of elbow injury, surgery, or anatomic abnormality and randomized into one of the two groups. Specimens were stored at – 20 °C and thawed at room temperature for 24 h before preparation. The humerus was disarticulated from the ulna and radial bone, and all soft tissue (including the collateral ligaments) except the common flexor origin (consisting of the flexor carpi radialis muscle, the flexor carpi ulnaris muscle, the palmaris longus muscle and the flexor digitorum superficialis muscle) and common extensor origin (consisting of the extensor carpi ulnaris muscle, the extensor carpi radialis brevis muscle, the extensor digitorum muscle, and the extensor digiti minimi muscle) was removed. The humerus was then potted in plaster (Moldasynth, Heraeus Kulzer GmbH, Hanau, Germany) to preserve the position during testing. Care was taken to keep an exact distance of 5 cm from the plaster to the most distal point of the humerus for each specimen (Fig. 1).

Surgical technique

Two orthopaedic surgeons (Philipp Proier and Andreas Lenich) performed all re-fixations of the extensors and flexors. Two different techniques were used to test fixation strength using a single row or double row technique. Prior to the placing of the anchors, the common flexors and extensors including the cortical bone of its origins were removed.

The single row construct (Fig. 2) consisted of one single- and one double-loaded 3.0 mm suture anchor (SutureTak, Arthrex, Inc., Naples, FL) with 2–0 fiber wires to secure the common tendons origin to the medial or lateral humeral bone. With the use of a suitable drill, two holes were positioned like follows: The double-loaded anchor was routinely placed 1 cm proximal to the cartilage-bone-border in the extended axis of the humeral shaft with the same distance to the anterior and posterior joint surface. The single-loaded anchor was subsequently placed 1 cm proximal to the first anchor in the same axis. The six suture limbs of both the double-loaded and single-loaded anchor were shuttled through the common tendon in a mattress technique leaving an approximately 1 cm gap from the tendons margin. Finally, each pair of suture limbs was tied down using seven alternating half hitches and the sutures were cut.

The double row construct (Fig. 1) was similar to the single row construct with the only difference that all six

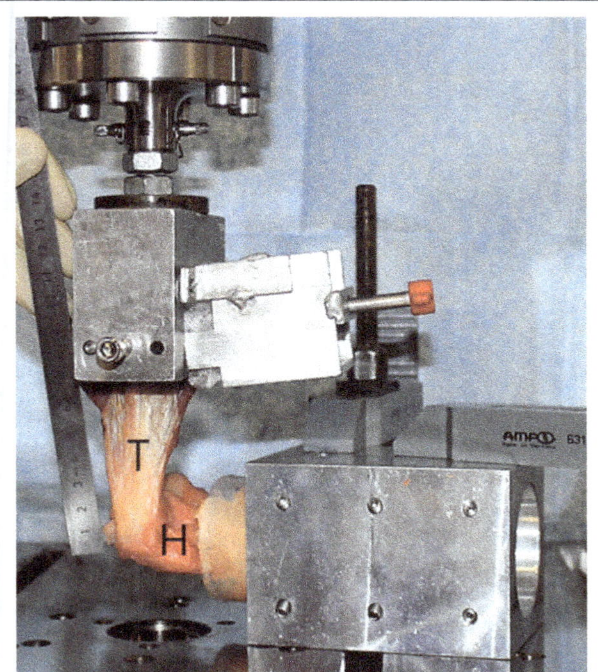

Fig. 1 Before testing, care was taken to ensure that the common tendon was aligned vertically to the humeral shaft axis. The distance from tendon insertion to the clamped and frozen muscles was routinely chosen to be 7 cm, while the distance between the most distal part of the humerus and the potted plaster was routinely about 5 cm (T = tendons, H = humerus)

suture limbs of both previously positioned 3.0 mm suture anchors were loaded into the eyelet of a 3.5 mm knotless suture anchor (SwiveLock, Arthrex, Inc., Naples, FL) after tying the knots. Subsequently, a bone socket was created with a punch 1 cm posterior and 0.5 cm proximal to the most proximal anchor of the single row anchors. The eyelet of the anchor was brought to the edge of the socket and the limbs of sutures were individually tensioned. The eyelet was then advanced into the socket until the anchor body contacted the bone, effectively tensioning the suture limbs. Once the anatomy of the common extensor or flexor footprint was restored, the body of the anchor was advanced clockwise into the bone socket to secure the sutures.

Biomechanical testing

Each construct was biomechanically assed using a dynamic tensile testing machine (Instron ElectroPuls E10000, Instron Systems, Norwood, MA). Before clamping the muscles in a custom fixture approximately 7 cm from the common tendons margin (Fig. 2), the clamps were treated with dry ice to prevent muscle slippage within the fixture during testing. The embedded humerus was securely fixed to the stationary base of the tensile testing machine. After preloading the muscles to 10 N (extensors) or 15 N (flexors), care was taken to ensure that the common tendon was aligned vertically (Fig. 2). The preload of the muscles was defined to be 10% of the natural load of the common extensors or flexors which has been described to be about 100 N for the extensors and 150 N

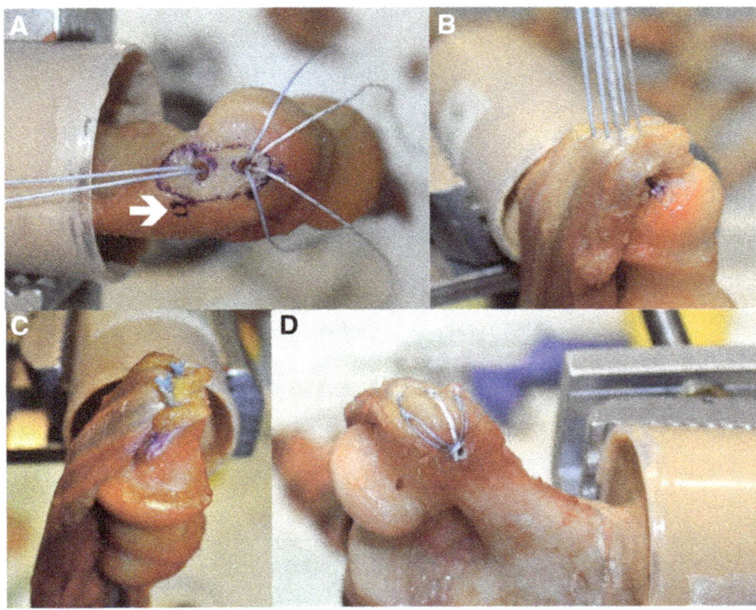

Fig. 2 Surgical technique: **a** One single- and one double-loaded suture anchor were placed for the single-row technique in the extended axis of the humeral shaft. If needed, a third anchor was placed posteriorly for the double-row construct (white arrow). **b** All suture limbs of the single-row anchors were shuttled through the tendon in a mattress configuration. **c** Final single-row construct. **d** Final double-row construct

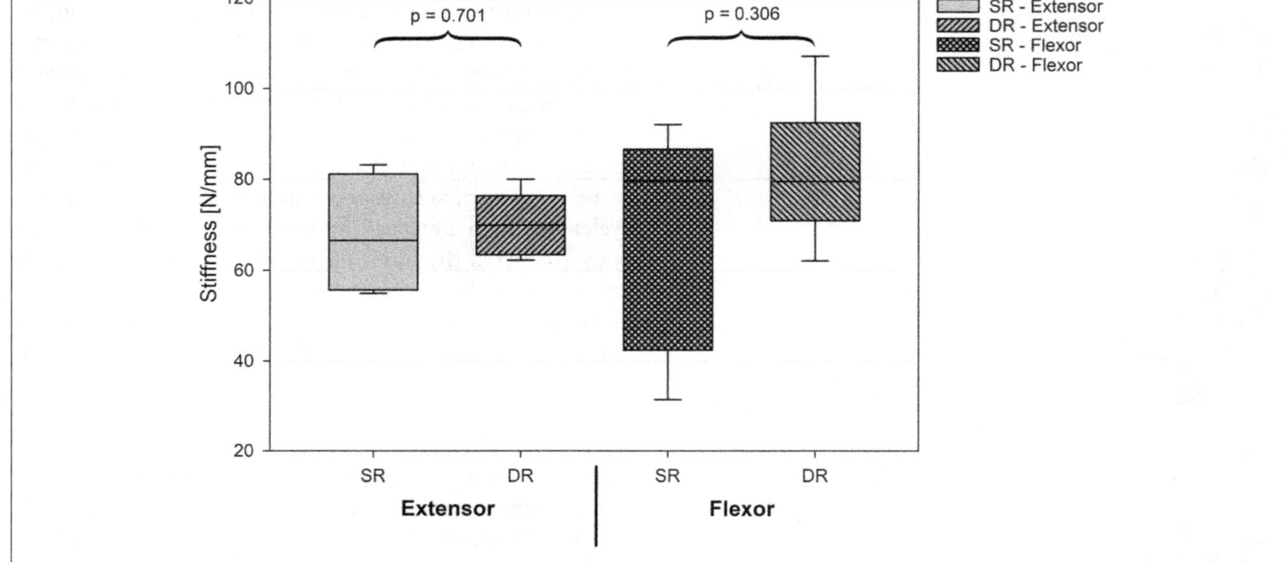

Fig. 3 No significant differences in stiffness could be detected between techniques and location of fixation. SR = single row technique. DR = double row technique

for the flexors [13]. Each construct was cyclically loaded at 1 Hz in 10 steps for five minutes each. The baseline load was 15 N for the extensors and 10 N for the flexors with a stepwise 15 N (extensors) or 10 N (flexors) increase after each step. If the construct was still intact after the 10 steps of cyclic loading, it was pulled to failure at 60 mm/min. Failure was defined as suture breakage or any perceived movement of the implanted anchors. Failure mode was observed and defined in each case by two reviewers. Stiffness as well as maximum load during the pull to failure and mode of failure were recorded and calculated. Stiffness of the repair was calculated as the slope of the load-versus-displacement curve at pull-to-failure (PTF) or the final cycle of cyclic loading if PTF was not reached.

Statistical analysis

An a priori power calculation was conducted and the usage of six specimens per group was found to be sufficient to detect an effect size of d = 1.2 with 80%

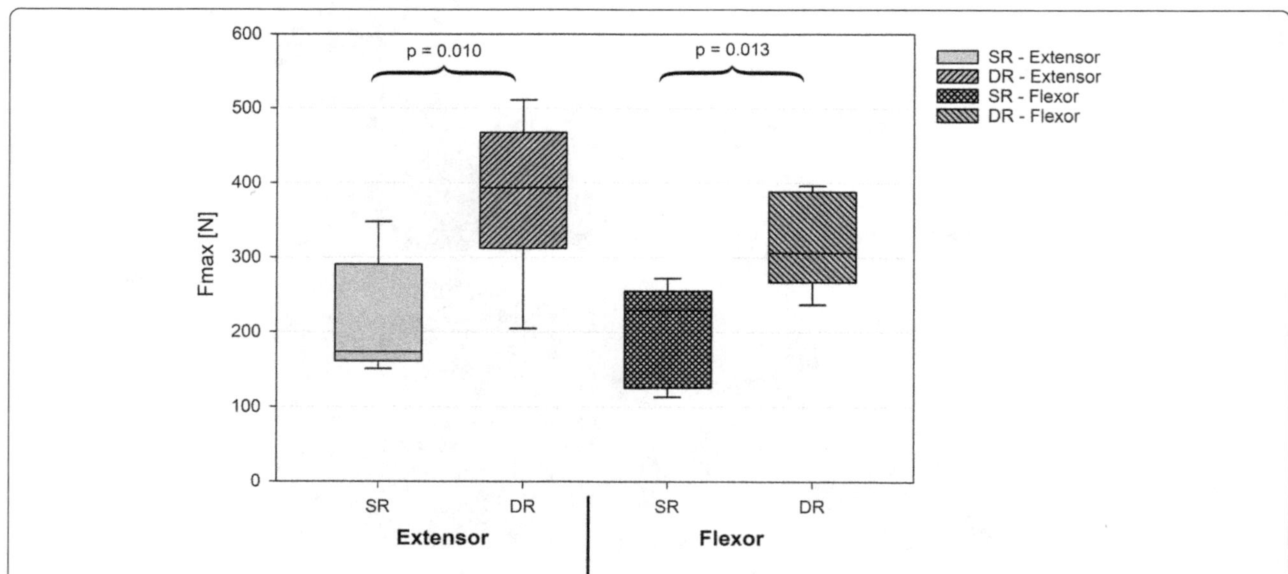

Fig. 4 The mean load to failure was significantly higher for the DR technique compared to the SR technique for both extensor and flexor refixation. SR = single row technique. DR = double row technique. Fmax = maximum force

Table 1 Overview of the results for testing the SR technique for re-fixation of the common extensor origin

Single Row Technique Extensor	Cycles to Failure	Stiffness of the repair (N/mm)	Maximum load (N)	Pull-to-failure	Failure Mode
Specimen 1	PTF	55.9	171.1	Yes	suture cut out through tendon
Specimen 2	PTF	54.9	150.8	Yes	suture cut out through tendon
Specimen 3	PTF	68.0	175.5	Yes	suture cut out through anchor
Specimen 4	PTF	80.5	348.0	Yes	suture cut out through anchor
Specimen 5	PTF	83.2	164.6	Yes	suture cut out through tendon
Specimen 6	PTF	65.2	271.4	Yes	suture cut out through tendon
Average ± SD		67.9 ± 11.9	213.6 ± 78.7		

Stiffness, maximum load pull-to-failure, and failure mode are presented for each specimen individually. PTF, pull-to-failure; Y = yes, N = Newton, mm = millimeter

statistical power. All continuous variables were not observed to be skewed or over dispersed, so parametric testing methods were used. Thus, t-test models were built to compare the two groups. All statistical analyses and graphics were produced using the statistical program SigmaPlot, version 13.0 (Systat, San Jose, CA).

Results

No significant differences in stiffness were observed between the two techniques for both the extensor and flexor refixation ($P = 0.701$ and $P = 0.306$, respectively; Fig. 3). The mean maximum load at failure indicated that the DR construct was significantly stronger than the SR construct. This was found to be true for both the extensor and flexor re-fixation (213.6; SD 78.7 N versus 384.1; SD 105.6 N, $P = 0.01$ and 203.7; SD 65.8 N versus 318.0; SD 64.6 N, $P = 0.013$, respectively; Fig. 4). Two constructs of the SR technique failed before reaching the pull-to-failure testing during cyclic loading while testing the pullout strength of the common flexor refixation (Table 3). None of the DR specimens failed during this phase.

The most commonly observed failure mode for both the SR and DR construct was suture cut out through the tendon. More detailed information of the results of the testing of each technique is given in Tables 1, 2, 3 and 4.

Discussion

The most important findings of the study were that stiffness was not significantly different between the two tested techniques and that the double row technique was significantly superior to the single row technique concerning maximum load to failure. These findings confirm our hypothesis and support the use of a double row technique for re-fixation of the common flexor or extensor origin to the medial or lateral epicondyle following acute elbow dislocation.

The use of suture anchors for re-fixation of primary or secondary stabilizers of the elbow is a common and proven technique in daily clinical practice [14, 15]. Although there exists a paucity of literature concerning controlled laboratory studies evaluating different types of fixation techniques for tendon-to-bone repairs of the elbow, multiple studies already assessed the biomechanical strengths of rotator cuff repairs. Assuming the results of the shoulder to be transferable to the elbow, the ideal repair construct has to provide sufficient contact pressures at the bone-tendon-interface over the greatest possible contact area [16]. As a result, the double row repair technique has been recently evolved [16, 17]. Moreover, to avoid a functional tenodesis of the repaired tendon and thus a compromised blood supply hampering the healing, knotless and self-reinforcing repair techniques have been developed [18, 19].

Table 2 Overview of the results for testing the DR technique for re-fixation of the common extensor origin

Double Row Technique Extensor	Cycles to Failure	Stiffness of the repair (N/mm)	Maximum load (N)	Pull-to-failure	Failure Mode
Specimen 1	PTF	73.3	511.2	Yes	anchor breakage
Specimen 2	PTF	62.2	348.2	Yes	suture cut out through tendon
Specimen 3	PTF	66.6	415.9	Yes	anchor breakage
Specimen 4	PTF	75.1	371.1	Yes	anchor cut out
Specimen 5	PTF	63.9	204.5	Yes	suture cut out through tendon
Specimen 6	PTF	80.0	453.8	Yes	suture cut out through tendon
Average ± SD		70.2 ± 7.0	384.1 ± 105.6		

Stiffness, maximum load pull-to-failure, and failure mode are presented for each specimen individually. PTF, pull-to-failure; Y = yes, N = Newton, mm = millimeter

Table 3 Overview of the results for testing the SR technique for re-fixation of the common flexor origin

Single Row Technique Flexor	Cycles to Failure	Stiffness of the repair (N/mm)	Maximum load (N)	Pull-to-failure	Failure Mode
Specimen 1	352	31.4	113.3	No	suture cut out through tendon
Specimen 2	PTF	84.8	248.8	Yes	suture cut out through tendon
Specimen 3	402	46.0	129.6	No	suture cut out through tendon
Specimen 4	PTF	92.0	232.6	Yes	suture cut out through tendon
Specimen 5	PTF	80.5	225.7	Yes	suture cut out through tendon
Specimen 6	PTF	78.7	272.0	Yes	suture cut out through tendon
Average ± SD		68.9 ± 9.9	203.7 ± 65.8		

Stiffness, maximum load pull-to-failure, and failure mode are presented for each specimen individually. PTF, pull-to-failure; Y = yes, N = Newton, mm = millimeter

The results of our controlled laboratory study support the assumption that the aforementioned findings from rotator cuff studies are valid for the elbow, too. We found the double row repair technique to be significantly stronger than the single row technique for both the common extensor and flexor origin repair. Even though reasons for this finding have not been assessed, several arguments can explain these findings. First of all, the use of an additional suture anchor has probably added further stability to the repair. Furthermore, the resultant double row construct allowed for a better distribution of the loading forces and thus were probably able to withstand significantly higher loads compared to the single row repair technique before failing [17]. Finally, a further known advantage of knotless fixation and thus a potential contributing factor to increased fixation strengths is the consistency in the fixation strengths, as previous studies have demonstrated that hand-tied knots have a high variability of strength [20, 21]. Of note, the vast majority of our constructs failed at the suture-tendon-interface with the sutures cutting out of the tendon. This mode of failure is typical for tendon-to-bone repairs and generally considered to be the weak spot of the repair [22].

Taking all of our findings into account, we believe that the double row construct is not only biomechanically but might also potentially be clinically superior to the single row construct as it allows for a reliable and early rehabilitation postoperatively. However, future comparative clinical studies have to confirm our assumption. Moreover, there exist some disadvantages of the double row repair technique in daily practice, which need to be mentioned as well. First of all, the extent of injury in case of a complex and acute elbow dislocation is most likely not limited to the flexor muscles and/or extensor muscles but also includes the primary stabilizers such as the collateral ligaments. As those might need to be re-fixated with suture anchors, too, the total amount of suture anchors used for the repair should be limited to avoid iatrogenic deterioration of the bone. Apart from that, the correct intraoperative positioning of the suture anchors gets more challenging with an increasing number of anchors used. Finally, the additional suture anchor adds surgery time and costs to the repair.

Overall, this biomechanical study provides utility by removing many external variables that may impact results, making a direct comparison of the two techniques more accurate. However, there are also inherent limitations to a cadaveric biomechanical study that cannot be controlled. The uniaxial forces applied to the common flexor or extensor tendon vertically from the humerus may not accurately reflect the dynamic loads experienced throughout a full range of motion of the elbow. More precisely, our setup did not take varus and valgus movements into account which play a substantial role in elbow dislocations. Moreover, without the contribution of healing, scarring, or muscle contractions, the measured fixation strength only simulates reconstruction immediately after surgery. Nonetheless, simulating the threshold of fixation strength

Table 4 Overview of the results for testing the DR technique for re-fixation of the common flexor origin

Double Row Technique Flexor	Cycles to Failure	Stiffness of the repair (N/mm)	Maximum load (N)	Pull-to-failure	Failure Mode
Specimen 1	PTF	84.7	276.9	Yes	suture cut out through tendon
Specimen 2	PTF	73.9	396.4	Yes	suture cut out through tendon
Specimen 3	PTF	107.0	385.7	Yes	suture cut out through tendon
Specimen 4	PTF	74.3	278.4	Yes	suture cut out through tendon
Specimen 5	PTF	62.0	236.6	Yes	suture cut out through tendon
Specimen 6	PTF	87.5	333.7	Yes	suture cut out through tendon
Average ± SD		81.5 ± 15.4	318.0 ± 64.6		

Stiffness, maximum load pull-to-failure, and failure mode are presented for each specimen individually. PTF, pull-to-failure; Y = yes, N = Newton, mm = millimeter immediately post-operatively may be useful information for developing appropriate rehabilitation protocols and may be useful for subsequent clinical studies.

Conclusion

The double row technique provides significant greater stability to the re-fixated common flexor or extensor origin to the medial or lateral epicondyle. Thus, it should be considered in the development of improved repair techniques for stabilizers of the elbow.

Abbreviations

IRB: Institutional Review Board; LCL: Lateral collateral ligament; MCL: Medial collateral ligament; N: Newton; PTF: Pull-to-failure; Y: Yes

Acknowledgements

The authors would like to thank Arthrex Inc. for providing the specimen and surgical supplies. Arthrex Inc. had no influence on the design of the study and collection, analysis, and interpretation of data and as well as writing the manuscript.

Funding

Not applicable.

Authors' contributions

AL: Study design, pilot testing, testing, data interpretation, writing the manuscript, editing the manuscript. CP: Study design, pilot testing, testing, editing the manuscript. PP: Study design, pilot testing, testing, editing the manuscript. RF: Pilot testing, testing, editing the manuscript. CW: Pilot testing, testing, data analysis, editing the manuscript. MR: Pilot testing, testing, data analysis, editing the manuscript. FM: Study design, data interpretation, editing the manuscript. JP: Study design, data interpretation, writing the manuscript, editing the manuscript. All authors read and approved the final manuscript.

Consent for publication

Not applicable. All specimen were provided by Arthrex Inc., Naples, Florida, USA.

Competing interests

CW and MR are employees of Arthrex Inc. AL and FM are consultants for Arthrex Inc. All other authors declare no competing interests.

Author details

[1]Department of Orthopedic Sports Medicine, Technical University of Munich, Klinikum rechts der Isar, Ismaninger Str. 22, 81675 Munich, Germany. [2]Helios Clinic Munich West, Department of Orthopedic Sports Medicine, Trauma Surgery and Hand Surgery, Steinerweg 5, 81241 Munich, Germany. [3]German Center for Shoulder Surgery, ATOS Clinic Munich, Effnerstraße 38, 81925 Munich, Germany. [4]Regensburg University Medical Center, Department of Trauma Surgery, Franz-Josef-Strauß-Allee 11, 93053 Regensburg, Germany. [5]Department of Research & Development, Arthrex GmbH, Munich, Germany.

References

1. Stoneback JW, Owens BD, Sykes J, Athwal GS, Pointer L, Wolf JM. Incidence of elbow dislocations in the United States population. J Bone Joint Surg Am. 2012;94(3):240–5.
2. Mehta JA, Bain GI. Elbow dislocations in adults and children. Clin Sports Med. 2004;23(4):609–27 ix.
3. O'Driscoll SW. Classification and evaluation of recurrent instability of the elbow. Clin Orthop Relat Res. 2000;370:34–43.
4. McGuire DT, Bain GI. Management of dislocations of the elbow in the athlete. Sports Med Arthrosc Rev. 2014;22(3):188–93.
5. Grazette AJ, Aquilina A. The assessment and Management of Simple Elbow Dislocations. Open Orthop J. 2017;11:1373–9.
6. Taylor F, Sims M, Theis JC, Herbison GP. Interventions for treating acute elbow dislocations in adults. Cochrane Database Syst Rev. 2012;4:CD007908.
7. Hildebrand KA, Patterson SD, King GJ. Acute elbow dislocations: simple and complex. Orthop Clin North Am. 1999;30(1):63–79.
8. Anderson DR, Haller JM, Anderson LA, Hailu S, Chala A, O'Driscoll SW. Surgical treatment of chronic elbow dislocation allowing for early range of motion: operative technique and clinical results. J Orthop Trauma. 2018; 32(4):196–203.
9. Jupiter JB, Ring D. Treatment of unreduced elbow dislocations with hinged external fixation. J Bone Joint Surg Am. 2002;84-A(9):1630–5.
10. Iordens GI, Van Lieshout EM, Schep NW, De Haan J, Tuinebreijer WE, Eygendaal D, et al. Early mobilisation versus plaster immobilisation of simple elbow dislocations: results of the FuncSiE multicentre randomised clinical trial. Br J Sports Med. 2017;51(6):531–8.
11. Bachman DR, Thaveepunsan S, Park S, Fitzsimmons JS, An KN, O'Driscoll SW. The effect of prosthetic radial head geometry on the distribution and magnitude of radiocapitellar joint contact pressures. J Hand Surg Am. 2015; 40(2):281–8.
12. Wake H, Hashizume H, Nishida K, Inoue H, Nagayama N. Biomechanical analysis of the mechanism of elbow fracture-dislocations by compression force. J Orthop Sci. 2004;9(1):44–50.
13. Brand PW, Beach RB, Thompson DE. Relative tension and potential excursion of muscles in the forearm and hand. J Hand Surg Am. 1981;6(3): 209–19.
14. O'Brien MJ, Lee Murphy R, Savoie FH 3rd. A preliminary report of acute and subacute arthroscopic repair of the radial ulnohumeral ligament after elbow dislocation in the high-demand patient. Arthroscopy. 2014;30(6):679–87.
15. Lee YC, Eng K, Keogh A, McLean JM, Bain GI. Repair of the acutely unstable elbow: use of tensionable anchors. Tech Hand Up Extrem Surg. 2012;16(4): 225–9.
16. Park MC, Cadet ER, Levine WN, Bigliani LU, Ahmad CS. Tendon-to-bone pressure distributions at a repaired rotator cuff footprint using transosseous suture and suture anchor fixation techniques. Am J Sports Med. 2005;33(8): 1154–9.
17. Kim DH, Elattrache NS, Tibone JE, Jun BJ, DeLaMora SN, Kvitne RS, et al. Biomechanical comparison of a single-row versus double-row suture anchor technique for rotator cuff repair. Am J Sports Med. 2006;34(3):407–14.
18. Park MC, Peterson AB, McGarry MH, Park CJ, Lee TQ. Knotless Transosseous-equivalent rotator cuff repair improves biomechanical self-reinforcement without diminishing footprint contact compared with medial knotted repair. Arthroscopy. 2017;33(8):1473–81.
19. Millett PJ, Hussain ZB, Fritz EM, Warth RJ, Katthagen JC, Pogorzelski J. Rotator cuff tears at the musculotendinous junction: classification and surgical options for repair and reconstruction. Arthrosc Tech. 2017;6(4): e1075–e85.
20. Hanypsiak BT, DeLong JM, Simmons L, Lowe W, Burkhart S. Knot strength varies widely among expert Arthroscopists. Am J Sports Med. 2014;42(8): 1978–84.
21. Pogorzelski J, Muckenhirn KJ, Mitchell JJ, Katthagen JC, Schon JM, Dahl KD, et al. Biomechanical comparison of 3 glenoid-side fixation techniques for superior capsular reconstruction. Am J Sports Med. 2018;46(4):801–8.
22. Sileo MJ, Ruotolo CR, Nelson CO, Serra-Hsu F, Panchal AP. A biomechanical comparison of the modified Mason-Allen stitch and massive cuff stitch in vitro. Arthroscopy. 2007;23(3):235–40.

12

Infection-free rates and Sequelae predict factors in bone transportation for infected tibia

Zhen Zhang[1,2], W. Benton Swanson[2], Yan-Hong Wang[3], Wei Lin[4] and Guanglin Wang[1*]

Abstract

Background: Tibia infected nonunion and chronic osteomyelitis are challenging clinical presentations. Bone transportation with external or hybrid fixators (combined external and internal fixators) is versatile to solve these problems. However, the infection-free rates of these fixator systems are unknown. Additionally, the prognosis factors for results of bone transportation are obscure. Therefore, this systematic review and meta-analysis was conducted to answer these questions.

Methods: A systematic review was conducted following the PRISMA-IPD guidelines. Relevant publications from January 1995 to September 2018 were compiled from Medline, Embase, and Cochrane. The infection-free rates of external and hybrid fixators were achieved by synthesizing aggregate data and individual participant data (IPD). IPD was analyzed by two-stage method with logistical regression to identify prognosis factors of sequelae.

Results: Twenty-two studies with 518 patients were identified, including 11 studies with 167 patients' IPD, and 11 studies with 351 patients' aggregate data. The infection-free rate of hybrid fixator group was 86% (95%CI: 79–94%), lower than that of external fixator which was 97% (95%CI: 95–98%,). The number of previous surgeries was found predict factor of bone union sequelae ($p = 0.04$) and function sequelae($p < 0.01$); The external fixation time was found predict factor of function sequelae ($p = 0.015$).

Conclusions: Hybrid fixators may be associated with a greater risk of infection-recurrence in the treatment of tibia infected nonunion and chronic osteomyelitis. The number of previous surgeries and external fixation time can be used as predictors of outcomes. Proper fixators and meticulously designed surgery are important to avoid unexpected operations and shorten external fixation time.

Keywords: Bone transportation, Infection-free rate, Predict factor of Sequelae

Background

Tibial infected nonunion and chronic posttraumatic osteomyelitis are common clinical presentations which pose substantial burdens on both patients and society [1, 2]. However, their treatment remains a large challenge; most cases are associated with infection caused by antibiotic-resistant bacteria, bone and soft tissue loss, deformities, and limb-length discrepancy [3, 4]. Many patients suffer from multiple operations due to more than one stage of treatment and associated complications [5, 6], especially the reoccurring infection which may be refractory and lead to amputation [7–9]. To achieve an infection-free result, radical debridement is necessary, but massive skeletal defects also result as a consequence [9]. Bone transport, based on principles of distraction osteogenesis, could tackle segmental bone defects and coexisting problems of lone bone infection simultaneously. The procedure of bone transportation could be divided into distraction and consolidation phases: After corticectomy in metaphysis, the lost tissue is compensated by gradual distraction of healthy bone segment towards the defect site, and consequent consolidation follows when bone

* Correspondence: wangglfrank@hotmail.com
[1]Department of Orthopedics, West China Hospital, Sichuan University, No. 37, Guoxue Lane, Wuhou District, Chengdu 610041, Sichuan Province, China
Full list of author information is available at the end of the article

ends meet [10, 11].During the phases of distraction and consolidation in bone transportation technique, osseous stability is provided by various fixator systems [12].

However, factors related to fixator choice for infected tibia is still obscure [8, 13]. Among fixators, the most commonly used are external frames including circular and mono-lateral fixators. The external frames allow for early weight bearing and maintenance of tibia length during treatment. Nevertheless, external fixators suffer from complications associated with long-time external fixation, such as pin site infection and joint stiffness [14]. To shorten the external fixation time, several researchers have combined internal fixators with external frames for bone transportation during distraction and/or consolidation phases [13, 15–19]. This "hybrid fixator" system facilitates early removal of the external frame, helps maintain alignment, and prevents refracture [17, 20]. Despite its advantages, the hybrid fixators are suspected to be associated with a greater risk of infection recurrence which is worrisome for both clinicians and patients [8, 21]. During treatment procedure, infection recurrence leads to repetitive debridement, prolonged treatment time, and increased psychological stress on patients. Patients suffered from multiple reinfection may even refuse further revision, demanding amputation as the final solution [22]. Even though the infection-free result is important in this scenario, the infection-free rates of external and hybrid fixators are still unknown.

Additionally, Ilizarov methods are associated with high rates of temporary complication and residual sequela which are difficult to avoid. As an application of distraction osteogenesis, bone transport technique were also reported with sequelae in many studies [6, 23]. Residual sequelae, which remain unsolved at the end of the treatment period, are used as indicators for criteria to grade outcomes of both bone union and function [3, 24, 25]. Despite the high rate of satisfactory results (excellent and good) reported in most studies, the rate of sequela-free result (excellent), is varied. Since prognosis factors are seldom studied, it is difficult to determine those factors leading to a sequela-free result.

Thus, this systematic review was conducted to addresses the question in the treatment of tibial infected nonunion and chronic osteomyelitis.: 1) Do hybrid fixators have lower incidence of infection-free results compared to external fixators? 2) What are predictive factors of sequelae in bone transportation technique?

Methods

Strategy

The systematic review was conducted according to Preferred Reported Items for Systematic Reviews of Meta-Analyses Statement for Individual Patient Data (PRISMA-IPD) [26]. Databases including Medline, Embase, and Cochrane were searched from January 1995 until September 2018. Key words "bone transport technique," "Ilizarov," "infectious non-union," "osteomyelitis," "distraction osteogenesis," and "tibia" were combined in the search procedure. The reference lists of included studies were manually searched to avoid omissions.

Eligibility criteria

After excluding duplicates, two independent reviewers screened all remaining records based on both titles and abstracts, then screened the full text of the potentially relevant studies. Studies were considered acceptable for inclusion if the following criteria were fulfilled: (1) studies treated adult patients (more than 16 years of age) diagnosed of tibia infectious non-union or osteomyelitis; (2) studies with a minimum sample of 5 aforementioned consecutive patients were treated with multifocal bone transport technique; For IPD collection, each subgroup of fixator systems should contain no less than 5 patients. (3) main outcome of bone union and function were graded to excellent, good, fair or poor according to Paley or ASAMI classification, and recurrence of osteomyelitis or deep bone infection was recorded; (4) original articles written in English. In the cases of research on the same patient group published at the same institution, the most complete or recent data was used. Disagreements were solved by consulting a third reviewer.

Data collection

Specific information from selected papers was compiled. According to the details of Paley or ASAMI classification, the outcomes are graded by the number of sequelae: "excellent" is the outcome without sequelae, while the "good," "fair," and "poor" outcomes are associated with increasing numbers of sequelae. Herein we define those patients who received excellent results in a "sequelae free" group, while the good, fair, and poor are considered "sequelae." IPD were compiled for the following variables where available: demographic information (age, gender), number of previous operations, type of fixator, size of bone defect, length of distraction osteogenesis, time of external fixation and consolidation, healing index (time between application of fixators and consolidation divided by the length of the defect), and external fixation index (external fixation time divided by the length of defect).

Statistical analysis

The rates of infection-free outcomes were synthesized in subgroups of external fixator group or hybrid fixator group with the variance-stabilizing double arcsine transformation [27]. Heterogeneity was quantified using the I^2 statistic. The I^2 heterogeneity was degreed as follows: < 25% low, 25 to 50% moderate and > 50% high. Fixed-effects models were used for low and moderate heterogeneity while random-effects models for high heterogeneity. To understand the factors which impact associated sequelae, two-step method with logistic regression was used to investigate the IPD (95% confidence interval). IPD from each study was independently analyzed in the first step to produce an estimate for each study, and then these data were analyzed. All analyses were performed using Stata (version 14.0, StataCorp, College Station, TX, USA).

Results

Based on our review, twenty-two studies with 518 patients met inclusion criteria: eleven studies with 167 patients' IPD, and 11 studies with 351 patients' aggregate data (Fig. 1). Hybrid fixators were applied on 63 patients, while external fixators were applied on 454 patients (Table 1). The overall infection-free rate of bone transportation for tibia infected nonunion and chronic osteomyelitis is 96% (95%CI: 94–98%, Fig. 2). Significant heterogeneity existed between the groups of hybrid and external fixators ($p = 0.01$, Fig. 2). The infection-free rate of hybrid fixator group was 86% (95%CI: 79–94%, Fig. 2), while that of external fixator was 97% (95%CI: 95–98%, Fig. 2).

For the IPD data, the mean age of patients was 38.25 years (range from 16 to 79 years), the mean number of previous surgeries was 3.49 (range from 1 to 20). The mean size of bone defect after debridement was 5.25 cm (range from 1 to 12 cm). The mean healing index was 1.74 months/cm (range from 0.8 to 15.8 months/cm), the mean external fixator index was 1.1 months/cm (range from 0.4 to 1.7 months/cm) (Table 2).

Among the variables of IPD, the number of previous operations before bone transportation had a significant impact on the sequelae of both bone union ($p = 0.04$) and function ($p < 0.01$). Longer external fixation ($p =$

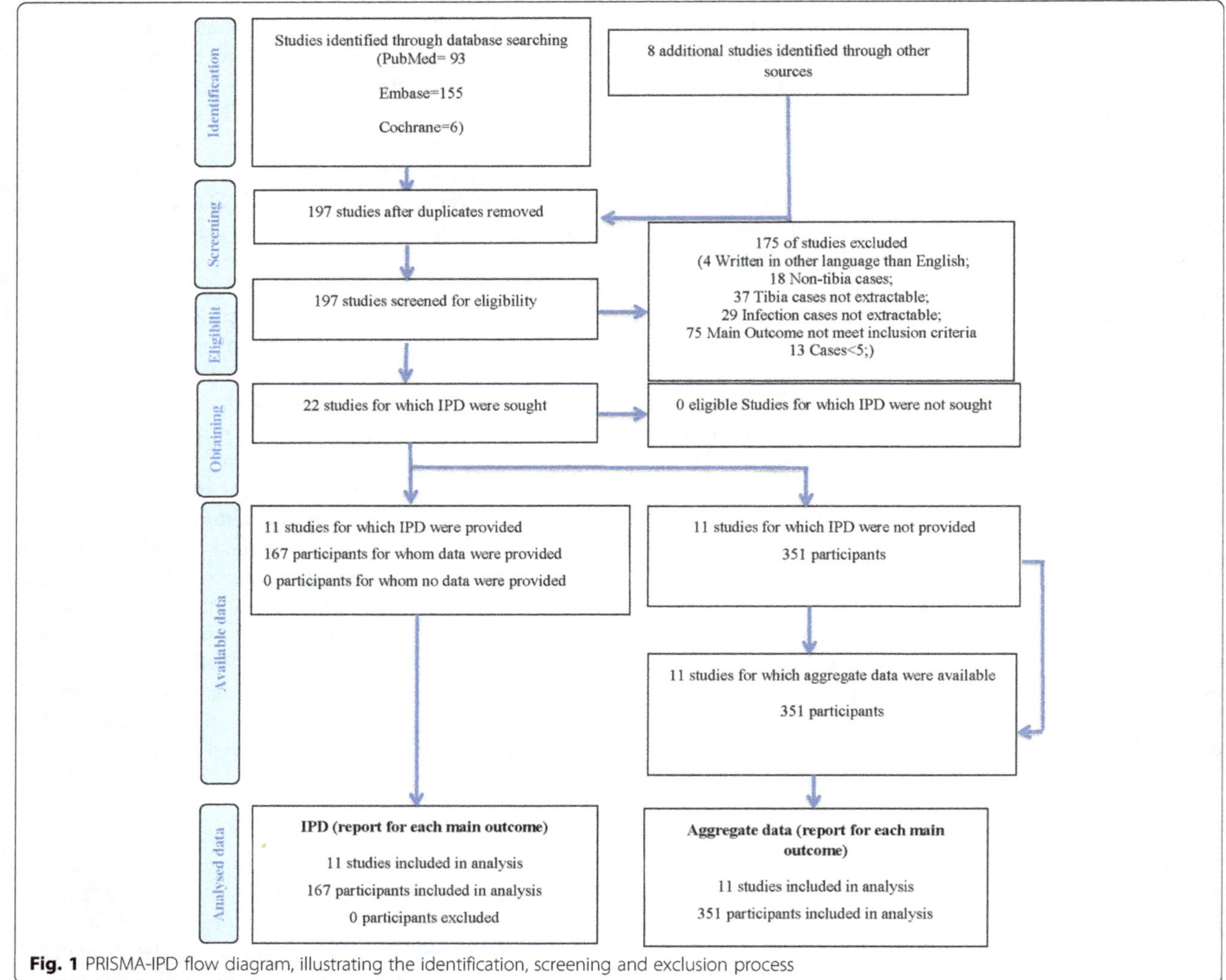

Fig. 1 PRISMA-IPD flow diagram, illustrating the identification, screening and exclusion process

Table 1 Summary of Included Studies

ID	Data type	Patients Number	Gender		Age(year)	Fixator System	Soft-tissue Reconstruction	Satisfactory Result		Sequelae-free		Infection Free
			Male	Female				Bone	Function	Bone	Function	
Dendrinos 1995 [38]	IPD	28	23	5	37.43(18~74)	Ilizarov EF	–	24	18	14	7	28
Eralp 2016 [43]	IPD	6	3	3	48.33(33~79)	Ilizarov EF; TSF	1[b]	–	4	–	2	6
Khan 2015 [44]	IPD	6	6	0	40.60(19~55)	Ilizarov EF	3[b]	4	4	0	1	5
Kocaoglu 2006 [17]	IPD	7	5	2	35.29(18~52)	Hybrid Fixator	2[b; c]	7	7	6	6	5
Lalit 2000 [40]	IPD	16	16	0	30.81(17~46)	Ilizarov EF	–	11	12	8	5	14
Liu 2012 [45]	IPD	35	25	10	37.29(18~64)	EF	5[b]	33	34	28	30	32
Marko 2010 [46]	IPD	30	29	1	30.57(20~49)	Ilizarov EF	–	29	27	19	13	30
Oh 2008 [16]	IPD	10	10	0	46.00(18~76)	Hybrid Fixator	5[b]	–	10	–	4	9
Oh 2013 [47]	IPD	10	9	1	40.40(16~64)	Hybrid Fixator	4[b]	10	9	10	6	10
Panagiotis 2010 [48]	IPD	6	5	1	34.50(21~52)	Ilizarov EF	2[b]	6	4	3	1	6
Zhang 2016 [19]	IPD	14	13	1	38.07(21~62)	Mono-lateral EF; Hybrid Fixators[a]	1[b];2[c]	14	11	12	8	5;6[a]
Emara 2008 [18]	AD	33	22	11	29	Ilizarov ring; Hybrid Fixators[a]	–	33	28	32	25	16;16[a]
McNally 2017 [22]	AD	18	–	–	–	Ilizarov ring	–	14	17	13	13	18
Peng 2015 [49]	AD	58	38	20	29.4(18~51)	Ilizarov ring	–	53	46	30	28	57
Rohilla 2016 [4]	AD	70	62	8	31.25(18~65)	Mono-lateral EF; Ring EF	0	62	55	35	28	35
Sadek 2016 [5]	AD	14	12	2	29.50	Ring EF	8	14	8	11	8	14
Tetsworth 2017 [7]	AD	21	18	3	38.2(18~66)	Ring/Ilizarov EF	–	20	20	15	14	21
Tong 2017 [50]	AD	13	–	–	–	Mono-lateral EF; Ilizarov EF	–	10	5	5	1	9
Yin 2014 [51]	AD	72	–	–	–	Ilizarov EF	–	63	52	46	25	72
Eralp 2012 [13]	AD	15	14	3	39(25~69)	Hybrid Fixator	–	14	15	10	10	14
Gupta 2018 [52]	AD	14	13	1	38.1	Hybrid Fixator	1[b]	14	14	14	8	13
Madhusudhan 2008 [53]	AD	22	–	–	–	Ilizarov EF	4[b]	13	5	5	1	16

AD Aggregate data, *IPD* Individual participant data, *EF* External Fixators, *TSF* Taylor Spatial Frame; a: Early change from external fixators to internal fixators; b: Soft-tissue flap; c: Skin graft

0.015) was associated with a greater chance of functional sequelae. Age, size of bone defect, and length of bone distraction did not have significant impacts on the sequelae of bone union or function (Table 3).

Discussion

Infection relapse of tibial infectious nonunion and chronic osteomyelitis is common, because most causative bacteria are antibiotic-resistant, making it difficult to completely eradicate their populations with common prophylaxis [28, 29]. The affected patients tend to incur more than one surgery before achieving a successful infection-free result. Bone transportation techniques with external or hybrid fixator systems have been proved versatile to deal with this clinical challenge. However, the infection-free rates of these two fixator systems remain unknown and seldom compared. In the present meta-analysis, hybrid fixators were found to have a higher rate of infection recurrence compared to external fixators (Fig. 2).

In bone transportation technique, the choice of fixator systems depends on the treatment philosophy of long bone infection [17]. However, this philosophy has evolved in recent decades, from "the infection would burn on the fire of the bone regeneration," by Ilizarov, to "the only cure for osteomyelitis is radical debridement,"

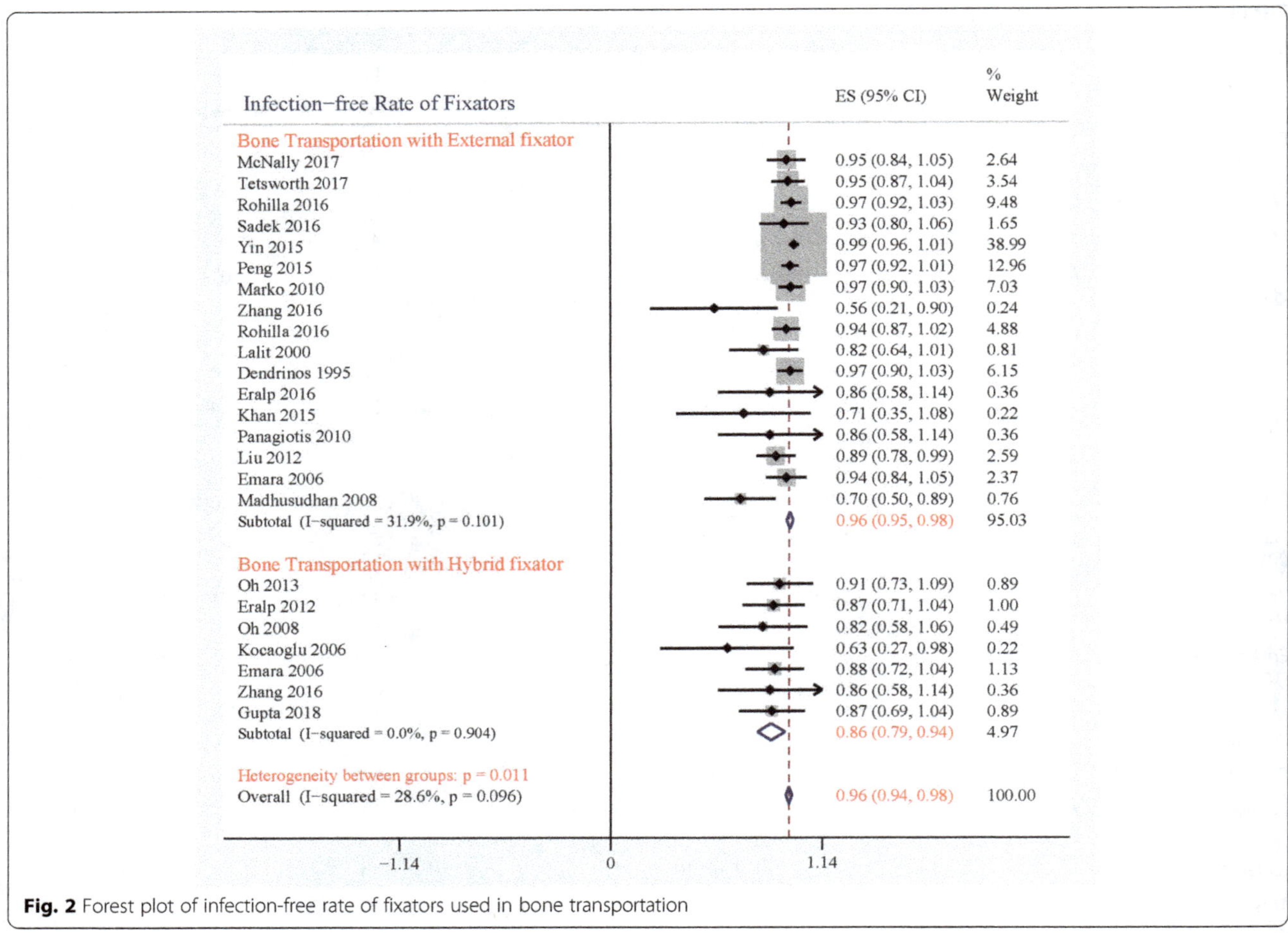

Fig. 2 Forest plot of infection-free rate of fixators used in bone transportation

by Cierny [30]. The later concept has greater amounts supportive evidence recently and is more widely accepted [31]. In most cases the infected tissue was extensively excised until live and bleeding bone (paprika sign), with which a large amount of bacterial burden would be removed. Based on this prerequisite it seems safe to implement internal fixators during or after the distraction period to overcome the disadvantage of external fixation [17]. However, the risk of infection recurrence comes along with internal fixators still exists. The reason is that debridement alone is not sufficient to sterilize the operative site. Small bacterial colonies can be displaced

Table 2 Summary of IPD

ID	Previous Surgery	Bone defect(cm)	Bone graft	Length of distraction(cm)	External Fixation Time (weeks)	External Fixation Index (months/cm)	Heal Time (weeks)	Heal Index (months/cm)
Dendrinos 1995	4.04(1~20)	6.14 ± 2.68	3	5.54 ± 2.46	41.46(21.50~77.40)	1.95 ± 0.74	27.77(17.20~43.00)	1.35 ± 0.64
Eralp 2016		–	–	3.00 ± 2.61	32.26(21.43~42.86)	1.04 ± 0.11	–	–
Khan 2015	2.00(1~3)	2.82 ± 0.95	–	2.82 ± 0.95	–	–	72.80(32.00~124.00)	7.77 ± 6.38
Kocaoglu 2006	5.29(1~20)	7.00 ± 1.83	7	–	12.63(8.00~20.00)	–	33.09(21.45~55.77)	1.07 ± 0.21
Lalit 2000	2.38(1~5)	7.71 ± 2.30	3	–	–	–	–	–
Liu 2012	2.69(1~6)	3.55 ± 1.47	2	7.81 ± 2.21	–	–	–	1.37 ± 0.12
Marko 2010	–	6.87 ± 1.76	1	6.53 ± 1.53	–	1.48 ± 0.07	17.86(14.00~20.00)	1.03 ± 0.06
Oh 2008	–	5.75 ± 2.89	10	–	–	0.80 ± 0.27	–	2.09 ± 0.61
Oh 2013	–	5.91 ± 1.96	10	–	–	0.45 ± 0.08	–	2.15 ± 0.23
Panagiotis 2010	5.00(1~6)	6.67 ± 3.20	–	–	33.67(17.00~59.00)	–	–	–
Zhang 2016	4.36(1~7)	–	6	5.91 ± 1.24	41.43(23.00~57.00)	–	44.86(31.00~61.00)	1.87 ± 0.59

Table 3 Factors on Sequelae-free Result of Bone and Function

Variables	Sequelae-free Bone Result				Sequelae-free Function Result			
	Num of studies	Odds Ratio (95% CI)	*P* value	I^2(%)	Num of studies	Odds Ratio (95% CI)	*P* value	I^2(%)
Age	7	0.995(0.961 to 1.031)	0.789	0.0%	10	0.969(0.936 to 1.003)	0.075	0.0%
Previous Surgery Times	5	0.687(0.480 to 0.984)	0.040	37.5%	4	0.338(0.189 to 0.603)	0.000	0.0%
Bone defect	6	1.030(0.842 to 1.260)	0.776	0.0%	7	0.828(0.657 to 1.043)	0.109	3.2%
Length of Distraction	4	0.979(0.605 to 1.583)	0.930	49.6%	5	0.919(0.664 to 1.273)	0.613	14.8%
Time of External Fixation	4	0.977(0.924 to 1.032)	0.404	0.0%	4	0.899(0.825 to 0.979)	0.015	0.0%
Time of Bone Union	4	0.962(0.872 to 1.060)	0.431	0.0%	4	0.836(0.740 to 0.954)	0.004	0.0%

during the debridement procedure even under most careful cleaning [32]. If internal fixator is subsequently implanted, the residual bacteria on the device surface could form a biofilm, leading to infection recurrence. Consistently, in this research hybrid fixators showed potential inferior infection-free result than external fixators, indicating the internal fixators may not be appropriate in this specific scenario.

Similarly, Bose suggested that external fixators are safer than internal fixation for an infected nonunion fracture. Though all the infected bone and unhealthy enveloping soft tissue were completely excised, four of six patients had infection recurrence after internal fixation [21]. Liodakis found that in cases where an intramedullary rod was involved, there was a greater rate of infection recurrence than in cases of external fixation when dealing with infected post-traumatic tibia. He recommended the post-traumatic bone defects with chronic infection should only be fixed by external frame [8]. Besides providing a potential harbor for residual bacteria, the intramedullary nails also facilitate the spread of the pin tract infection along implants [33].To avoid internal-related infection recurrence, internal fixators can be applied at a later time, not immediately after debridement. In this way, when the distraction phase is over, the external fixators are removed and replaced by internal fixators. Zhang conducted early osteosynthesis with plate or intramedullary nail once two bone ends meet at the dock site. and no reinfection was noted [19]. However, Emara suggested this method still has risk of infection recurrence; in his study infection recurrence occurred in one patient who received early nailing, and the intramedullary nail was changed to an Ilizarov fixator until final union [18]. Last but not least, patients' immunologic status has an impact on the infection-free rates. Within the hybrid fixator treatment group in Oh's study, a diabetes mellitus patient was complicated with infectious recurrence [15]. Even though no statistical conclusion is draw due to the small sample size, patients with inferior immunologic function likely have a greater risk of infection recurrence and may be better suited for treatment by external fixator, which is safer.

Complete coverage of soft tissue is important to control and prevent infection. The early coverage of soft tissue may provide nutrition, obliterate dead space, facilitate local immunologic defense, and antibiotic delivery [22]. In most cases, soft tissue reconstruction was done empirically according to surgeons' evaluation and preference. In the current review musculocutaneous flaps and skin grafts were the most commonly used methods to compensate for lost soft tissue and achieve satisfactory coverage (Table 1). However, due to the insufficient reported data, the hypothesis that soft reconstruction could increase infection-free rates, and the implementation of internal fixators could undermine the soft tissue, cause poor vascularity, and consequently reduce infection-free rates, remains to be investigated. Oh believed implantation of a locking plate would not compromise the surrounding soft tissue because of minimally invasive or percutaneous techniques [27]. Even though more thorough evidence is warranted to draw a conclusion for the role of soft tissue, proper reconstruction of surrounding soft tissue is still a great concern when surgical plans are made.

Despite these observations, the advantages of hybrid fixators are still remarkable. The external fixator could be removed once defect ends meet with combined fixation. This shortens the timeframe for potential distraction-related complications. Additionally, early removal of external fixators is more comfortable for the patients [17]. It is well known that the long-time external fixation imposes psychosocial hardships and disruption in daily lives to patients. The bulky external fixators interrupt activities of daily living (ADL) as well as leisure and sport activities [24]. Combining internal fixators facilitates the early return to ADL without the need for wearing external apparatus. Similarly, it can also allow early rehabilitation and prevent related joint stiffness [17]. Hybrid fixators demonstrated the highest success rate compared with external fixators alone for bone healing in the case of limb salvage of long bone defects [12]. However, for the infected cases, the higher potential risk of infection recurrence is more worrisome and serious than uncomfortableness. Notably, internal fixators used in all included studies were traditional internal implants without antibiotic surface modification.

Antibiotic-coated implants have gained increasing interest recently. These novel surface coatings have been successfully used in the treatment of osteomyelitis and long bone infectious nonunion [28, 34–37]. This method could provide both infection control, or prophylaxis, and osseous stability simultaneously [28, 34]. Further research in this area is necessary towards a more comprehensive understanding of the long-term success of such surface coatings.

Infection recurrence leads to multiple operations [17, 38]. Many patients with tibia infection suffer from repeated surgeries before seeking the final bone transport treatment. In the present analysis, the number of previous operations is a predictive factor of prognosis for bony union ($p = 0.04$, Table 3) and functional restoration ($p < 0.01$, Table 3): a greater number of previous surgeries are correlated with a greater chance of sequelae. Several reason could explain this result. First, the repeatedly debridement and surgery would lead to prolonged hospital stays, loss of soft and bone tissue, impaired function of the affected limbs, increased pain, and a poor quality of life [39]. Additionally, the repeated operation could cause more scar tissue and subsequently poor soft tissue flexibility, which cause difficult exposure for the subsequent procedures [40, 41]. The consequent surgeries pose a high risk of poor outcome, as well as financial and psychological burdens to patients. Number of previous surgeries is a useful indicator to predict the treatment outcome for the patients with repeated revision. Therefore, it is important to meticulously design a surgery treatment plan and conduct limb salvage by an experienced multidisciplinary team in order to minimize the need for further unexpected operations.

The duration of external fixation has been suspected to be associated with a worse functional result. However, it is hard to make a definitive conclusion because of small sample sizes in previous research. In the present study, by pooling the IPD to increase sample size, the time of external fixation is found to be associated a greater risk of functional sequelae ($p = 0.015$, Table 3). In cases of extended duration of external fixation patients tend to suffer more joint stiffness, muscle dystrophy and significant pain. Additionally, more pin-related infections are also involved [6]. Hence, a shortened external frame time is necessary to reduce functional complications related to external fixators and improve patient outcomes [14, 16, 17]. To shorten external frame time of distraction, one option is to add more transport segments in large bone defects. Paley and Maar suggested trifocal bone transport when the bone defect is larger than 10 cm [24], while Rozbruch and Zhang set the criterion for trifocal transport at greater than 6 cm [42]. All trifocal patients in their studies had reduced distraction times. The trifocal bone transport could double the distraction speed because two-level osteotomies divided lengthening (and healing) into two locations [14]. To shorten the duration of dock consolidation, combining an internal implant could facilitate the early removal of external fixators and rehabilitation. However, there is a potential risk of infections recurrence, which should be considered in treatment and surgical planning. If the antibiotic-coated internal implants could achieve satisfactory control and prophylaxis of infection, it is an effective choice to manage cases of tibia infectious nonunion and osteomyelitis.

This is the first study to summary the infection-free results of bone transport techniques with external and hybrid fixators for tibia infectious nonunion and chronic osteomyelitis, and the first to determine factors which predict bone and function sequela. Here, hybrid technique involved traditional internal fixators showed more potential risk of infection recurrence than external groups. The number of previous operations and the duration of external fixation were confirmed associated with greater risk of sequelae. However, the results of this analysis should be interpreted carefully because of the limitations of this study. First, most of the included studies are retrospective with small sample sizes. Second, though the principle of the criterion of the ASIMI and Paley classifications are the same, in which classifications are graded by number of sequelae, difference exists in their criterion. Third, the included studies have obvious heterogeneity even though selection criteria were set. In the future prospective and large-scale clinical research is necessary to better understand the factors influencing patient outcomes.

Conclusions

Bone transport technique is an established treatment to deal with segmental bone defects due to infection. Hybrid fixator system combining traditional internal and external fixators may be associated with a greater risk of infection recurrence; antibiotic-coated internal implants maybe a promising choice to circumvent this well-known issue. Additionally, we have demonstrated that number of previous operations as well as duration of external fixation are useful prognostic indicators for predicting outcomes. To achieve successful healing and functional results, meticulous surgical planning is necessary in order to avoid additional surgeries and long external fixation times.

Abbreviations

AD: Aggregate Data; ADL: Activities of Daily Living; EF: External Fixator; IPD: Individual Patient Data; PRISMA-IPD: Preferred Reported Items for Systematic Reviews of Meta-Analyses Statement for Individual Patient Data; TSF: Taylor Spatial Frame

Acknowledgements

Not applicable.

Funding

This research was supported by Sichuan Science and Technology Department (2018SZ0145) and Sichuan Health and Family Planning Commission (17PJ128).

The funding body did not take part in the design of the study and collection, analysis, and interpretation of data and in writing the manuscript.

Authors' contributions

ZZ and Y-H W searched and screened papers as well as abstracted data. ZZ and WBS did statistic work and wrote the paper. WL solved disagreement of paper's selection. WL and GW designed the whole study and guided the whole research. All authors have read and approved the manuscript and agree to publish.

Consent for publication

Not applicable.

Competing interests

The authors declare that they have no competing interests.

Author details

[1]Department of Orthopedics, West China Hospital, Sichuan University, No. 37, Guoxue Lane, Wuhou District, Chengdu 610041, Sichuan Province, China. [2]Department of Biologic and Materials Sciences, School of Dentistry, University of Michigan, Ann Arbor, USA. [3]Department of Neonatology, Beijing Gynecology & Obstetrics Hospital, Capital Medical University, Beijing, China. [4]Department of Gynecology, West China Second Hospital, Sichuan University, Chengdu, China.

Reference

1. Hak DJ, Fitzpatrick D, Bishop JA, Marsh JL, Tilp S, Schnettler R, Simpson H, Alt V. Delayed union and nonunions: epidemiology, clinical issues, and financial aspects. Injury. 2014;45(Suppl 2):S3–7.
2. Brinker MR, Hanus BD, Sen M, O'Connor DP. The devastating effects of tibial nonunion on health-related quality of life. J Bone Joint Surg Am. 2013; 95(24):2170–6.
3. Yin P, Li T, Zhang L, Wang G, Li J, Liu J, Zhou J, Zhang Q, Tang P. Infected nonunion of tibia and femur treated by bone transport. J Orthop Surg Res. 2015;10:49.
4. Rohilla R, Wadhwani J, Devgan A, Singh R, Khanna M. Prospective randomised comparison of ring versus rail fixator in infected gap nonunion of tibia treated with distraction osteogenesis. Bone Joint J. 2016;98-B(10): 1399–405.
5. Sadek AF, Laklok MA, Fouly EH, Elshafie M. Two stage reconstruction versus bone transport in management of resistant infected tibial diaphyseal nonunion with a gap. Arch Orthop Trauma Surg. 2016;136(9):1233–41.
6. Paley D. Problems, obstacles, and complications of limb lengthening by the Ilizarov technique. Clin Orthop Relat Res. 1990;(250):81-104.
7. Tetsworth K, Paley D, Sen C, Jaffe M, Maar DC, Glatt V, Hohmann E, Herzenberg JE. Bone transport versus acute shortening for the management of infected tibial non-unions with bone defects. Injury. 2017;48(10):2276–84.
8. Liodakis E, Kenawey M, Krettek C, Wiebking U, Hankemeier S. Comparison of 39 post-traumatic tibia bone transports performed with and without the use of an intramedullary rod: the long-term outcomes. Int Orthop. 2011; 35(9):1397–402.
9. Patzakis MJ, Zalavras CG. Chronic posttraumatic osteomyelitis and infected nonunion of the tibia: current management concepts. J Am Acad Orthop Surg. 2005;13(6):417–27.
10. Paley D. Treatment of tibial nonunion and bone loss with the Ilizarov technique. Instr Course Lect. 1990;39:185–97.
11. Gubin AV, Borzunov DY, Malkova TA. The Ilizarov paradigm: thirty years with the Ilizarov method, current concerns and future research. Int Orthop. 2013; 37(8):1533–9.
12. Kadhim M, Holmes L Jr, Gesheff MG, Conway JD. Treatment options for nonunion with segmental bone defects: systematic review and quantitative evidence synthesis. J Orthop Trauma. 2017;31(2):111–9.
13. Eralp L, Kocaoglu M, Polat G, Bas A, Dirican A, Azam ME. A comparison of external fixation alone or combined with intramedullary nailing in the treatment of segmental tibial defects. Acta Orthop Belg. 2012;78(5):652–9.
14. Zhang Y, Wang Y, Di J, Peng A. Double-level bone transport for large post-traumatic tibial bone defects: a single Centre experience of sixteen cases. Int Orthop. 2018;42(5):1157–64.
15. Oh CW, Apivatthakakul T, Oh JK, Kim JW, Lee HJ, Kyung HS, Baek SG, Jung GH. Bone transport with an external fixator and a locking plate for segmental tibial defects. Bone Joint J. 2013;95-B(12):1667–72.
16. Oh CW, Song HR, Roh JY, Oh JK, Min WK, Kyung HS, Kim JW, Kim PT, Ihn JC. Bone transport over an intramedullary nail for reconstruction of long bone defects in tibia. Arch Orthop Trauma Surg. 2008;128(8):801–8.
17. Kocaoglu M, Eralp L, Rashid HU, Sen C, Bilsel K. Reconstruction of segmental bone defects due to chronic osteomyelitis with use of an external fixator and an intramedullary nail.[Reprint in J Bone Joint Surg Am. 2007 Sep;89 Suppl 2 Pt.2:183–95; PMID: 17768214]. *J Bone Joint Surg Am.* 2006;88(10):2137–45.
18. Emara KM, Allam MF. Ilizarov external fixation and then nailing in management of infected nonunions of the tibial shaft. J Trauma. 2008; 65:685–91.
19. Zhang S, Wang H, Zhao J, Xu P, Shi H, Mu W. Treatment of post-traumatic chronic osteomyelitis of lower limbs by bone transport technique using mono-lateral external fixator: follow-up study of 18 cases. J Orthop Sci. 2016;21(4):493–9.
20. Li Z, Zhang X, Duan L, Chen X. Distraction osteogenesis technique using an intramedullary nail and a monolateral external fixator in the reconstruction of massive postosteomyelitis skeletal defects of the femur. Canadian journal of surgery Journal canadien de chirurgie. 2009; 52(2):103–11.
21. Bose D, Kugan R, Stubbs D, McNally M. Management of infected nonunion of the long bones by a multidisciplinary team. Bone Joint J. 2015;97-B(6):814–7.
22. McNally M, Ferguson J, Kugan R, Stubbs D. Ilizarov treatment protocols in the Management of Infected Nonunion of the tibia. J Orthop Trauma. 2017; 31(Suppl 5):S47–54.
23. Yin P, Ji Q, Li T, Li J, Li Z, Liu J, Wang G, Wang S, Zhang L, Mao Z, et al. A systematic review and meta-analysis of Ilizarov methods in the treatment of infected nonunion of tibia and femur. PLoS One. 2015;10(11):e0141973.
24. Paley D, Maar DC. Ilizarov bone transport treatment for tibial defects. J Orthop Trauma. 2000;14(2):76–85.
25. Paley D, Catagni MA, Argnani F, Villa A, Benedetti GB, Cattaneo R. Ilizarov treatment of tibial nonunions with bone loss. Clin Orthop Relat Res. 1989; (241):146–65.
26. Stewart LA, Clarke M, Rovers M, Riley RD, Simmonds M, Stewart G, Tierney JF. Group P-ID: preferred reporting items for systematic review and meta-analyses of individual participant data: the PRISMA-IPD statement. Jama. 2015;313(16):1657–65.
27. Freeman MF, Tukey JW. Transformations related to the angular and the square root. The Annals of Mathematical Statistics. 1950;21(4):607–11.
28. Barger J, Fragomen AT, Rozbruch SR. Antibiotic-coated interlocking intramedullary nail for the treatment of long-bone osteomyelitis. JBJS Rev. 2017;5(7):e5.
29. Metsemakers WJ, Kuehl R, Moriarty TF, Richards RG, Verhofstad MHJ, Borens O, Kates S, Morgenstern M. Infection after fracture fixation: current surgical and microbiological concepts. Injury. 2018;49(3):511–22.
30. Cierny G 3rd. Infected tibial nonunions (1981-1995). The evolution of change. Clin Orthop Relat Res. 1999;360:97–105.
31. Simpson AH, Deakin M, Latham JM. Chronic osteomyelitis. The effect of the extent of surgical resection on infection-free survival. J Bone Joint Surg Br. 2001;83(3):403–7.
32. Winkler H, Haiden P. Treatment of chronic bone infection. Oper Tech Orthop. 2016;26(1):2–11.
33. Clasper JC, Stapley SA, Bowley DM, Kenward CE, Taylor V, Watkins PE. Spread of infection, in an animal model, after intramedullary nailing of an infected external fixator pin track. J Orthop Res. 2001;19(1):155–9.
34. Yu X, Wu H, Li J, Xie Z. Antibiotic cement-coated locking plate as a temporary internal fixator for femoral osteomyelitis defects. Int Orthop. 2017;41(9):1851–7.
35. Koury KL, Hwang JS, Sirkin M. The antibiotic nail in the treatment of long bone infection: technique and results. The Orthopedic clinics of North America. 2017;48(2):155–65.
36. Thonse R, Conway JD. Antibiotic cement-coated nails for the treatment of infected nonunions and segmental bone defects. J Bone Joint Surg Am. 2008;90(Suppl 4):163–74.
37. Qiang Z, Jun PZ, Jie XJ, Hang L, Bing LJ, Cai LF. Use of antibiotic cement rod to treat intramedullary infection after nailing: preliminary study in 19 patients. Arch Orthop Trauma Surg. 2007;127(10):945–51.

38. Dendrinos GK, Kontos S, Lyritsis E. Use of the Ilizarov technique for treatment of non-union of the tibia associated with infection. J Bone Joint Surg Am. 1995;77(6):835–46.
39. Barker KL, Lamb SE, Simpson AH. Functional recovery in patients with nonunion treated with the Ilizarov technique. J Bone Joint Surg Br. 2004;86(1):81–5.
40. Maini L, Chadha M, Vishwanath J, Kapoor S, Mehtani A, Dhaon BK. The Ilizarov method in infected nonunion of fractures. Injury. 2000;31(7):509–17.
41. Ma CH, Chiu YC, Tsai KL, Tu YK, Yen CY, Wu CH. Masquelet technique with external locking plate for recalcitrant distal tibial nonunion. Injury. 2017; 48(12):2847–52.
42. Robert Rozbruch S, Weitzman AM, Tracey Watson J, Freudigman P, Katz HV, Ilizarov S. Simultaneous treatment of tibial bone and soft-tissue defects with the Ilizarov method. J Orthop Trauma. 2006;20(3):197–205.
43. Eralp IL, Kocaoglu M, Dikmen G, Azam ME, Balci HI, Bilen FE. Treatment of infected nonunion of the juxta-articular region of the distal tibia. Acta Orthop Traumatol Turc. 2016;50(2):139–46.
44. Khan MS, Rashid H, Umer M, Qadir I, Hafeez K, Iqbal A. Salvage of infected non-union of the tibia with an Ilizarov ring fixator. J Orthop Surg (Hong Kong). 2015;23(1):52–5.
45. Liu T, Yu X, Zhang X, Li Z, Zeng W. One-stage management of post-traumatic tibial infected nonunion using bone transport after debridement. Turkish Journal of Medical Sciences. 2012;42(6):1111–20.
46. Bumbasirevic M, Tomic S, Lesic A, Milosevic I, Atkinson HD. War-related infected tibial nonunion with bone and soft-tissue loss treated with bone transport using the Ilizarov method. Arch Orthop Trauma Surg. 2010; 130(6):739–49.
47. Oh CW, Apivatthakakul T, Oh JK, Kim JW, Lee HJ, Kyung HS, Baek SG, Jung GH: Bone transport with an external fixator and a locking plate for segmental tibial defects. Bone and Joint Journal 2013, 95 B(12):1667–1672.
48. Megas P, Saridis A, Kouzelis A, Kallivokas A, Mylonas S, Tyllianakis M. The treatment of infected nonunion of the tibia following intramedullary nailing by the Ilizarov method. Injury. 2010;41(3):294–9.
49. Peng J, Min L, Xiang Z, Huang F, Tu C, Zhang H. Ilizarov bone transport combined with antibiotic cement spacer for infected tibial nonunion. Int J Clin Exp Med. 2015;8(6):10058–65.
50. Tong K, Zhong Z, Peng Y, Lin C, Cao S, Yang YP, Wang G. Masquelet technique versus Ilizarov bone transport for reconstruction of lower extremity bone defects following posttraumatic osteomyelitis. Injury. 2017.
51. Yin P, Zhang Q, Mao Z, Li T, Zhang L, Tang P. The treatment of infected tibial nonunion by bone transport using the Ilizarov external fixator and a systematic review of infected tibial nonunion treated by Ilizarov methods. Acta Orthop Belg. 2014;80(3):426–35.
52. Gupta S, Malhotra A, Mittal N, Garg SK, Jindal R, Kansay R. The management of infected nonunion of tibia with a segmental defect using simultaneous fixation with a monorail fixator and a locked plate. Bone Joint J. 2018;100-b(8):1094–9.
53. Madhusudhan TR, Ramesh B, Manjunath K, Shah HM, Sundaresh DC, Krishnappa N. Outcomes of Ilizarov ring fixation in recalcitrant infected tibial non-unions - a prospective study. Journal of trauma management & outcomes. 2008;2(1):6.

13

Anatomic double-bundle medial patellofemoral ligament reconstruction with aperture fixation using an adjustable-length loop device: a 2-year follow-up study

Jae-Ang Sim[1], Jin-Kyu Lim[2] and Byung Hoon Lee[2*]

Abstract

Background: To assess the clinical availability of an adjustable-length loop device for use in the double-bundle technique with aperture fixation at the patella and femur during anatomic double-bundle medial patellofemoral ligament reconstruction (DB-MPFLR) for recurrent patellar dislocation.

Methods: We retrospectively investigated 11 patients (12 knees) with recurrent patellar dislocation who underwent anatomic DB-MPFLR with an ipsilateral semitendinosus tendon autograft. The graft was folded in half, and its central portion was hanged using the adjustable-length loop device. Both free ends of the graft were fixed at the proximal and distal ends of the medial edge of the patella by using suture anchors, and the hanged graft loop was pulled into the femoral tunnel while maintaining equal tension on both bundles. Manual traction of the suture loops was applied to fix the graft appropriately in full range of motion (ROM) of the knee joint under arthroscopic guidance. Clinical outcomes such as re-dislocation, ROM, clinical scores (Kujala score, Lysholm score, and visual analogue scale score for anterior knee pain), and complications were assessed preoperatively and at 2 years postoperatively. Radiographic parameters indicating patellar position, including congruence angle and lateral patellofemoral angle, were measured at 4 different angles of knee flexion (30°, 45°, 60°, and 90°).

Results: At 4 different flexion angles of the knee joint, the preoperative congruence angle decreased significantly and the lateral patellofemoral angle increased significantly at the final follow-up ($P < 0.001$). Notably, the improvements in these angles were maintained with no significant differences at the 4 different flexion angles. None of the patients experienced subluxation or re-dislocation after surgery. The patellar instability symptoms improved, as confirmed on the basis of radiographic and other clinical outcomes.

Conclusion: New DB technique with aperture fixation at the patella and femur by using an adjustable-length loop device offers high stability with full ROM of the knee joint, can be considered as a feasible procedure and technique for recurrent patellar dislocation.

Keywords: Medial patellofemoral ligament, Patella, Recurrent patellar dislocation, Double bundle, Aperture fixation, Adjustable-length loop device

* Correspondence: oselite@naver.com
[2]Department of Orthopedic Surgery, Kang-Dong Sacred Heart Hospital, Hallym University Medical School, 134-701, Gil-dong, Seoul, South Korea
Full list of author information is available at the end of the article

Background

Recurrent patellar dislocation (RPD) is related to various pathological abnormalities [1–10]. The medial patellofemoral ligament (MPFL) provides a primary restraint against the lateral dislocation of the patella [11, 12], and MPFL insufficiency is considered to be the main cause of traumatic RPD or patellar instability [13]. During MPFL reconstruction, graft fixation is critical to ensure the restoration of MPFL function. Several techniques have been introduced to fix the graft to the patellar MPFL attachment site, including the patellar bone tunnel technique [14–16] and the suture anchor technique [14, 17].

Non-anatomic reconstruction of the MPFL can lead to non-physiologic patellofemoral pressure and abnormal patellar tracking [18]. Therefore, recent techniques for reconstruction of the medial patellofemoral complex seek to restore the identical footprint of both the patellar and femoral attachments for biomechanical matching. The anatomic attachment site and anatomic shape of the native MPFL was previously defined. Double-bundle (DB) reconstruction at the patellar side may be a reasonable method for restoring the native ligamentous morphologic and biomechanical properties [17]. Therefore, increased interest has been directed toward anatomic DB reconstruction, which replicates 2 functional bundles, to more closely restore the normal patellofemoral stability and kinematics.

Nevertheless, the biomechanical rationale of anatomic DB reconstruction is not well established [19]. During DB anterior cruciate ligament reconstruction, both the anteromedial and posterolateral bundles are stretched and loaded in the extended knee position [20]. Therefore, graft fixation in this stretched and loaded position avoids elongation of the graft, potentially facilitating early rehabilitation with full range of motion (ROM). However, the DB MPFL reconstruction (DB-MPFLR) does not take into consideration the length change pattern of the respective bundles.

The aperture fixation technique introduced by Schöttle et al. [21] may not apply the length change patterns at each knee flexion of the MPFL, a complex of functionally varying fibers, with some taut and others slack, throughout the range of knee motion [19]. Therefore, direct anatomic/aperture fixation [22] to restore the triangular form of the MPFL for anatomic reconstruction can result in uneven and non-isometric graft tensioning and might induce non-physiologic patellofemoral loads and kinematics [23] with full ROM. Furthermore, micro-motion of the graft during knee flexion-extension can increase the risk of delayed or insufficient tendon-to-bone healing [24].

We hypothesized that the adjustable-length loop device used in femoral cortical suspension systems, which are the most convenient devices for use in ligament reconstruction with soft tissue graft [25], will be applicable in anatomic DB-MPFLR, with 2 clinical benefits. First, certain reciprocal movement of the looped graft into the femoral tunnel may allow the even tension to restrain the lateral force throughout the ROM. Second, graft fixation with appropriate tension in full ROM of the knee joint can be easily achieved by manual traction using lead sutures under arthroscopic guidance. Here, we describe a DB technique with aperture fixation at the patella and femur by using an adjustable-length loop device, which offers high stability in full ROM of the knee joint.

Materials and methods

Between 2014 and 2015, 18 patients underwent surgery for the treatment of RPD depending on individual pathologic abnormalities. All surgeries were done by the same senior orthopedic surgeon. All patients who underwent surgery during this period were screened. The indication for operation was RPD (defined as at least 2 episodes of patellar dislocation despite non-operative treatment). Lateral patellar dislocations were diagnosed on the basis of history taking, physical examination, simple radiographs, computed tomography, and magnetic resonance imaging. Seven patients who required additional procedures for RPD and had various pathologic abnormalities [1, 2], such as bony pathologies on the femoral or tibial side, were excluded, as follows: trochlear dysplasia (Dejour classification C) [3, 4, 26] ($n = 1$), increased tibial tuberosity to trochlear groove (TT-TG) distance (> 20 mm) [4, 5] ($n = 4$), patella alta (Insall-Salvati [IS] ratio > 1.5) [27] ($n = 1$), and combined genu valgum deformity (criteria: > ± 3° mechanical femorotibial angle [MFTA] on anteroposterior long-leg weight-bearing lower-extremity scanographs) [28] ($n = 1$). Patellar height, TT-TG distance, and MFTA were preoperatively assessed by the same surgeon. Patients with a minimum postoperative follow-up of 2 years were considered eligible. Eventually, a total of 11 patients (12 knees) with RPD were treated using our approach of anatomic DB-MPFLR. The current study obtained institutional review board approval (GAIRB 2017–236) before the study onset, and informed consent was obtained from all patients. The patients' demographic data are presented in Table 1.

Surgical technique

Before RPD correction, diagnostic arthroscopic examination was performed in all patients. After the completion of arthroscopy, a 2-cm-long oblique incision was performed at the pes anserinus. After incising the sartorius aponeurosis, the semitendinous tendon was harvested and used as an autograft. The usable part of the tendon needed to be at least 20 cm long. After the tendon was harvested using a stripper and the muscle tissue was removed, the doubled tendon diameter was determined and both ends were whip stitched using an absorbable braided suture over a length of 15 mm. The graft was then folded in half, and its central portion was hanged

Table 1 Demographic Data on Patients

No	Sex/Age	Episode	Patellar position	F/u period (months)	MFTA (°)	TT-TG distance (mm)	IS Ratio[a]		ROM (°) [a]		pVAS score[a]		Kujala score[a]		Lysholm score[a]	
							Preop	Postop	Preop	Postop	Preop	Postop	Preop	Postop	Preop	Postop
1	F/18	2	SL	25	1.6	17.1	1.2	1.1	130	130	6	3	54	88	70	91
2	F/13	4	SL	26	0.6	11.2	1.4	1.0	135	140	4	0	62	94	65	99
3	M/14	3	SL	26	2.7	12.2	1.1	1.1	130	130	5	1	75	98	70	100
4	M/16	2	SL	25	−3.0	10.2	1.3	1.2	130	130	5	2	56	90	75	90
5	F/28	> 10	SL	24	1.1	16	1.0	0.9	120	125	7	2	56	84	74	85
6	F/16 (Lt)	2	SL	24	0.7	10.1	1.1	1.1	150	150	4	1	70	86	72	90
	(Rt)	2	SL	26	−1.7	15.4	1.2	1.0	140	140	4	1	72	86	70	90
7	M/22	2	SL	35	1.1	14.5	1.2	1.1	130	130	6	2	75	92	72	94
8	M/19	5	SL	34	3.0	19.9	1.0	1.0	130	130	4	3	80	98	76	100
9	F/26	4	SL	31	−2.7	13.1	1.4	1.3	135	130	5	0	63	93	76	100
10	M/18	2	SL	36	−3.0	18.2	1.1	1.0	120	125	3	1	75	95	70	95
11	F/18	2	SL	27	−0.2	16.2	1.3	1.3	135	135	3	0	70	80	70	85

IS Ratio Insall-Salvati ratio, *MFTA* mechanical femorotibial angle, *pVAS score* Visual analogue scale for the anterior knee pain, *ROM* range of motion, *SL* Subluxation, *TT-TG* tibial tuberosity to trochlear groove

[a]IS Ratio and clinical scores (Kujala, Lysholm, and pVAS score) were evaluated at preoperatively and postoperative 2-year follow-up

using the adjustable-length loop device (TightRope RT; Arthrex Inc., Naples, FL, USA). The diameter of all doubled tendons was 7 or 8 mm (Fig. 1).

Preparation for patellar fixation

A 2-cm incision was made at the medial border of the patella. The superomedial aspect of the patella was approached. To achieve aperture fixation on the patellar side, the free graft ends were directly fixed to the patella. A longitudinal periosteal incision was made about 1 cm lateral from the medial borderline of the patella, and the periosteum was detached and reflected medially. After the MPFL footprint was exposed, minimal decortication of the reconstruction area was performed for better bone-to-graft healing. Two guidewires were drilled tangentially into the patella at the proximal and distal ends of the medial edge, and 2 suture anchors (Bio Mini-Revo®; Linvatec, Largo, FL, USA) were inserted into the proximal margin and center of the medial aspect of the patella (Fig. 2). The free graft ends were sutured to the inserted grafts after flipping them over through the detached periosteum. Thereafter, the medial patellar periosteal tissue was sutured, covering the embedded graft and avoiding subcutaneous irritation by the knots.

Femoral tunneling and graft tensioning

In each femur, the femoral tunnel was made at the Schöttle point [29] in the proximal and anterior direction under C-arm guidance, in order to prevent iatrogenic peroneal nerve injury (Fig. 3a). Then, the tunnel was created to pass the button of the adjustable-length loop device, for which a 4.0-mm cannulated reamer was used. The length of the tunnel was measured using a depth gauge, and the femoral tunnel was drilled to have the same diameter as the graft until there was an 8-mm bone stock from the lateral femoral cortex (Fig. 3b). The graft was pulled into the femoral tunnel by using the lead suture inserted from the outside to the inside of the tunnel while maintaining equal tension on both bundles. The 2 strands of the graft passed between the first and second layers. The graft was fixed using the button of the device after it was flipped over the lateral cortex. After confirming that the button was on the cortex, manual traction of the suture loops was applied to fix the graft appropriately in full ROM of the knee joint with the lateral patellar edge positioned in line with the lateral trochlear border, under arthroscopic guidance (Fig. 4). The lateral retinaculum was released if the patient experienced lateral tightness. By using electrocautery under arthroscopic visualization, the capsular structure was released longitudinally along the lateral margin of the patella. The release was performed from 2 cm proximal to the superior patellar pole and extended distally for 1.5 to 2 cm.

Postoperative rehabilitation

Tolerable weight bearing was allowed and quadriceps setting exercises could be started immediately with free ROM, if tolerated. Running or cycling was permitted at 6 weeks after the operation; full activity was permitted at 3 months after the operation.

Outcome evaluation

Clinical outcomes related to recurrence of dislocation, apprehension test, ROM, clinical scores (Kujala score [30], Lysholm score [31], and visual analogue scale for anterior knee pain [pVAS]), complications, and radiological outcomes (congruence angle, lateral patellofemoral angle [32], and IS ratio) were assessed before and after the operation, and at the final 2-year follow-up.

Our primary outcomes of interest were radiographic parameters indicating patellar position, including congruence angle [2] and lateral patellofemoral angle [32]. The sulcus angle is the angle between a line between the lateral femoral condyle and intercondylar sulcus midpoint and a line between the medial femoral condyle and intercondylar sulcus midpoint. Each parameter was measured at 4 different angles of knee flexion (30°, 45°, 60°, and 90°).

Statistical considerations

Statistical tests were performed using IBM SPSS version 22 (IBM, Armonk, NY, USA). Continuous variables were described as mean ± standard deviation (SD). A priori power analysis was performed to determine the sample size with the 2-sided hypothesis test considering an α error of 0.05 and power of 0.90. The calculations involving our sample size of 11 patients indicated adequate power (0.85–0.95) to detect a significant difference of 5 degrees in

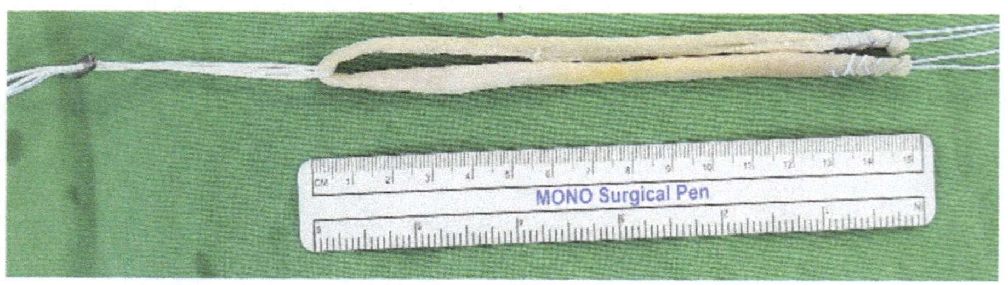

Fig. 1 Graft preparation

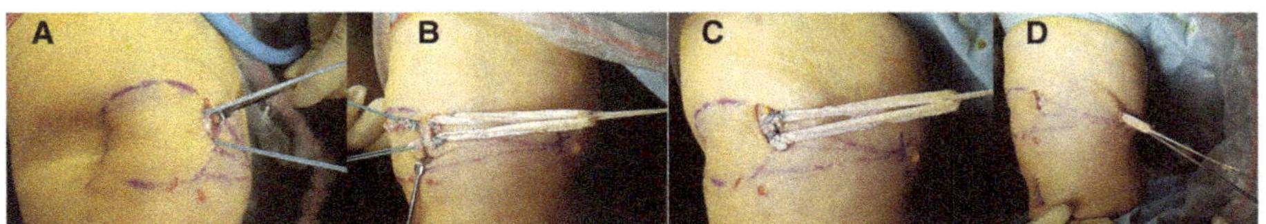

Fig. 2 A 2-cm longitudinal incision was made at the medial border of the patella. The deep fascia and periosteum were detached and reflected medially. After minimal decortication of the reconstruction area, 2 suture anchors were inserted into the proximal margin and center of the medial aspect of the patella (**a**). The free graft ends were sutured to the inserted grafts after flipping them over through the detached periosteum (**b** and **c**). Looped graft with the adjustable-length loop device at the ending was brought into the separated layer between the vastus medialis obliquus (VMO) and the joint capsule, using long curved Kelly with caution to avoid any injury to the joint (**d**)

the measurement outcomes of congruence angle and lateral patellofemoral angle in the present study. Wilcoxon signed-rank tests were used to compare the pVAS, Lysholm, and Kujala scores; IS ratio; congruence angle; and lateral patellofemoral and sulcus angles before and after the operation. A P-value of < 0.05 was considered statistically significant. The intra-class correlation coefficient (ICC) was determined to rule out observation bias between the 2 separate orthopedic surgeons. The parameters were measured twice, at an interval of 2 weeks.

Results

The patients' mean age at surgery was 18.6 ± 4.4 years (range: 13–28 years). The median follow-up period was 28.8 months (range: 24–48 months). The average value of the IS ratio was 1.2 (SD: 0.1) and the TT-TG distance was 14.5 cm (SD: 3.2). All measured ICCs were almost good to perfect, ranging from 0.726 to 0.991.

At the time of the final assessment, ROM was restored to the preoperative level and anterior knee pain improved in all patients, indicated by a decrease in the mean pVAS score from 4.7 ± 1.2 to 1.3 ± 1.1 ($P < 0.001$). No patients experienced surgical complications, including patellar fracture and re-dislocation. The patellar instability symptoms improved, as confirmed on the basis of the radiographic outcomes as well as the Lysholm and Kujala scores. The mean Lysholm score improved from 71.7 ± 3.2 preoperatively to 93.3 ± 5.6 postoperatively ($P < 0.001$), and the Kujala score improved from 67.3 ± 8.8 preoperatively to 90.3 ± 5.7 postoperatively ($P < 0.001$) (Table 1).

On merchant view with the patient supine, the knees flexed 30 degrees [33], the preoperative lateral patellofemoral angle (-7.6 ± 10.6 to 7.6 ± 3.1, $p < 0.001$) and congruence angle (30.1 ± 13.9 to 3.6 ± 1.5, $p < 0.001$) were improved after reconstruction. The congruence angle and the lateral patellofemoral angle were also improved significantly at 4 different flexion angles (30°, 45°, 60°, and 90°) of the knee joint ($p < 0.001$). The improvements in these angles were maintained with no significant differences at the 4 different flexion angles (Table 2) (Fig. 5). Analysis of the measured radiographic parameters showed that patellar height, determined from the IS ratio, decreased slightly from 1.2 ± 0.1 to 1.1 ± 0.1 after the operation ($P < 0.001$).

Discussion

The most important findings of the present study were that the aperture fixation technique using the adjustable-length loop device from femoral cortical suspension systems improved the alignment parameters (congruence angle and

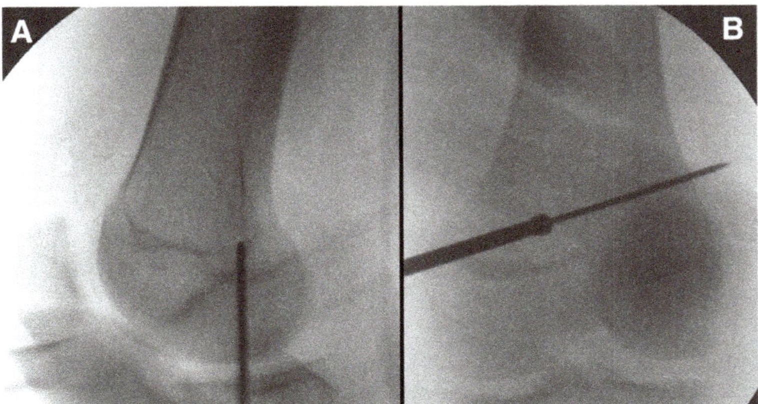

Fig. 3 A femoral tunnel was made at the Schöttle point [2] (**a**) in the proximal and anterior direction in order to prevent iatrogenic peroneal nerve injury. **b** Intraoperative control was achieved using an image intensifier

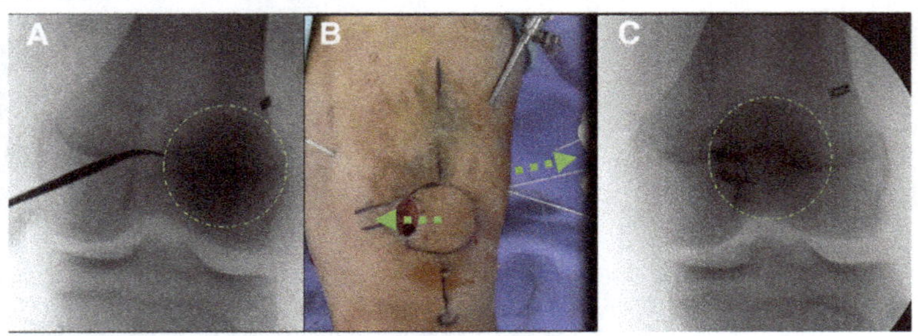

Fig. 4 The patellar position was tracked and fixed simultaneously by manual traction of the suture loops (**b**), and the graft was appropriately fixed in full range of motion of the knee joint with the lateral patellar edge positioned in line with the lateral trochlear border, under arthroscopic guidance (**a**, **c**)

Table 2 Preoperative, Immediate Postoperative, and Two-year Follow-Up Radiologic Parameters[a]

Knee flexion angle		Preop		Postop		F/U
Lateral patellofemoral angle (°)	30 °	−7.6 ± 10.6		7.6 ± 3.1		8.8 ± 4.1
			< 0.001		*0.260*	
	45 °	−6.2 ± 6.5		9.2 ± 0.4		10.4 ± 4.6
			0.001		*0.285*	
	60 °	−0.9 ± 5.6		11.0 ± 2.5		13.0 ± 3.2
			0.006		*0.140*	
	90 °	6.6 ± 3.4		12.2 ± 2.4		15.6 ± 3.2
			0.033		*0.093*	
Congruence angle (°)	30 °	30.1 ± 13.9		3.6 ± 1.5		2.9 ± 1.3
			< 0.001		*0.221*	
	45 °	26.1 ± 15.2		2.9 ± 1.0		2.7 ± 1.0
			0.001		*0.233*	
	60 °	18.4 ± 11.0		2.8 ± 1.6		2.7 ± 1.4
			0.014		*0.008*	
	90 °	11.5 ± 7.4		1.7 ± 1.1		1.7 ± 1.0
			0.010		*0.483*	
Sulcus angle (°)	30 °	146.9 ± 7.4		145.3 ± 6.4		145.4 ± 5.5
			0.491		*0.442*	
	45 °	146.6 ± 2.4		145.5 ± 1.7		146.0 ± 4.8
			0.549		*0.255*	
	60 °	146.1 ± 4.5		145.2 ± 5.9		146.5 ± 5.4
			0.870		*0.302*	
	90 °	146.4 ± 3.4		145.8 ± 5.5		144.8 ± 5.0
			0.634		*0.322*	
IS Ratio		1.2 ± 0.1				1.1 ± 0.1
				< 0.001		

IS Ratio Insall-Salvati ratio
[a]Value are mean ± standard deviation
P-value was expressed in Italic
Values of $P < 0.05$ are displayed in bold

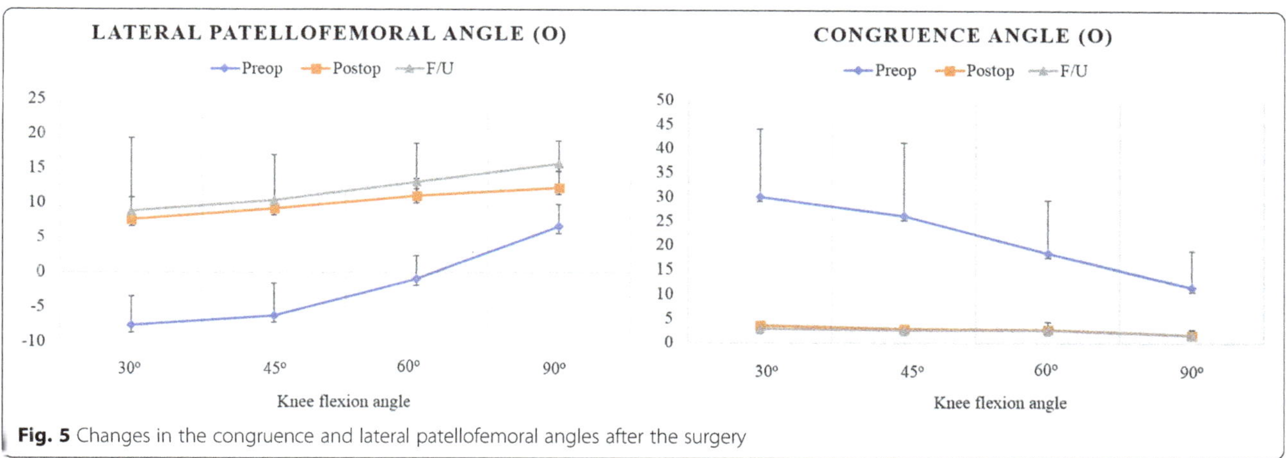

Fig. 5 Changes in the congruence and lateral patellofemoral angles after the surgery

patellar tilt angle) and yielded high stability in full ROM of the knee joint for 2 years after the operation.

Reconstruction techniques with the DB structure for restoring the anatomic shape of the MPFL have been recently highlighted [34, 35]. The MPFL is not a single-bundle structure but a complex of functionally varying fibers, some of which are taut and some are slack, throughout the range of knee motion [19]. Superior patellar fixation may cause patellar instability at mid to high knee angles, and conversely, inferior patellar fixation may produce excessive laxity at low flexion angles [19]. Anatomic DB-MPFLR lowers patellar rotation during the flexion-extension movement that may occur during single-bundle reconstruction.

Undoubtedly, the aperture fixation technique has clinical benefits in terms of the effort required to decrease the risk of delayed or insufficient tendon-to-bone healing [21, 24]. Schöttle et al. indicated that it provides high stability, as the proximal bundle seems to stabilize in extension while the distal bundle stabilizes in flexion.

However, as described in the Introduction, we hypothesized that certain reciprocal movement of the looped graft into the femoral tunnel may ensure more biocompatible reconstruction, rather than leaving the tension of each bundle to the discretion of the surgeon without a thorough understanding of the length change or the biomechanics of the 2 bundles of the MPFL throughout the range of knee motion. We did not directly evaluate the permissible amount of the reciprocal movement of the looped graft into the femoral tunnel. We sought to determine the clinical significance of the technique on the basis of our finding that improvements in radiographic parameters representing patellar position were noted irrespective of the angle of knee flexion (30°, 45°, 60°, or 90°). We also found that at the 2-year follow-up, no graft slackening, graft failure, or reduction failure from elongation of the graft or the "bungee" effect in the femoral socket had occurred in any case. However, it remains to be determined whether a kinematic isometric length change of about 6–9 mm throughout the range of knee motion [19] affects the radiological and clinical outcomes in clinical practice.

Other studies described several techniques for anatomic DB-MPFLR. White and Sherman [17] used an absorbable soft tissue interference screw for femoral fixation in 30° of knee flexion. Colvin and West [36] also used absorbable interference screws for femoral fixation of the 2 free ends of the graft in 30° of knee flexion, and performed combined bone groove and suture anchor fixation at the patella. Dejour et al. [37] used a "Y"-shaped graft for reconstruction. An absorbable soft tissue interference screw was used for femoral fixation, and the lateral bone bridge tie was used for patellar fixation. Additionally, they introduced the surgical technique of lateral retinaculum plasty to release eccentric dynamic loading through the ROM.

Graft fixation is recommended with appropriate tension at 20–30° of knee flexion and with the patella aligned in the trochlear groove throughout the entire ROM of the knee. However, it is not easy to determine the appropriate graft tension during graft fixation. Previous arbitrary techniques that rely on the surgeon's subjective skill carry the risk of over-tensioning of the MPFL graft, which can increase the patellofemoral pressure [38]. Goutallier et al. [39] reported that anterior knee pain persisted after the operation in up to 38–40% of patients. Our technique using the adjustable-length loop device has clinical applicability in this aspect. The patellar position, which can easily be determined under arthroscopic guidance throughout flexion, was tracked and fixed simultaneously by a simple pulling of the suture loops. Moreover, the possible reciprocal movement of the looped graft into the femoral tunnel might release eccentric loading through the ROM. It can also diminish the learning curve to achieve appropriate graft tensioning during MPFL reconstruction. In the present study, we found that anterior knee pain was relieved in all patients, the patients had full ROM immediately after the surgery, and there was no reduction loss at follow-up with early rehabilitation.

Our study has some inherent limitations because of its retrospective design. The relatively short follow-up period and small sample size were also limitations in judging the postoperative outcomes. However, a 2-year follow-up period is sufficient to determine clinical outcomes such as re-dislocation. Furthermore, a lack of comparison with other aperture techniques is a major limitation of the present study. In addition, this study did not directly compare the patellofemoral kinematic changes by using additional biomechanical measurement tools. Thus, the findings may not be adequate to determine the clinical relevance of using the adjustable-length loop device with regard to patellofemoral kinematics.

Conclusion

New DB technique with aperture fixation at the patella and femur by using an adjustable-length loop device offers high stability with full ROM of the knee joint, can be considered as a feasible procedure and technique for recurrent patellar dislocation.

Abbreviations

ACLR: Anterior cruciate ligament reconstruction; AP: Anteroposterior; DB-MPFLR: Double-bundle medial patellofemoral ligament reconstruction; ICC: Intra-class correlation coefficient; MFTA: Mechanical femorotibial angle; MPFL: Medial patellofemoral ligament; pVAS: Pain visual analogue scale; ROM: Range of motion; RPD: Recurrent patellar dislocation; SD: Standard deviation; TT-TG: Tibial tuberosity to trochlear groove

Acknowledgments

The authors thank all members of the Sports Medicine Center, Gil Hospital, for their great scientific debates.

Authors' contributions

JAS and BHL participated in the study design and helped in drafting the manuscript. BHL, as a statistical consultant, performed the statistical analysis. JAS and JKL conceived the study, participated in its design and coordination, and helped draft the manuscript. All authors participated in the development of and approved the final manuscript, and agreed to be accountable for the integrity of the content.

Consent for publication

Not applicable.

Competing interests

The authors declare that they have no competing interests.

Author details

[1]Department of Orthopaedic Surgery, Gil Hospital, Gachon University of Medicine and Science, Inchon, South Korea. [2]Department of Orthopedic Surgery, Kang-Dong Sacred Heart Hospital, Hallym University Medical School, 134-701, Gil-dong, Seoul, South Korea.

References

1. White BJ, Sherman OH. Patellofemoral instability. Bull NYU Hosp Jt Dis. 2009; 67:22-9.
2. Colvin AC, West RV. Patellar instability. J Bone Joint Surg Am. 2008;90:2751–62.
3. Dejour H, Walch G, Neyret P, Adeleine P: [dysplasia of the femoral trochlea]. Rev Chir Orthop Reparatrice Appar Mot 1990, 76:45–54.
4. Dejour H, Walch G, Nove-Josserand L, Guier C. Factors of patellar instability: an anatomic radiographic study. Knee Surg Sports Traumatol Arthrosc. 1994;2:19–26.
5. Goutallier D, Bernageau J, Lecudonnec B. the measurement of the tibial tuberosity. Patella groove distanced technique and results (author's transl). Rev Chir Orthop Reparatrice Appar Mot. 1978;64:423–8.
6. Geenen E, Molenaers G, Martens M. Patella alta in patellofemoral instability. Acta Orthop Belg. 1989;55:387–93.
7. Neyret P, Robinson AH, Le Coultre B, Lapra C, Chambat P. Patellar tendon length--the factor in patellar instability? Knee. 2002;9:3–6.
8. Simmons E Jr, Cameron JC. Patella Alta and recurrent dislocation of the patella. Clin Orthop Relat Res. 1992;(274):265–9.
9. Ward SR, Terk MR, Powers CM. Patella Alta: association with patellofemoral alignment and changes in contact area during weight-bearing. J Bone Joint Surg Am. 2007;89:1749–55.
10. Guerrero P, Li X, Patel K, Brown M, Busconi B. Medial patellofemoral ligament injury patterns and associated pathology in lateral patella dislocation: an MRI study. Sports Med Arthrosc Rehabil Ther Technol. 2009;1:17.
11. Conlan T, Garth WP,J, Lemons JE. Evaluation of the medial soft-tissue restraints of the extensor mechanism of the knee. J Bone Joint Surg Am. 1993;75:682–93.
12. Burks RT, Desio SM, Bachus KN, Tyson L, Springer K. Biomechanical evaluation of lateral patellar dislocations. Am J Knee Surg. 1998;11:24–31.
13. Buckens CF, Saris DB. Reconstruction of the medial patellofemoral ligament for treatment of patellofemoral instability: a systematic review. Am J Sports Med. 2010;38:181–8.
14. Christiansen SE, Jacobsen BW, Lund B, Lind M. Reconstruction of the medial patellofemoral ligament with gracilis tendon autograft in transverse patellar drill holes. Arthroscopy. 2008;24:82–7.
15. Han H, Xia Y, Yun X, Wu M. Anatomical transverse patella double tunnel reconstruction of medial patellofemoral ligament with a hamstring tendon autograft for recurrent patellar dislocation. Arch Orthop Trauma Surg. 2011;131:343–51.
16. Panni AS, Alam M, Cerciello S, Vasso M, Maffulli N. Medial patellofemoral ligament reconstruction with a divergent patellar transverse 2-tunnel technique. Am J Sports Med. 2011;39:2647–55.
17. Schottle PB, Fucentese SF, Romero J. Clinical and radiological outcome of medial patellofemoral ligament reconstruction with a semitendinosus autograft for patella instability. Knee Surg Sports Traumatol Arthrosc. 2005;13:516–21.
18. Amis AA, Firer P, Mountney J, Senavongse W, Thomas NP. Anatomy and biomechanics of the medial patellofemoral ligament. Knee. 2003;10:215–20.
19. Song SY, Pang CH, Kim CH, Kim J, Choi ML, Seo YJ. Length change behavior of virtual medial patellofemoral ligament fibers during in vivo knee flexion. Am J Sports Med. 2015;43:1165–71.
20. Wang JH, Kato Y, Ingham SJ, Maeyama A, Linde-Rosen M, Smolinski P, Fu FH. Measurement of the end-to-end distances between the femoral and tibial insertion sites of the anterior cruciate ligament during knee flexion and with rotational torque. Arthroscopy. 2012;28:1524–32.
21. Schottle PB, Schmeling A, Rosenstiel N, Weiler A. Radiographic landmarks for femoral tunnel placement in medial patellofemoral ligament reconstruction. Am J Sports Med. 2007;35:801–4.
22. Brand J Jr, Weiler A, Caborn DN, Brown CH Jr, Johnson DL. Graft fixation in cruciate ligament reconstruction. Am J Sports Med. 2000;28:761–74.
23. Steensen RN, Dopirak RM, WG MD 3rd. The anatomy and isometry of the medial patellofemoral ligament: implications for reconstruction. Am J Sports Med. 2004;32:1509–13.
24. Li J, Li Y, Wei J, Wang J, Gao S, Shen Y. A simple technique for reconstruction of medial patellofemoral ligament with bone-fascia tunnel fixation at the medial margin of the patella: a 6-year-minimum follow-up study. J Orthop Surg Res. 2014;9:66.
25. Lubowitz JH, Schwartzberg R, Smith P. Cortical suspensory button versus aperture interference screw fixation for knee anterior cruciate ligament soft-tissue allograft: a prospective, randomized controlled trial. Arthroscopy. 2015;31:1733–9.

26. Dejour D, Le Coultre B. Osteotomies in patello-femoral instabilities. Sports Med Arthrosc. 2007;15:39–46.
27. Shabshin N, Schweitzer ME, Morrison WB, Parker L. MRI criteria for patella Alta and Baja. Skelet Radiol. 2004;33:445–50.
28. Haviv B, Bronak S, Thein R, Thein R. The results of corrective osteotomy for valgus arthritic knees. Knee Surg Sports Traumatol Arthrosc. 2013;21:49–56.
29. Barnett AJ, Howells NR, Burston BJ, Ansari A, Clark D, Eldridge JD. Radiographic landmarks for tunnel placement in reconstruction of the medial patellofemoral ligament. Knee Surg Sports Traumatol Arthrosc. 2012;20:2380–4.
30. Kujala UM, Jaakkola LH, Koskinen SK, Taimela S, Hurme M, Nelimarkka O. Scoring of patellofemoral disorders. Arthroscopy. 1993;9:159–63.
31. Tegner Y, Lysholm J. Rating systems in the evaluation of knee ligament injuries. Clin Orthop Relat Res. 1985;(198):43–9.
32. Lee CH, Wu CC, Pan RY, Lu HT, Shen HC. Medial retinacular flap advancement and arthroscopic lateral release for symptomatic chronic patellar lateral subluxation with tilting. Knee Surg Sports Traumatol Arthrosc. 2014;22:2499–504.
33. Laurin CA, Levesque HP, Dussault R, Labelle H, Peides JP. The abnormal lateral patellofemoral angle: a diagnostic roentgenographic sign of recurrent patellar subluxation. J Bone Joint Surg Am. 1978;60:55–60.
34. Schottle PB, Romero J, Schmeling A, Weiler A. Technical note: anatomical reconstruction of the medial patellofemoral ligament using a free gracilis autograft. Arch Orthop Trauma Surg. 2008;128:479–84.
35. Thaunat M, Erasmus PJ. The favourable anisometry: an original concept for medial patellofemoral ligament reconstruction. Knee. 2007;14:424–8.
36. Wang HD, Dong JT, Gao SJ. Medial patellofemoral ligament reconstruction using a bone groove and a suture anchor at patellar: a safe and firm fixation technique and 3-year follow-up study. J Orthop Surg Res. 2016;11:138.
37. Niu Y, Wang X, Liu C, Wang X, Dong Z, Niu J, Wang F. Double-bundle anatomical medial patellofemoral ligament reconstruction with lateral retinaculum plasty can lead to good outcomes in patients with patellar dislocation. Knee Surg Sports Traumatol Arthrosc. 2017.
38. Stephen JM, Lumpaopong P, Dodds AL, Williams A, Amis AA. The effect of tibial tuberosity medialization and lateralization on patellofemoral joint kinematics, contact mechanics, and stability. Am J Sports Med. 2015;43:186–94.
39. Feller JA, Richmond AK, Wasiak J. Medial patellofemoral ligament reconstruction as an isolated or combined procedure for recurrent patellar instability. Knee Surg Sports Traumatol Arthrosc. 2014;22:2470–6.

Effects of mesenchymal stromal cells versus serum on tendon healing in a controlled experimental trial in an equine model

A. B. Ahrberg[1,2*†], C. Horstmeier[2,3,4†], D. Berner[5], W. Brehm[2,3,4], C. Gittel[4], A. Hillmann[2,3], C. Josten[1], G. Rossi[6], S. Schubert[2,3,7], K. Winter[4,8] and J. Burk[2,3,7,9]

Abstract

Background: Mesenchymal stromal cells (MSC) have shown promising results in the treatment of tendinopathy in equine medicine, making this therapeutic approach seem favorable for translation to human medicine. Having demonstrated that MSC engraft within the tendon lesions after local injection in an equine model, we hypothesized that they would improve tendon healing superior to serum injection alone.

Methods: Quadrilateral tendon lesions were induced in six horses by mechanical tissue disruption combined with collagenase application 3 weeks before treatment. Adipose-derived MSC suspended in serum or serum alone were then injected intralesionally. Clinical examinations, ultrasound and magnetic resonance imaging were performed over 24 weeks. Tendon biopsies for histological assessment were taken from the hindlimbs 3 weeks after treatment. Horses were sacrificed after 24 weeks and forelimb tendons were subjected to macroscopic and histological examination as well as analysis of musculoskeletal marker expression.

Results: Tendons injected with MSC showed a transient increase in inflammation and lesion size, as indicated by clinical and imaging parameters between week 3 and 6 ($p < 0.05$). Thereafter, symptoms decreased in both groups and, except that in MSC-treated tendons, mean lesion signal intensity as seen in T2w magnetic resonance imaging and cellularity as seen in the histology ($p < 0.05$) were lower, no major differences could be found at week 24.

Conclusions: These data suggest that MSC have influenced the inflammatory reaction in a way not described in tendinopathy studies before. However, at the endpoint of the current study, 24 weeks after treatment, no distinct improvement was observed in MSC-treated tendons compared to the serum-injected controls. Future studies are necessary to elucidate whether and under which conditions MSC are beneficial for tendon healing before translation into human medicine.

Keywords: MSC, Serum, Animal model, Tendon, Horse

Background

In orthopedic surgery and sports medicine, tendinopathy has become one of the most challenging conditions. Achilles tendinopathy, for example, is a growing problem with a high incidence [1]. Various therapies have been tried without lasting success [2–8]. This underlines the need for a new curative therapy from the field of regenerative medicine. The horse, which could be referred to as animal athlete, suffers from a natural tendinopathy in its superficial digital flexor tendon (SDFT) which is similar to the Achilles tendon in its structure, function and pathophysiology [9–12]. Therefore, horses are considered as highly suitable model animals for orthopedic research and have been recommended by authorities such as the U.S. Food and Drug Administration (FDA) and the European Medicines Agency (EMA) [13, 14]. Contrary to human medicine, regenerative cell therapies have already been used in equine medicine for more than a decade, with most

* Correspondence: annette.ahrberg@medizin.uni-leipzig.de
†A. B. Ahrberg and C. Horstmeier contributed equally to this work.
[1]Department of Orthopedics, Traumatology and Plastic Surgery, University of Leipzig, Liebigstr. 20, 04103 Leipzig, Germany
[2]Translational Center for Regenerative Medicine (TRM), University of Leipzig, Leipzig, Germany
Full list of author information is available at the end of the article

experiences in multipotent mesenchymal stromal cells (MSC) therapy for tendon disease [15]. Clinical results are promising, although the mechanisms of action leading to improved tendon healing are not yet fully understood [11, 16, 17].

MSC are adult progenitor cells displaying plastic-adherence and multipotent differentiation potential in vitro and can be further characterized by a set of surface marker antigens [18]. They can be extracted from various tissues, e.G. adipose tissue or bone marrow and are thought to support tissue regeneration not only by cell replacement, but also via trophic and modulatory effects which are mediated by cell-cell contact or paracrine mechanisms [19–21].

The promising results of MSC therapy in equine patients make a translation into human medicine appear reasonable. Recently we were able to show that adipose-derived MSC engrafted within tendon lesions after local injection in an equine model although there was also systemic distribution of a small number of cells [22]. These results were obtained on the basis of labeling the MSC with superparamagnetic iron oxide (SPIO) and rhodamine. After demonstrating long-term MSC persistence we aimed to evaluate the effect of these MSC on tendon healing within the same set of animals as presented in the current study. We hypothesized that local injection of adipose-derived MSC improves outcome parameters obtained by clinical imaging and histological assessment as well as gene expression analysis over a follow-up period of 24 weeks.

Methods

Study design

Tendinopathy of the SDFT was induced in all limbs of 6 horses and autologous adipose tissue was harvested (week − 3). MSC were expanded and labeled with SPIO. MSC resuspended in serum or serum alone were injected into the left and right tendon lesions 3 weeks after their induction (week 0). Clinical examinations and diagnostic imaging were performed over 24 weeks (week 0, 1, 2, 3, 4, 6, 8, 12 and 24). Tendon biopsies were taken after 3 weeks from the hindlimb SDFT for early histological evaluation (week 3). After euthanasia at week 24, forelimb SDFT were harvested for macroscopic and late histological evaluation and for analysis of musculoskeletal marker expression. Approval of the local ethics committee (TVV 34/13) had been given beforehand.

Animals

Six horses (standardbred; mean age: 6 years; age range: 3–10 years; 3 female, 3 male; body weight: 400–550 kg) were included in the study. The horses were obtained from trot racing courts in accordance with the local authority. Clinical evaluation, ultrasound (US) and Magnetic Resonance Imaging (MRI) of all extremities were performed prior to the first surgery to ensure the animals were healthy. The horses were housed in the hospital's stables. All procedures were performed within the facility, so no transport of the horses was needed.

Induction of tendinopathy and adipose tissue collection

Tendinopathy was induced by minor mechanical tissue disruption combined with a low-dose injection of collagenase type I (4.8 mg/mL, Life Technologies GmbH, Darmstadt, Germany) in the SDFT of all 4 extremities under general anesthesia (week − 3). With the horse placed in lateral position, the skin was clipped and prepared aseptically. An 11-gauge bone marrow aspiration needle was introduced into the SDFT in the middle of the metatarsal/metacarpal region via a skin incision. 0.4 mL collagenase type I (250 IU per tendon lesion) were injected while removing the needle from 2 cm proximal to 1 cm proximal from its entry point without further damage of the epitenon. The incisions in the peritendineum and skin were closed by suture and a dressing was applied. Subcutaneous adipose tissue was obtained from the supragluteal region of the horse in the same surgery. The same orthopedic surgeon performed all surgeries.

Post-surgery regime

After induction of tendinopathy, horses were restricted to stall rest for 5 weeks (2 weeks after MSC injection) and then managed according to the rehabilitation protocol previously described [23].

The horses were checked 3 times a day using standardized pain scores until 10 days post-surgery. For pain relief, they received flunixin-meglumine (CP-Pharma Handelsgesellschaft mbH, Burgdorf, Germany), 1.1 mg/kg bwt twice daily on the day of surgery and 0.55 mg/kg bwt twice daily on day 1 to 4 post surgery, followed by 0.55 mg/kg once daily on day 5 and 6, as well as additional single 1.1 mg/kg bwt doses when required according to pain scoring results.

Cell isolation and injection

The adipose tissue was subjected to cell isolation by collagenase digestion and plastic-adherent cells were isolated and expanded as described previously [24]. The cells were cultivated in a standard culture medium with Dulbecco's Modified Eagle's Medium (DMEM, Life Technologies GmbH, Darmstadt, Germany), 20% Fetal Bovine Serum (FBS, Sigma-Aldrich Chemie GmbH, Steinheim, Germany), 1% Penicillin (10.000 IE/ml)/Streptomycin (10.000 μg/ml, Life Technologies GmbH, Darmstadt, Germany) and 0,1% Gentamicin (50 mg/ml, Life Technologies GmbH, Darmstadt, Germany). At passage 2 and 80% confluency, MSC were labeled with SPIO particles (Molday ION Rhodamine B™, BioPAL, Inc.™, Worcester, MA, USA) at 25 μg Fe per ml for 20 h and harvested. Part of the cells from each animal was used to confirm MSC characteristics such as trilineage differentiation and expression of CD29, CD44, CD90 and CD105 as described before [24, 25].

Three weeks after lesion induction (week 0), the freshly harvested and labeled MSC were injected into the lesions under ultrasonographic guidance. Horses were sedated and received an ulnar nerve block (forelimbs) or a high plantar nerve block (hindlimbs) with additional local anesthesia (Lidocain 2%, bela-pharm GmbH & Ko. KG, Vechta, Germany). With the horses standing, the skin was clipped and prepared aseptically. In a randomized manner, one hindlimb and one forelimb were injected with MSC (10^7 cells in 1 ml autologous serum) and the contralateral side with 1 ml autologous serum. All injections were performed in a standardized procedure by the same veterinary surgeon blinded to the content of the syringes.

Clinical and imaging evaluation

Two veterinarians blinded for the treatment performed all examinations in a standardized procedure.

Clinical parameters comprised a palpation score and a lameness score. The palpation score included diffuse and local swelling, heat and pain to palpation, the total score points ranging from 4 (normal) to 16 (severe). The lameness score included weight bearing/lameness when standing, walking, trotting, and turning, the total score points ranging from 7 (normal) to 29 (severe).

Ultrasonographic examinations of the SDFT were performed using a 10 MHz linear transducer (LOGIQ 5 Expert, GE Healthcare, Munich, Germany) with a standoff probe. The SDFT was divided into zones and at least one transverse and one longitudinal image was recorded at every level [26]. Echogenicity of the lesion, peritendinous edema and fiber pattern were evaluated for each zone by 2 blinded observers in consensus, using a semi quantitative score [27]. Furthermore, the cross-sectional areas of the tendon lesion and the whole tendon were measured in each transverse image and used to calculate the percentage of the tendon lesion.

MRI of the SDFT region was performed in the standing sedated horse using a 0.27 Tesla dedicated equine low-field MRI system (Hallmarq EQ2, Hallmarq Veterinary Imaging, Guildford, Surrey, UK). T2-weighted (T2w) fast spin echo sequences acquired in transverse plane at weeks 0, 3, 12 and 24 were used to determine lesion signal and lesion areas. Lesion volume was approximated by multiplying the sum of the lesion areas in all images by 6 mm (5 mm slice thickness + 1 mm gap). Image processing was performed using Mathematica (Wolfram Research, Inc., Mathematica, Version 10.3.0.0, Champaign, IL). Tendon regions were manually drawn onto the images and converted into binary image masks. Background-corrected MRI images were segmented, and segmentations were multiplied with the corresponding binary image masks to detect lesion areas within the tendons. Positive regions in the resulting binary images were smoothed and final binary lesion masks were obtained. Grayscale values for tendon and lesion regions were extracted from the background-corrected images using the generated masks.

For all parameters obtained from ultrasonographic images as well as lesion signal intensity obtained from MRI images, mean values of images obtained from the different tendon levels were calculated and used for further analysis, in order to account for the proximo-distal dimensions of the lesions.

Collection of tendon samples

Three weeks after MSC injection, tendon biopsies of the maximum lesion, which had been identified by MRI before, were taken from the hindlimbs under general anesthesia. The tendon was approached via a skin incision of 3 cm and 0.2 × 0.3 × 2 cm tendon tissue was collected and fixed in paraformaldehyde (Carl Roth, Karlsruhe, Germany) for histological examination. Tendon, peritendineum, subcutis and skin were sutured, and dressings were applied. Post-operative management and pain medication were performed as described above. After taking this biopsy, the hindlimbs were excluded from all further assessments.

24 weeks after MSC injection, the animals were euthanized in general anesthesia using Romifidin 0,06 mg/kg bwt i.v. (Sedivet®, 10 mg/ml, Boehringer Ingelheim Vetmedica GmbH, Ingelheim am Rhein, Germany) and Butorphanol 0,03 mg/kg bwt i.v (Alvegesic®, 10 mg/ml, CP-Pharma Handelsgesellschaft mbH, Burgdorf, Germany) for sedation, Diazepam 0,08 mg/kg bwt i.v. (Diazepam-® Lipuro, 5 mg/ml, B. Braun Melsungen AG, Melsungen, Germany) and Ketamin 2,2 mg/kg bwt i.v (Ursotamin®, 100 mg/ml, Serumwerk Bernburg AG, Bernburg, Germany) for the induction of anesthesia and T61® 6 ml/50 kg bwt i.v. (Intervet Deutschland GmbH, Unterschleißheim, Germany) for euthanasia. The whole metacarpal region of both forelimb SDFT was collected. First, macroscopic evaluation was performed, at which all parameters (swelling, edema, adhesions, redness) were summarized in a score ranging from 0 (normal) to 15 (severe). Afterwards, the tendons were sectioned into 2 cm long pieces, of which the lateral part was fixed in paraformaldehyde for histological examination and the medial part was frozen for gene expression analysis.

Histology

For histological examination, 3 μm paraffin sections were prepared from the hindlimb biopsies and from the forelimb tendons, stained and assessed as described below. Regarding the forelimb tendons, unless stated otherwise, mean values were calculated from all dissected tendon pieces, representing the whole metacarpal region including proximal and distal healthy areas, for further analysis.

The parameters evaluated in hematoxylin-eosin (HE) staining were polymorphonuclear leukocytes, lymphocytes, macrophages, perivasculitis, necrosis, edema, calcification, collagen disposition, fibrinosis and fiber organization. The microscopic assessment was done by a blinded veterinary pathologist, the score ranging from 0 (normal) to 30 (severe) as described before [28].

Masson's Trichrome staining was used for evaluation of the percentage of Fuchsin staining corresponding to uninjured or regenerated tendon regions [29]. The percentages of Fuchsin-stained red areas were measured based on whole slide scans obtained in a slide scanner (Pannoramic SCAN, 3DHISTECH, Budapest, Hungary). Red and blue color channels were extracted from the acquired images and respective stained regions were segmented by the Kittler-Illingworth minimum error thresholding method using Mathematica software [30].

Picrosirius red staining and polarized light microscopy were used to assess the occurrence of crimp. Three images from randomly chosen fields of view were obtained per slide using a 10× objective (Olympus BX41 Laboratory microscope equipped with a U-pot drop in polarizer; Olympus GmbH, Hamburg, Germany). The percentages of large crimp (> 15 μm distance) representing healthy, mature crimp, or small and no crimp (< 15 μm distance) representing immature or missing crimp were measured manually by 2 blinded investigators using ImageJ open source software.

DAPI (4′,6-diamidino-2-phenylindole, Carl Roth GmbH + Co. KG, Karlsruhe, Germany) nuclear staining was used to evaluate cellularity based on the nucleated cell fraction. Whole slide scans from the maximum lesion levels were obtained in the slide scanner evaluated in analogy to the Masson's Trichrome stained slides. The occurrence of nucleated cells represented by the percentage of blue staining (DAPI filter channel) was determined relative to the total area of each section. Similarly, as an indicator for vascularization, the occurrence of erythrocytes was calculated as the percentage of red fluorescence (Rhodamine filter channel), representing erythrocyte autofluorescence, per total section area.

Collagen I immunohistochemical staining was performed on representative sections from the proximal lesion, maximum lesion, and distal lesion for each forelimb tendon and one section of each hindlimb biopsy. Staining was done with anti-collagen I antibody (rabbit polyclonal, Abcam, Cambridge, UK) and a detection kit (EXPOSE Mouse and Rabbit Specific AP, Abcam) according to the manufacturer's instructions. Two blinded investigators evaluated the absence or presence of collagen I with 0 representing absence, 1 representing mild and 2 representing marked presence of immunostaining.

Musculoskeletal marker expression

Musculoskeletal marker expression was analyzed by real-time reverse-transcription polymerase chain reaction (RT-PCR) in each forelimb tendon sample piece.

Table 1 Primers used for RT-PCR analysis of musculoskeletal marker expression

Gene	Primer pair sequences	GenBank accession number	PCR product in bp
ACTB	For: ATCCACGAAACTACCTTCAAC	NM_001081838.1	174
	Rev: CGCAATGATCTTGATCTTCATC		
GAPDH	For: TGGAGAAAGCTGCCAAATACG	NM_001163856.1	309
	Rev: GGCCTTTCTCCTTCTCTTGC		
Collagen 1A2	For: CAACCGGAGATAGAGGACCA	XM_001492939.1	243
	Rev: CAGGTCCTTGGAAACCTTGA		
Collagen 2A1	For: ATTGTAGGACCCAAAGGACC	XM_001496152	199
	Rev: CAGCAAAGTTTCCACCAAGG		
Collagen 3A1	For: AGGGGACCTGGTTACTGCTT	XM_001917620.2	216
	Rev: TCTCTGGGTTGGGACAGTCT		
Decorin	For: ACCCACTGAAGAGCTCAGGA	NM_001081925.2	239
	Rev: GCCATTGTCAACAGCAGAGA		
Tenascin-C	For: CTAGAGTGTCTCACTATCAGG	XM_001916622.2	163
	Rev: CTAGAGTGTCTCACTATCAGG		
Scleraxis	For: TACCTGGGTTTTCTTCTGGTCACT	NM_001105150.1	51
	Rev: TATCAAAGACACAAGATGCCAGC		
Osteopontin	For: TGAAGACCAGTATCCTGATGC	XM_001496152	158
	Rev: GCTGACTTGTTTCCTGACTG		

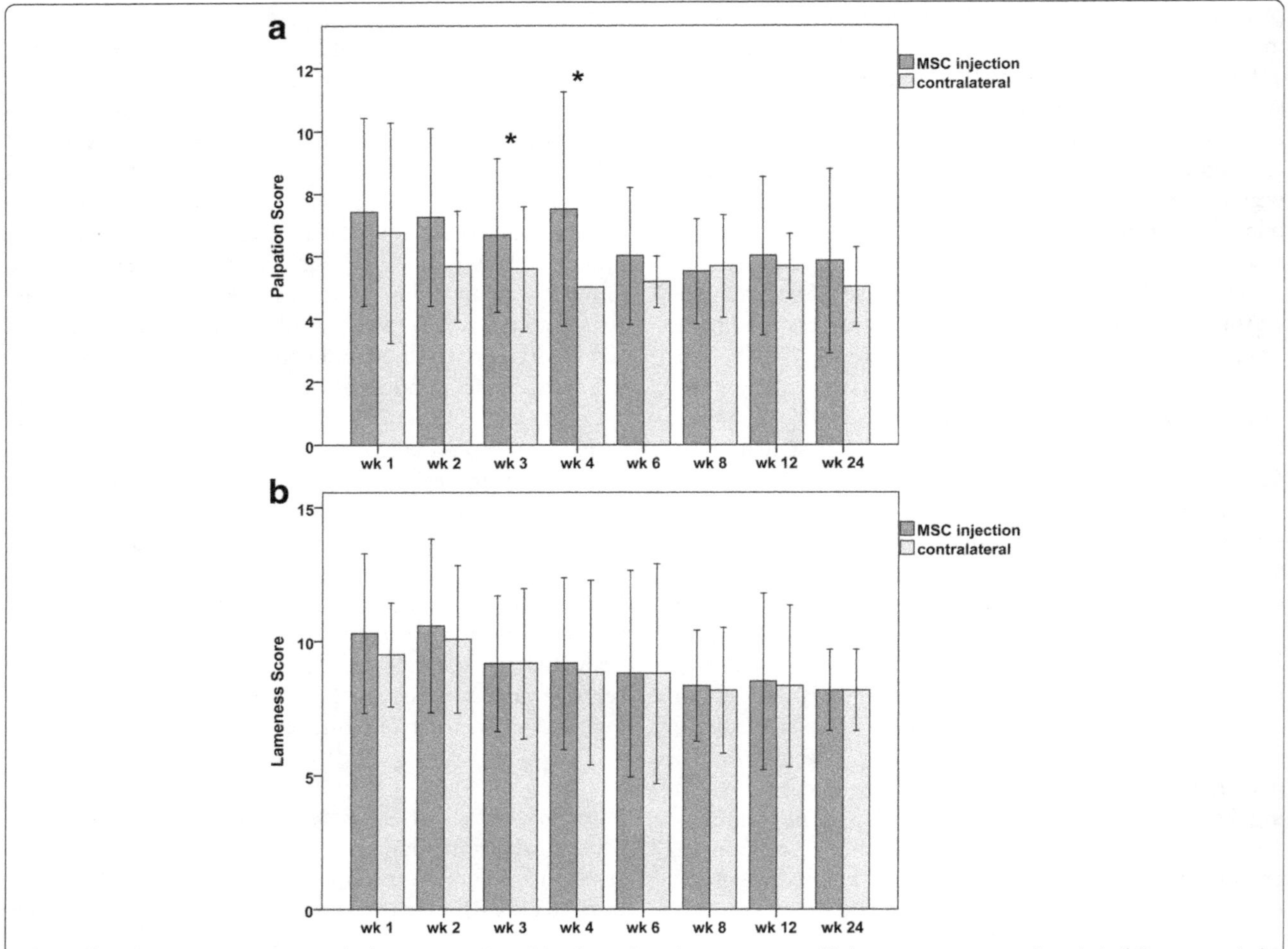

Fig. 1 Clinical parameters: Diagrams displaying mean (± 2 SD) values of **a** palpation score and **b** lameness score over the whole follow-up period; stars indicate significant differences between MSC-injected and contralateral tendons ($p < 0.05$); wk.: week post MSC injection

Mean values, representing the whole metacarpal region of the tendon, were used for further analysis.

Frozen tendon samples were homogenized, and total RNA was isolated, purified and transcribed into cDNA using the RevertAid H Minus First Strand cDNA Synthesis Kit (Thermo Fisher Scientific). RT-PCR was performed with a 7500 Real Time PCR System (Applied Biosystems, Foster City, USA) as described previously [31]. Primers used are listed in Table 1, ACTB and GAPDH were used as housekeeping genes for relative quantification [32].

Statistical analysis

Using SPSS 20 statistics software (IBM, Ehningen, Germany), Shapiro-Wilk tests were executed to test the hypothesis of normal distribution of data. If this hypothesis was not rejected, paired t-tests were performed to compare MSC-treated tendons with the contralateral controls, otherwise Wilcoxon-tests were performed. *P*-values < 0.05 were considered significant.

Results

Clinical and imaging results

Induction of tendon lesions was demonstrable in all tendons. No significant differences between the left and right tendons were observed prior to cell injection, neither clinically nor in imaging. The procedures, including the recovery from tendon biopsies, were tolerated well using the medication described above.

During the first 2 weeks after cell injection, no significant differences could be detected between the two groups. However, there was a tendency that the MSC-injected tendons showed prolonged clinical signs of inflammation including swelling, heat, and pain. This became manifest in the palpation scores, which remained higher in the MSC group until week 6, with the difference being significant at weeks 3 ($p = 0.015$) and 4 ($p = 0.022$) (Fig. 1). Correspondingly, as seen in ultrasonography, in the MSC group, the cross-sectional area of the tendon was higher at weeks 3 ($p = 0.016$) and 4 ($p = 0.022$), the percentage of the tendon lesion was

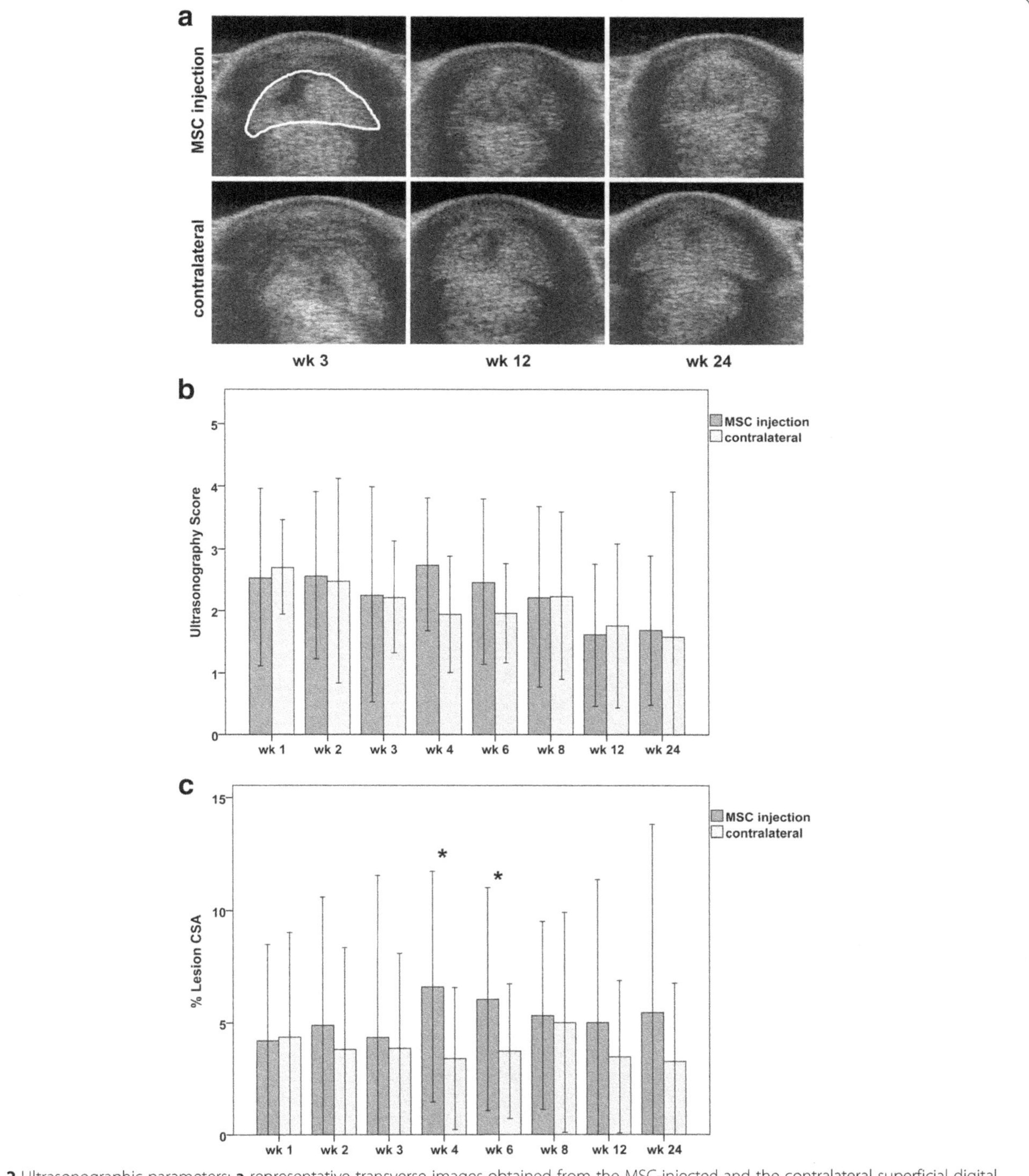

Fig. 2 Ultrasonographic parameters: **a** representative transverse images obtained from the MSC-injected and the contralateral superficial digital flexor tendons 3, 12 and 24 weeks after MSC injection; the respective tendon is indicated by the white line in the first upper image; note the hypoechoic (dark) lesions within the tendons, which are decreasing over time. Diagrams displaying mean (± 2 SD) values of **b** ultrasonography score and **c** percentage of the lesion within the cross-sectional area (CSA) of the tendon over the whole follow-up period; stars indicate significant differences between MSC-injected and contralateral tendons ($p < 0.05$); wk.: week post MSC injection

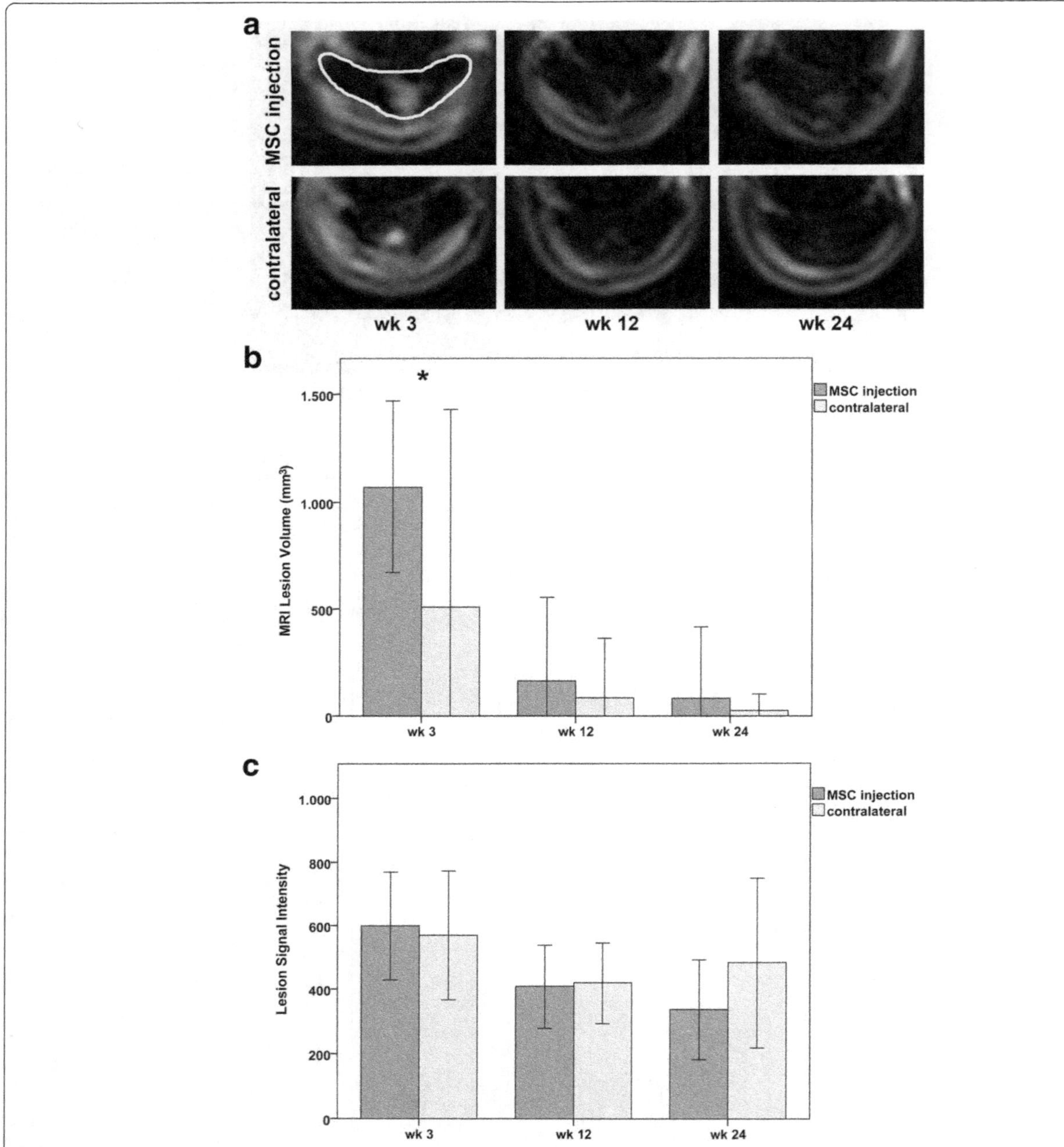

Fig. 3 Magnetic resonance imaging parameters: **a** representative transverse T2-weighted images obtained from the MSC-injected and the contralateral superficial digital flexor tendons 3, 12 and 24 weeks after MSC injection; the respective tendon is indicated by the white line in the first upper image; note the lesions within the tendons, displaying high signal intensity at week 3, which is decreasing over time. Diagrams displaying mean (± 2 SD) values of **b** lesion volume determined based on MRI images in mm^3 and **c** lesion signal intensity obtained from MRI images; star indicates significant difference between MSC-injected and contralateral tendons ($p < 0.05$); wk.: week post MSC injection; at week 24, instead of $n = 6$ tendons per group, only 2 tendons are shown in the MSC group and 3 in the contralateral control group, due to the fact that the remaining lesions were not detected anymore

higher at weeks 4 ($p = 0.042$) and 6 ($p = 0.039$), and the mean ultrasonography scores were higher at weeks 4 and 6, although the latter was not significant (Fig. 2). In MRI, lesion volume at week 3 was higher in the MSC group ($p = 0.02$) (Fig. 3).

However, after the first weeks, the clinical and imaging findings improved and were more similar in both groups. At week 24, based on the T2-weighted MRI image series, the tendon lesions had resolved in 4 out of 6 cases in the MSC group and in 3 out of 6 cases in

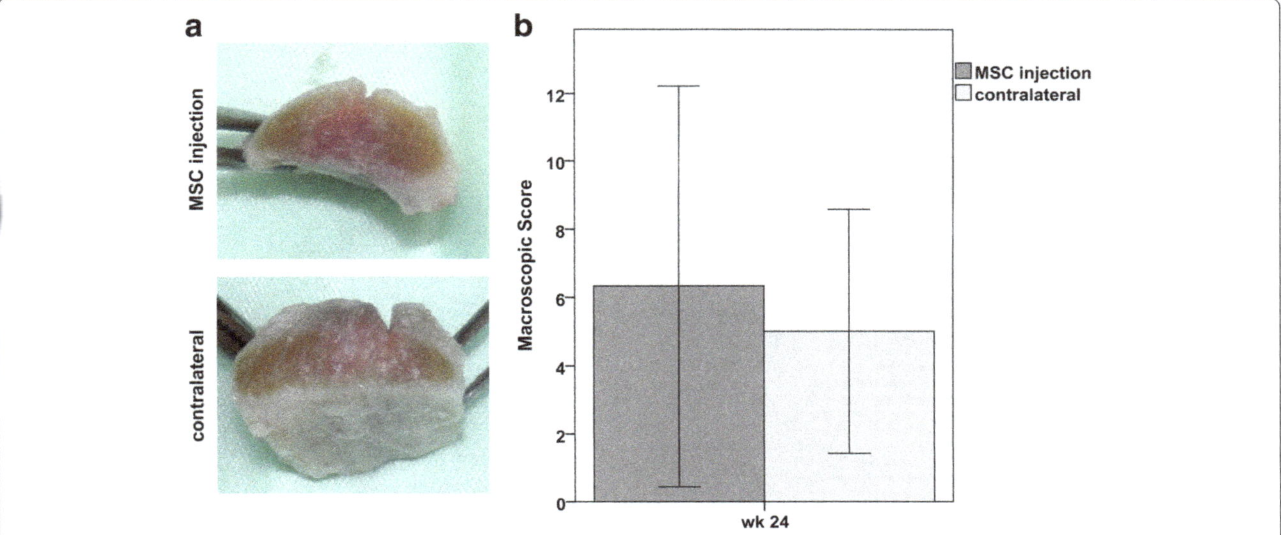

Fig. 4 Macroscopic parameters: **a** representative images of the dissected superficial digital flexor tendons at maximum lesion level, displaying reddish and whitish injured areas within the tendon cross-section and **b** diagram displaying mean (± 2 SD) values of score points obtained at macroscopic assessment; wk.: week post MSC injection

the control group. In the remaining lesions, the mean lesion signal intensity was lower in the MSC group, suggesting better tendon healing. Further clinical or imaging parameters did not indicate improvement compared to the controls. Correspondingly, macroscopic assessment after euthanasia did not reveal any significant differences (Fig. 4).

Histology

Histologic findings largely reflected the clinical and imaging findings.

At week 3, hindlimb biopsies displayed a more frequent occurrence of macrophages and perivasculitis, resulting in a higher HE score, a lower percentage of healthy crimp and a higher percentage of erythrocytes in the MSC group, suggesting increased inflammation and vascularization. However, these differences were not significant, and the percentage of Fuchsin staining, the percentage of nuclei as well as collagen I immunostaining were similar in both groups (Fig. 5).

At week 24, such differences did not exist anymore, most stainings and parameters assessed being similar in both groups (Fig. 6). However, the percentage of nuclei was lower in the MSC group ($p = 0.022$), reflecting lower cellularity (Fig. 5).

Musculoskeletal marker expression

All tendon markers including collagen 1A2, collagen 3A1, decorin, tenascin-C and scleraxis, as well as the putative early osteogenic marker osteopontin, were expressed at detectable but variable levels (Fig. 7). Collagen 2A1 was not expressed at detectable levels. No significant differences could be observed between both groups.

Discussion

Only few differences in tendon healing could be found between MSC and control group at week 24. Differences included that lesion resolution, as seen in T2w MRI, was more advanced and cellularity was lower in MSC-treated tendons at week 24. Furthermore, a transient increase in inflammatory reaction and lesion size was observed in the MSC-treated tendons during the first weeks. However, at week 24, clinical parameters, ultrasound, macroscopic and histological scores as well as musculoskeletal marker expression were not different between treated and control tendons. Based on the fact that MSC had engrafted within the tendon lesions [22] and having designed this study with a relatively long follow-up of 24 weeks, more significant differences between the two groups had been expected based on the previous literature. Yet, the current data fail to provide distinctive evidence to support the hypothesis that MSC improve tendon healing.

The therapeutic approach pursued in the current study was to locally inject adipose-derived MSC 3 weeks after the induction of the tendon lesions. Applying the MSC 3 weeks after induction of the lesion is realistic, because neither in human nor in equine medicine, the patient would receive this autologous therapy within days after the first onset of tendinopathy. Furthermore, the time frame of 3 weeks between induction and treatment should be adequate to support tendon healing, as Crovace et al. found better histological results in the treated groups after

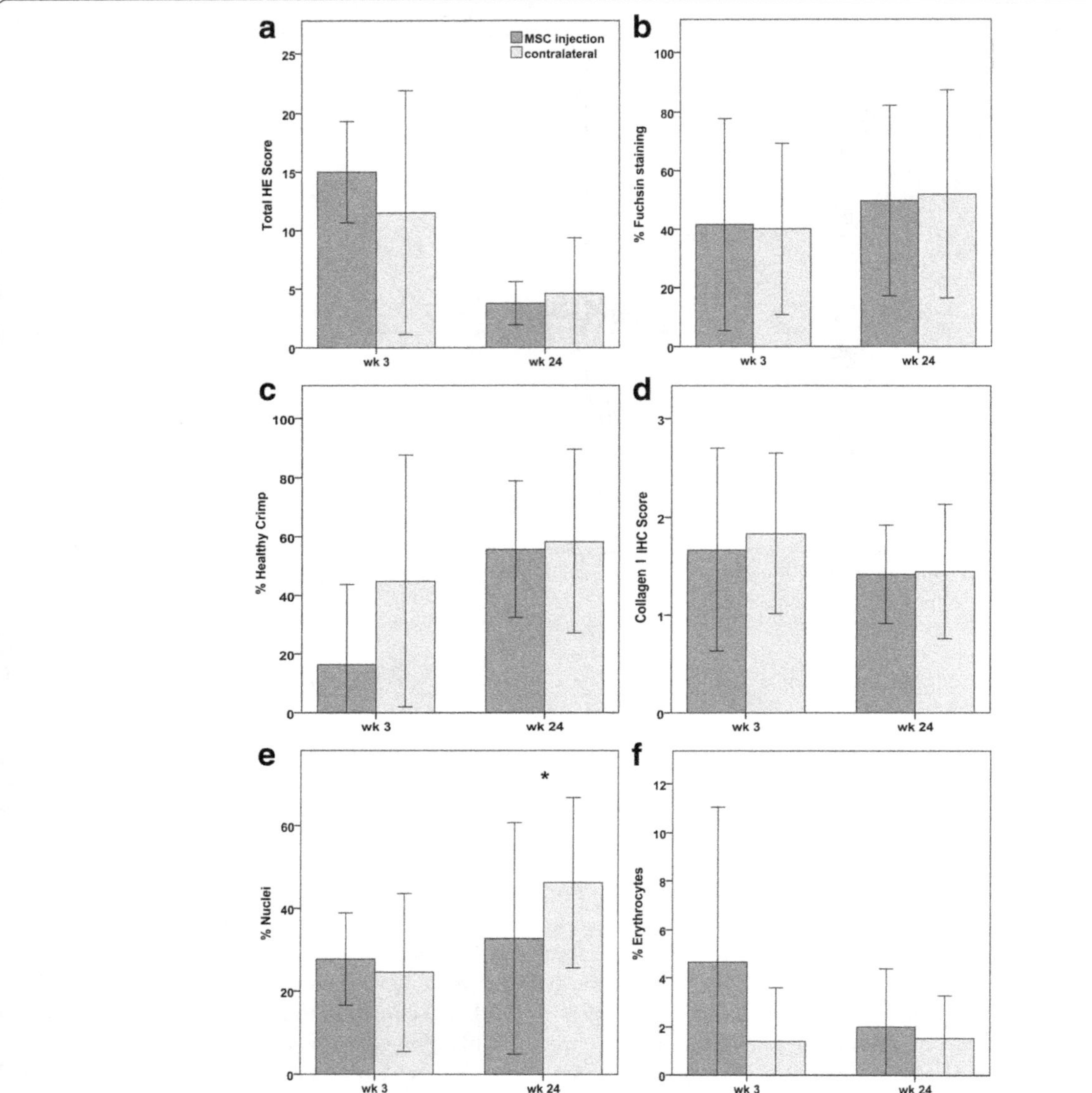

Fig. 5 Histology parameters: Diagrams displaying mean (± 2 SD) values of **a** score points obtained at evaluation of hematoxylin-eosin (HE) stained slides, **b** percentage of fuchsin staining representing uninjured or regenerated tendon tissue, **c** percentage of areas displaying healthy crimp, **d** intensity of collagen I immunohistochemical (IHC) staining, **e** percentage of DAPI-stained nuclei indicating cellularity and **f** percentage of erythrocytes indicating vascularization; star indicates significant difference between MSC-injected and contralateral tendons ($p < 0.05$); wk.: week post MSC injection

choosing an interval of 3 weeks as well [28]. The latter as well as most other studies in horses were conducted with bone marrow-derived MSC [11, 16, 28, 33]. However, the potential of adipose-derived cells is increasingly recognized [34] and adipose-derived cells have also been used for regenerative therapy of tendon lesions with good results [35, 36]. Furthermore, Burk et al. have shown that adipose-derived MSC might be superior to bone marrow-derived MSC regarding their potential to positively influence tendon matrix reorganization [37]. Therefore, the decision to use adipose-derived MSC was favorable, as adipose tissue is easily available with minor surgery in both horses and humans compared to bone marrow, and it remains unlikely that this cell source is the reason for the absence of more significant improvements.

However, the MSC used in the current study had been labeled with SPIO, aiming to track the injected cells and monitor their contribution to tendon healing at the same time. Favorably, these SPIO-labeled MSC have been demonstrated to integrate at the site of intralesional injection [22], in accordance with a similar recent study [38]. It has also been shown in vivo and in vitro that SPIO labeling influences neither stemness nor viability nor proliferation of stem cells [39–42]. In an ovine osteoarthritis model using

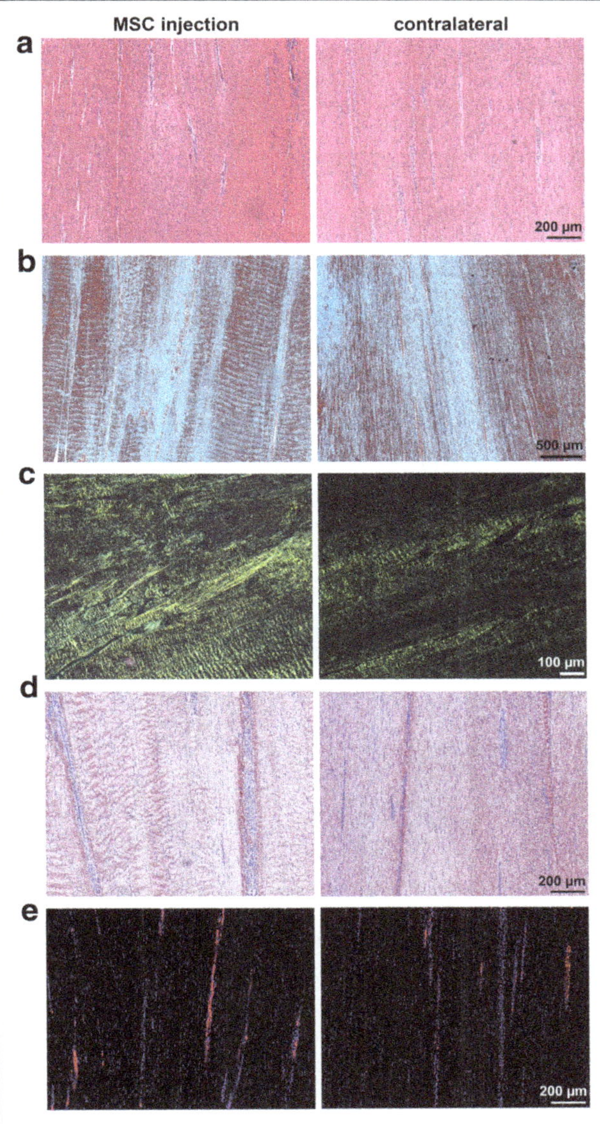

Fig. 6 Histology images: Representative images from paraffin sections stained with **a** hematoxylin-eosin, **b** Masson's Trichrome, **c** Picrosirius red, images obtained using polarized light, **d** anti-collagen I antibody and alkaline phosphatase (red) detection kit and **e** DAPI staining of nuclei (blue), the erythrocytes displaying red autofluorescence

SPIO-labeled as well as SPIO-negative control MSC, no adverse side effects of SPIO-labeled MSC have been demonstrated [43]. However, current literature also suggests that SPIO influences immune reactions in the surrounding tissue and inhibits endothelial nitric oxide synthase [44, 45]. Therefore, it cannot be excluded that SPIO-labeling of the MSC used in the current study might have compromised their regenerative capacity and/or that released SPIO particles have triggered inflammation.

In this study, the tendon defect was created by a low dose of collagenase injected with a 11 G bone marrow aspiration needle. This large needle creates a mechanical defect in addition to the enzymatical defect. The rationale behind this approach was to combine the advantages of the two most commonly used techniques, collagenase injection and surgical induction, mimicking natural core lesions more closely [46, 47]. This defect is therefore different from those in other studies using higher doses of collagenase and ultrasound-guided injection via smaller needles [28, 33, 48], which is likely to impact on responsiveness to MSC treatment.

Furthermore, the inclusion of adequate controls is crucial. In this study, we chose to use the contralateral tendons as intra-individual controls and to inject these tendons with serum, as serum was used as vehicle to deliver the MSC in the treatment group. The vehicle for MSC delivery should ideally maintain MSC viability prior to injection and support their regenerative effect. While for bone marrow MSC, bone marrow supernatant is most commonly used, serum is a good alternative for other MSC sources. However, saline or phosphate buffered saline (PBS) have frequently been chosen for injection into the control tendons [11, 33, 36], which is not indicative as to whether any observed effect is due to MSC treatment or the delivery vehicle. In this line, Geburek et al. used autologous conditioned serum (ACS) without MSC for treatment of naturally occurring tendinopathy and reported on significant reduction of lameness and swelling in the ACS group compared to saline [17]. This suggests that serum itself may have beneficial effects on tendon healing. Consequently, differences found in studies using PBS or saline for control injections but serum or bone marrow supernatant as MSC delivery vehicle [11, 33, 36] cannot without doubt be attributed solely to the MSC. This could partly explain that fewer beneficial effects were detected in the current study, in which serum was used as a more rigorous control regarding MSC efficacy.

The use of the contralateral tendon of the same animal as control limits interference of inter-individual differences with the results, reduces the numbers of animals required, and has been described by several groups [28, 33, 38]. However, MSC could enter the blood circulation after injection and migrate to other sites of injury or inflammation as well, e.g. the contralateral defect, a process referred to as homing [49, 50]. MSC have been shown to circulate in peripheral blood after intralesional injection but had not been found in untreated lesions so far [51, 52]. Yet, in the previously published part of the current study, MSC could be shown to be present in the contralateral tendon lesions as well, albeit in small numbers [22]. Based on that, the effect of MSC distribution after intralesional injection might have been underestimated when the current study was designed. However, we still consider a strong impact on the results as unlikely, as significantly fewer cells were found in the control lesions compared to the treated lesions.

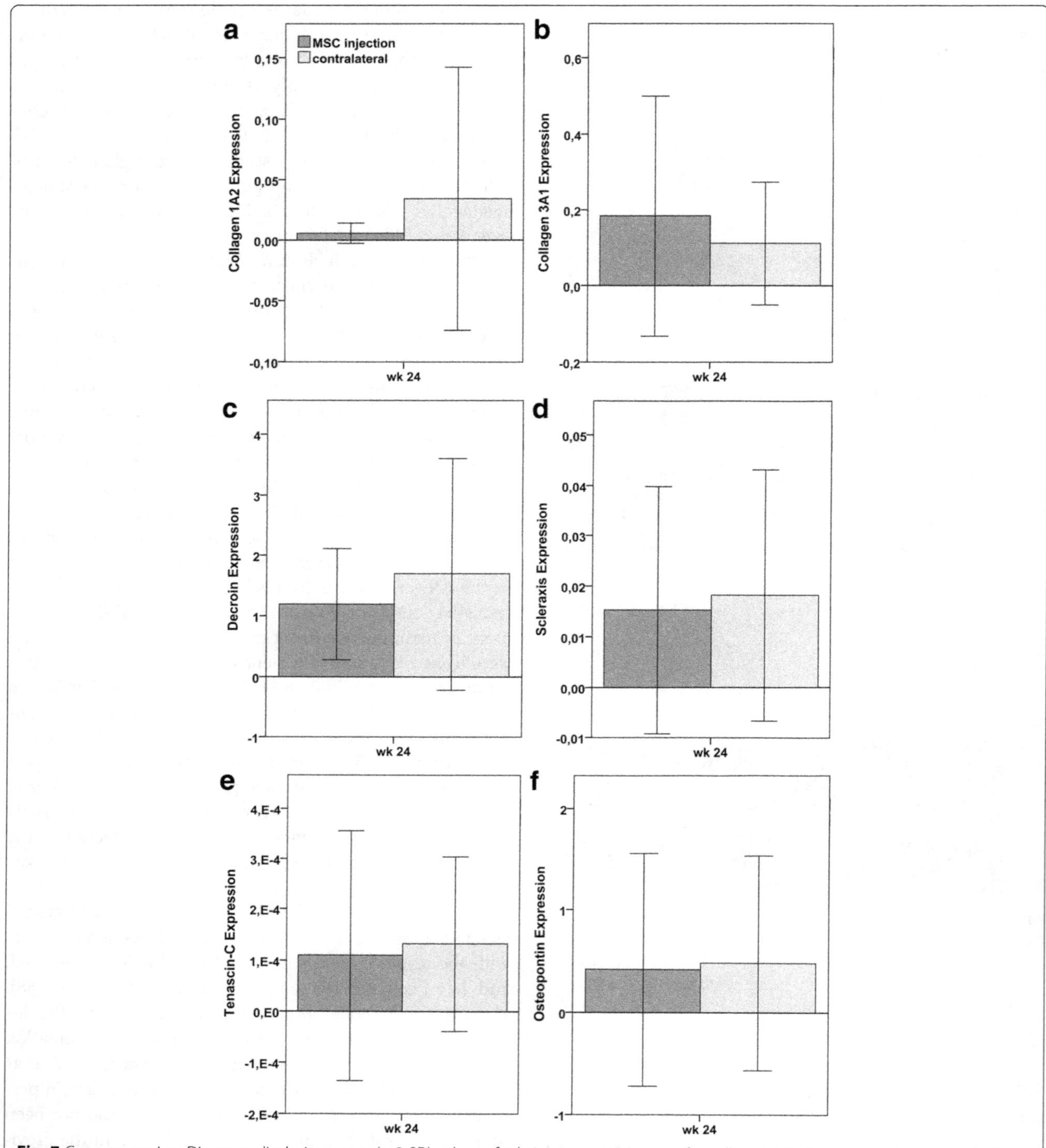

Fig. 7 Gene expression: Diagrams displaying mean (± 2 SD) values of relative gene expression of **a** collagen 1A2, **b** collagen 3A1, **c** decorin, **d** scleraxis, **e** tenascin-C and **f** osteopontin, 24 weeks (wk) after MSC injection

Regarding sample and data analysis, while other studies used only the maximum lesion zone for imaging assessment and the macroscopically affected areas of the tendon for histological examination [28, 33, 48], we analyzed the whole metacarpal area of the tendon. This may have hampered the detection of differences potentially existing at the maximum lesion sites only. However, this method is more rigorous as it takes the whole longitudinal extension of the defect into account, and there is no potential bias as subjective identification of maximum lesion site is not required.

Possibly elucidating which of the discussed factors and differences between studies might most likely explain the outcome, two previous studies are particularly interesting for comparison. A recent carefully designed study, investigating the effect of autologous adipose-derived MSC suspended in inactivated serum in surgically created tendon lesions in the horse, over a follow-up period of 22 weeks, also revealed few improvements. The authors did not find significant differences in histology, biochemical or biomechanical parameters between MSC-treated lesions and serum-injected contralateral control tendon lesions, although hydroxylysylpyridinoline content in the MSC group was closer to that of healthy tendon tissue, potentially indicating better crosslinking [38]. In a different study, the effect of bone marrow-MSC suspended in bone marrow supernatant for treatment of naturally occurring tendon lesions was investigated. After a follow-up of 6 months post injection, treatment outcome was favourable, with improved tissue structure, lower cellularity, vascularity, water and glycosaminoglycan content as well as matrix metalloproteinase-13 activity. While it should be considered that controls were based on saline injections, this study stands out because naturally occurring tendon lesions were used, instead of artificially creating them [11].

Considering the outcome of these two studies in line with the current results, it appears most likely that MSC are not capable to repair mechanically induced tendon lesions, potentially due to the associated loss of tissue that cannot be replaced adequately over a follow-up period of 22 or 24 weeks, respectively. The choice of the animal model is crucial in clinical translation and can strongly impact on the results of preclinical studies. Although we aimed to overcome the limitations of collagenase-based and surgical lesion induction by combining mild approaches of both techniques, the current model might still not reflect naturally occurring tendinopathy. Therefore, taking advantage of the fact that horses are equally prone to natural tendon disease as humans, to use them as natural models as reported by Smith et al. still represents the most reliable option- albeit not without challenges [11]. With equal importance, it remains possible that MSC are not significantly more effective than delivery vehicles such as bone marrow supernatant or serum, even if inactivated, indicating that this fundamental question has yet to be answered.

Yet, we observed significant differences during the early healing phase between weeks 3 and 6, at which clinical assessment and imaging suggested a stronger but transient inflammatory reaction in MSC-treated tendons. Although based on the current data, it cannot be excluded that SPIO might have induced this inflammatory response, our results correspond to a previous study, in which a transient increase in vascularization after injection of MSC was observed, while the latter were not labeled with SPIO [35]. This could be part of the immunomodulatory effects of MSC, which could be important for debridement and lesion resolution and to prevent fibrotic repair, thus there is reason to consider that this transient inflammatory reaction could be beneficial [53]. However, except for the lower cellularity of treated tendons, no distinctive evidence to support this hypothesis was found in this study, thus further studies need to elucidate the immunomodulatory effects of MSC in tendon healing.

Conclusions

Intralesional injection of adipose-derived MSC led only to minor improvements of tendon healing within the observed time frame of 24 weeks, indicating that MSC were not capable of repairing the mechanically disrupted tissue within the tendon lesions during the observed period. Future studies, ideally based on using naturally occurring tendon lesions as a model and using the adequate controls, still have to answer the fundamental question whether the effect of MSC is superior to that of biologically active body fluids such as serum. However, we observed that MSC induced a transient inflammation during early healing, followed by reduced cellularity in treated tendons at week 24, which suggests a modulatory effect warranting further investigations.

Abbreviations

ACS: Autologous Conditioned Serum; ACTB: Actin Beta; BMBF: German Federal Ministry of Education and Research; cDNA: Complementary Deoxyribonucleic Acid; cm: Centimeters; DAPI: 4′,6-diamidino-2-phenylindole; DMEM: Dulbecco's Modified Eagle's Medium; EMA: European Medicines Agency; FBS: Fetal Bovine Serum; FDA: Food and Drug Administration; Fe: Iron (Ferrum); G: Gauge; GAPDH: Glyceraldehyde 3-phosphate dehydrogenase; HE: Hematoxylin-Eosin; IHC: Immunohistochemical; IU: International Unit; mg/kg bwt: Milligrams per Kilogram body weight; ml: Milliliters; mm: Millimeters; MRI: Magnetic Resonance Imaging; MSC: Mesenchymal stromal cells; PBS: Phosphate Buffered Saline; RNA: Ribonucleic Acid; RT-PCR: Real-time reverse-transcription polymerase chain reaction; SD: Standard Deviation; SDFT: Superficial Digital Flexor Tendon; SMWK: Saxon Ministry of Science and the Fine Arts; SPIO: Superparamagnetic Iron Oxide; T2w: T2-weighted; US: Ultrasound; wk: Week

Acknowledgments

The authors would like to thank the team of the Large Animal Clinic for Surgery, University of Leipzig, for helping with the in vivo experiments, as well as the team of the Institute of Veterinary Pathology, University of Leipzig, for preparing the histological sections.

Funding

The work presented in this paper was made possible by funding from the German Federal Ministry of Education and Research (BMBF 1315883) and the Saxon Ministry of Science and the Fine Arts (SMWK). We acknowledge support from the German Research Foundation (DFG) and Leipzig University within the program of Open Access Publishing.

Authors' contributions

ABA, CH and JB made substantial contributions to research design, acquisition, analysis, and interpretation of data, to drafting the paper and revising it critically. DB, CG, AH and SS made substantial contributions to acquisition and interpretation of data and to revising the paper critically. WB and CJ made substantial contributions to research design and to revising the paper. GR and KW made substantial contributions to analysis and interpretation of data and to revising the paper critically. All authors read and approved the final manuscript.

Consent for publication

Not applicable.

Competing interests

The authors declare that they have no competing interests.

Author details

[1]Department of Orthopedics, Traumatology and Plastic Surgery, University of Leipzig, Liebigstr. 20, 04103 Leipzig, Germany. [2]Translational Center for Regenerative Medicine (TRM), University of Leipzig, Leipzig, Germany. [3]Saxon Incubator for Clinical Translation (SIKT), University of Leipzig, Leipzig, Germany. [4]University Equine Hospital, University of Leipzig, Leipzig, Germany. [5]Department of Clinical Science and Services, The Royal Veterinary College, University of London, London, UK. [6]School of Biosciences and Veterinary Medicine, University of Camerino, Camerino, Italy. [7]Institute of Veterinary Physiology, University of Leipzig, Leipzig, Germany. [8]Institute of Anatomy, Medical Faculty, University of Leipzig, Leipzig, Germany. [9]Department of Biotechnology, University of Natural Resources and Life Sciences, Vienna, Austria.

References

1. de Jonge S, van den Berg C, de Vos RJ, van der Heide HJL, Weir A, Verhaar JAN, et al. Incidence of midportion Achilles tendinopathy in the general population. Br J Sports Med. 2011;45:1026–8.
2. Alfredson H. Ultrasound and Doppler-guided mini-surgery to treat midportion Achilles tendinosis: results of a large material and a randomised study comparing two scraping techniques. Br J Sports Med. 2011;45:407–10.
3. de Jonge S, de Vos RJ, Weir A, van Schie HTM, Bierma-Zeinstra SMA, Verhaar JAN, et al. One-year follow-up of platelet-rich plasma treatment in chronic Achilles tendinopathy: a double-blind randomized placebo-controlled trial. Am J Sports Med. 2011;39:1623–9.
4. Sadoghi P, Rosso C, Valderrabano V, Leithner A, Vavken P. The role of platelets in the treatment of Achilles tendon injuries. J Orthop Res Off Publ Orthop Res Soc. 2013;31:111–8.
5. Willberg L, Sunding K, Ohberg L, Forssblad M, Fahlström M, Alfredson H. Sclerosing injections to treat midportion Achilles tendinosis: a randomised controlled study evaluating two different concentrations of Polidocanol. Knee Surg Sports Traumatol Arthrosc Off J ESSKA. 2008;16:859–64.
6. Vannini F, Di Matteo B, Filardo G, Kon E, Marcacci M, Giannini S. Platelet-rich plasma for foot and ankle pathologies: a systematic review. Foot Ankle Surg Off J Eur Soc Foot Ankle Surg. 2014;20:2–9.
7. Kearney RS, Parsons N, Metcalfe D, Costa ML. Injection therapies for Achilles tendinopathy. Cochrane Database Syst Rev. 2015;(5):CD010960.
8. Filardo G, Di Matteo B, Kon E, Merli G, Marcacci M. Platelet-rich plasma in tendon-related disorders: results and indications. Knee Surg Sports Traumatol Arthrosc. 2018;26(7):1984–99.
9. Avella CS, Ely ER, Verheyen KLP, Price JS, Wood JLN, Smith RKW. Ultrasonographic assessment of the superficial digital flexor tendons of National Hunt racehorses in training over two racing seasons. Equine Vet J. 2009;41:449–54.
10. Patterson-Kane JC, Becker DL, Rich T. The pathogenesis of tendon microdamage in athletes: the horse as a natural model for basic cellular research. J Comp Pathol. 2012;147:227–47.
11. Smith RKW, Werling NJ, Dakin SG, Alam R, Goodship AE, Dudhia J. Beneficial effects of autologous bone marrow-derived mesenchymal stem cells in naturally occurring tendinopathy. PLoS One. 2013;8:e75697.
12. Williams RB, Harkins LS, Hammond CJ, Wood JL. Racehorse injuries, clinical problems and fatalities recorded on British racecourses from flat racing and National Hunt racing during 1996, 1997 and 1998. Equine Vet J. 2001;33:478–86.
13. U.S. Department of Health and Human Services; Food and Drug Administration; Center for Biologics Evaluation and Research. Guidance for Industry: Preparation of IDEs and INDs for Products Intended to Repair or Replace Knee Cartilage [Internet]. 2011. Available from: https://www.fda.gov/downloads/ucm288011.pdf.
14. European Medicines Agency; Committee For Advanced Therapies (CAT). Reflection paper on in-vitro cultured chondrocyte containing products for cartilage repair of the knee. [Internet]. 2010. Available from: http://www.ema.europa.eu/docs/en_GB/document_library/Scientific_guideline/2010/05/WC500090887.pdf.
15. Smith RKW, Korda M, Blunn GW, Goodship AE. Isolation and implantation of autologous equine mesenchymal stem cells from bone marrow into the superficial digital flexor tendon as a potential novel treatment. Equine Vet J. 2003;35:99–102.
16. Godwin EE, Young NJ, Dudhia J, Beamish IC, Smith RKW. Implantation of bone marrow-derived mesenchymal stem cells demonstrates improved outcome in horses with overstrain injury of the superficial digital flexor tendon. Equine Vet J. 2012;44:25–32.
17. Geburek F, Lietzau M, Beineke A, Rohn K, Stadler PM. Effect of a single injection of autologous conditioned serum (ACS) on tendon healing in equine naturally occurring tendinopathies. Stem Cell Res Ther. 2015;6:126.
18. Dominici M, Le Blanc K, Mueller I, Slaper-Cortenbach I, Marini F, Krause D, et al. Minimal criteria for defining multipotent mesenchymal stromal cells. The International Society for Cellular Therapy position statement. Cytotherapy. 2006;8:315–7.
19. Richardson LE, Dudhia J, Clegg PD, Smith R. Stem cells in veterinary medicine–attempts at regenerating equine tendon after injury. Trends Biotechnol. 2007;25:409–16.
20. Brehm W, Burk J, Delling U, Gittel C, Ribitsch I. Stem cell-based tissue engineering in veterinary orthopaedics. Cell Tissue Res. 2012;347:677–88.
21. Uder C, Brückner S, Winkler S, Tautenhahn HM, Christ B. Mammalian MSC from selected species: Features and applications. Cytometry A. 2018;93(1):32–49.
22. Burk J, Berner D, Brehm W, Hillmann A, Horstmeier C, Josten C, et al. Long-term cell tracking following local injection of mesenchymal stromal cells in the equine model of induced tendon disease. Cell Transplant. 2016;25:2199–211.
23. Smith RKW, McIlwraith CW. Consensus on equine tendon disease: building on the 2007 Havemeyer symposium: consensus on equine tendon disease. Equine Vet J. 2012;44:2–6.
24. Burk J, Ribitsch I, Gittel C, Juelke H, Kasper C, Staszyk C, et al. Growth and differentiation characteristics of equine mesenchymal stromal cells derived from different sources. Vet J. 2013;195:98–106.
25. Paebst F, Piehler D, Brehm W, Heller S, Schroeck C, Tárnok A, et al. Comparative immunophenotyping of equine multipotent mesenchymal stromal cells: an approach toward a standardized definition. Cytom Part J Int Soc Anal Cytol. 2014;85:678–87.
26. Rantanen N, Jorgensen J, Genovese R. Ultrasonographic Evaluation of the Equine Limb: Technique. Ross MW, Dyson SJ Ed Diagn Manag Lameness Horse. 2nd ed. 2011. p. 182–205.
27. Vallance SA, Vidal MA, Whitcomb MB, Murphy BG, Spriet M, Galuppo LD. Evaluation of a diode laser for use in induction of tendinopathy in the superficial digital flexor tendon of horses. Am J Vet Res. 2012;73:1435–44.
28. Crovace A, Lacitignola L, Rossi G, Francioso E. Histological and Immunohistochemical Evaluation of Autologous Cultured Bone Marrow Mesenchymal Stem Cells and Bone Marrow Mononucleated Cells in Collagenase-Induced Tendinitis of Equine Superficial Digital Flexor Tendon. Vet Med Int [Internet]. 2010 [cited 2015 Dec 2]; 2010. Available from: http://www.ncbi.nlm.nih.gov/pmc/articles/PMC2859019/
29. Martinello T, Pascoli F, Caporale G, Perazzi A, Iacopetti I, Patruno M. Might the Masson trichrome stain be considered a useful method for categorizing experimental tendon lesions? Histol Histopathol. 2015;30:963–9.
30. Kittler J, Illingworth J. Minimum error thresholding. Pattern Recogn. 1986;19:41–7.
31. Hillmann A, Ahrberg AB, Brehm W, Heller S, Josten C, Paebst F, et al. Comparative characterization of human and equine mesenchymal stromal cells: a basis for translational studies in the equine model. Cell Transplant. 2016;25:109–24.
32. Pfaffl MW. Transcriptional biomarkers. Methods San Diego Calif. 2013;59:1–2.
33. Schnabel LV, Lynch ME, van der Meulen MCH, Yeager AE, Kornatowski MA, Nixon AJ. Mesenchymal stem cells and insulin-like growth factor-I gene-

enhanced mesenchymal stem cells improve structural aspects of healing in equine flexor digitorum superficialis tendons. J Orthop Res Off Publ Orthop Res Soc. 2009;27:1392–8.

34. Bourin P, Bunnell BA, Casteilla L, Dominici M, Katz AJ, March KL, et al. Stromal cells from the adipose tissue-derived stromal vascular fraction and culture expanded adipose tissue-derived stromal/stem cells: a joint statement of the International Federation for Adipose Therapeutics and Science (IFATS) and the International Society for Cellular Therapy (ISCT). Cytotherapy. 2013;15:641–8.
35. Conze P, van Schie HT, van WR, Staszyk C, Conrad S, Skutella T, et al. Effect of autologous adipose tissue-derived mesenchymal stem cells on neovascularization of artificial equine tendon lesions. Regen Med. 2014;9:743–57.
36. Carvalho A de M, Badial PR, Álvarez LEC, Yamada ALM, Borges AS, Deffune E, et al. Equine tendonitis therapy using mesenchymal stem cells and platelet concentrates: a randomized controlled trial. Stem Cell Res Ther. 2013;4:85.
37. Burk J, Gittel C, Heller S, Pfeiffer B, Paebst F, Ahrberg AB, et al. Gene expression of tendon markers in mesenchymal stromal cells derived from different sources. BMC Res Notes. 2014;7:826.
38. Geburek F, Mundle K, Conrad S, Hellige M, Walliser U, van Schie HTM, et al. Tracking of autologous adipose tissue-derived mesenchymal stromal cells with in vivo magnetic resonance imaging and histology after intralesional treatment of artificial equine tendon lesions - a pilot study. Stem Cell Res Ther. 2016;7:21.
39. Yang Y, Zhang J, Qian Y, Dong S, Huang H, Boada FE, et al. Superparamagnetic Iron oxide is suitable to label tendon stem cells and track them in vivo with MR imaging. Ann Biomed Eng. 2013;41:2109–19.
40. Addicott B, Willman M, Rodriguez J, Padgett K, Han D, Berman D, et al. Mesenchymal stem cell labeling and in vitro MR characterization at 1.5 T of new SPIO contrast agent: Molday ION rhodamine-BTM. Contrast Media Mol Imaging. 2011;6:7–18.
41. Bourzac CA, Koenig JB, Link KA, Nykamp SG, Koch TG. Evaluation of ultrasmall superparamagnetic iron oxide contrast agent labeling of equine cord blood and bone marrow mesenchymal stromal cells. Am J Vet Res. 2014;75:1010–7.
42. Wang L, Deng J, Wang J, Xiang B, Yang T, Gruwel M, et al. Superparamagnetic iron oxide does not affect the viability and function of adipose-derived stem cells, and superparamagnetic iron oxide-enhanced magnetic resonance imaging identifies viable cells. Magn Reson Imaging. 2009;27:108–19.
43. Delling U, Brehm W, Metzger M, Ludewig E, Winter K, Jülke H. In vivo tracking and fate of intra-Articularly injected superparamagnetic Iron oxide particle-labeled multipotent stromal cells in an ovine model of osteoarthritis. Cell Transplant. 2015;24:2379–90.
44. Astanina K, Simon Y, Cavelius C, Petry S, Kraegeloh A, Kiemer AK. Superparamagnetic iron oxide nanoparticles impair endothelial integrity and inhibit nitric oxide production. Acta Biomater. 2014;10:4896–911.
45. Schäfer R, Ayturan M, Bantleon R, Kehlbach R, Siegel G, Pintaske J, et al. The use of clinically approved small particles of iron oxide (SPIO) for labeling of mesenchymal stem cells aggravates clinical symptoms in experimental autoimmune encephalomyelitis and influences their in vivo distribution. Cell Transplant. 2008;17:923–41.
46. Williams IF, McCullagh KG, Goodship AE, Silver IA. Studies on the pathogenesis of equine tendonitis following collagenase injury. Res Vet Sci. 1984;36:326–38.
47. Little D, Schramme M. Ultrasonographic and MRI evaluation of a novel tendonitis model in the horse. Vet Surg. 2006;35:E15.
48. Nixon AJ, Dahlgren LA, Haupt JL, Yeager AE, Ward DL. Effect of adipose-derived nucleated cell fractions on tendon repair in horses with collagenase-induced tendinitis. Am J Vet Res. 2008;69:928–37.
49. De Becker A, Riet IV. Homing and migration of mesenchymal stromal cells: how to improve the efficacy of cell therapy? World J Stem Cells. 2016;8:73–87.
50. Chapel A, Bertho JM, Bensidhoum M, Fouillard L, Young RG, Frick J, et al. Mesenchymal stem cells home to injured tissues when co-infused with hematopoietic cells to treat a radiation-induced multi-organ failure syndrome. J Gene Med. 2003;5:1028–38.
51. Carvalho AM, Yamada ALM, Golim MA, Álvarez LEC, Hussni CA, Alves ALG. Evaluation of mesenchymal stem cell migration after equine tendonitis therapy. Equine Vet J. 2014;46:635–8.
52. Guest DJ, Smith MRW, Allen WR. Equine embryonic stem-like cells and mesenchymal stromal cells have different survival rates and migration patterns following their injection into damaged superficial digital flexor tendon. Equine Vet J. 2010;42:636–42.
53. Dakin SG, Dudhia J, Smith RKW. Resolving an inflammatory concept: the importance of inflammation and resolution in tendinopathy. Vet Immunol Immunopathol. 2014;158:121–7.

Early rehabilitation for volumetric muscle loss injury augments endogenous regenerative aspects of muscle strength and oxidative capacity

Sarah M. Greising[1*†], Gordon L. Warren[2], W. Michael Southern[3], Anna S. Nichenko[3], Anita E. Qualls[3], Benjamin T. Corona[1] and Jarrod A. Call[3,4†]

Abstract

Background: Volumetric muscle loss (VML) injuries occur due to orthopaedic trauma or the surgical removal of skeletal muscle and result in debilitating long-term functional deficits. Current treatment strategies do not promote significant restoration of function; additionally appropriate evidenced-based practice physical therapy paradigms have yet to be established. The objective of this study was to develop and evaluate early rehabilitation paradigms of passive range of motion and electrical stimulation in isolation or combination to understand the genetic and functional response in the tissue remaining after a multi-muscle VML injury.

Methods: Adult male mice underwent an ~ 20% multi-muscle VML injury to the posterior compartment (gastrocnemius, soleus, and plantaris muscle) unilaterally and were randomized to rehabilitation paradigm twice per week beginning 2 days post-injury or no treatment.

Results: The most salient findings of this work are: 1) that the remaining muscle tissue after VML injury was adaptable in terms of improved muscle strength and mitigation of stiffness; but 2) not adaptable to improvements in metabolic capacity. Furthermore, biochemical (i.e., collagen content) and gene (i.e., gene arrays) assays suggest that functional adaptations may reflect changes in the biomechanical properties of the remaining tissue due to the cellular deposition of non-contractile tissue in the void left by the VML injury and/or differentiation of gene expression with early rehabilitation.

Conclusions: Collectively this work provides evidence of genetic and functional plasticity in the remaining skeletal muscle with early rehabilitation approaches, which may facilitate future evidenced-based practice of early rehabilitation at the clinical level.

Keywords: Electrical stimulation, Neuromusculoskeletal injury, Regenerative medicine, Orthopaedic trauma, Skeletal muscle injury, Range of motion

* Correspondence: grei0064@umn.edu; smgreising@msn.com
†Sarah M. Greising and Jarrod A. Call contributed equally to this work.
[1]Extremity Trauma and Regenerative Medicine, United States Army Institute of Surgical Research, Fort Sam Houston, Texas 78234, USA
Full list of author information is available at the end of the article

Background

Volumetric muscle loss (VML) is a debilitating orthopaedic condition that results in chronic functional deficits and disability [1–3]. With no current surgical or rehabilitative standard of care to address the soft tissue loss, VML injures are left to follow the natural sequela of injury that ultimately results in the replacement of contractile skeletal muscle with non-contractile pathologic fibrotic tissue [4]. Furthermore, functional capacity after VML injury continues to deteriorate over time [5]. As such, interventions and treatment approaches are urgently needed to ameliorate the progressive functional disability related to VML injury [6].

Physical therapy and rehabilitation are an important component of functional improvements following all neuromusculoskeletal injuries, but there is currently a dearth of experimental studies to support any evidenced-based practice for VML injury. In part, the lack of clinical rehabilitation guidelines could be related to heterogeneous injury pattern and the prevalence of the multiple concomitant injuries to VML, such as fracture [7]. A limited number of VML injury case studies have consistently observed chronic functional deficits and disability that were not ameliorated by delayed, prolonged, intensive physical therapy [2, 8–10]. Lack of human-based experimental studies have been addressed using small and large animal models [6]. In fact, a small number of pre-clinical studies involving rodent models have demonstrated beneficial functional remodeling of skeletal muscle with running as a physical therapy modality [11–14]. However, quadruped running may rely upon and engage muscles differently than biped running, so more refined experimental designs are necessary to validate actively engaging VML injured muscle as part of a rehabilitation approach.

Understanding of early rehabilitative interventions in VML patients has yet to be fully established. Early mobilization and rehabilitation initiated in the hospital setting for various other clinical conditions results in shorter admission times and improved function [15]. Passive range of motion exercise are non-weight bearing rehabilitation techniques that do not rely on functionally innervated muscle fibers. The tolerance and effectiveness of range of motion rehabilitation to assist in recovery from conditions ranging from contraction-induced muscle injury [16] to rotator cuff repair [17] has been documented. It is expected that passive movement may mitigate the muscle stiffness following VML injury, but the approach has not been tested. Interestingly, in Duchenne muscular dystrophy, a condition presenting with pathologic fibrosis, muscle weakness and stiffness, muscle activation regimens in combination with range of motion therapy are reportedly more effective in improving limb endurance and function compared to range of motion therapy alone clinically [18]. VML injuries may present with motor unit recruitment issues, either from loss of consciousness (e.g., prolonged comatose state), peripheral nerve damage, or damaged neural tracks, and therefore a potential rehabilitation technique to circumvent these limitations is intermittent electrical stimulation. Intermittent electrical stimulation will recruit the muscle fibers remaining following injury via subdermal stimulation. Electrical stimulation has been shown to promote motor and sensory reinnervation and regeneration following nerve injury [19], and induce hyperopic overload [20, 21]. Both range of motion and intermittent electrical stimulation techniques represent rehabilitation paradigms that conceivably could be conducted in a hospital setting, even while patients were non-weight bearing.

This work sought to develop and evaluate two early rehabilitation paradigms of passive range of motion and electrical stimulation to understand the genetic and functional response in the tissue remaining following a multi-muscle VML injury. We developed the rehabilitation protocols broadly off of previous work [16, 18, 20, 21]. We hypothesized that early intervention following VML injury would enhance the endogenous regenerative and oxidative capacity of the muscle remaining following VML injury, ultimately improving muscle function.

Methods

Animals

Adult male C5BL/6 mice ($n = 96$) were purchased from Jackson Laboratories (Bar Harbor, ME). Animals were maintained on a 12 h light-dark schedule under specific pathogen-free conditions with ad libitum food and water in a vivarium accredited by the American Association for the Accreditation of Laboratory Animal Care. Upon arrival, all mice were given at least 1 week to acclimate to the facility prior to any experimentation. All protocols and animal care guidelines were approved by the Institutional Animal Care and Use Committee at the United States Army Institute of Surgical Research (A16–036) or the University of Georgia (A2017 08–004), in compliance with National Institute of Health Guidelines. All components were conducted in compliance with the Animal Welfare Act, the Implementing Animal Welfare Regulations and in accordance with the principles of the Guide for the Care and Use of Laboratory Animals.

At ~ 12.5 weeks of age mice underwent a VML injury to the posterior compartment of the hindlimb and were randomized to various treatment groups. Specific groups received no-treatment (VML), rehabilitation interventions of range of motion exercise (ROM) or range of motion and intermittent electrical stimulation (ROM-E). All rehabilitation bouts were conducted two times per week, beginning 2 days post-injury for up to 14 days post-injury for the acute study or 4 months for the chronic study. A subset of uninjured (naïve, no surgical intervention) control mice was used for various analyses throughout the project. Tissue harvest was conducted ~ 24 h following the final rehabilitation bout while mice were deeply anesthetized with isoflurane (1.5–2.0%) and mice were euthanized with an injection of Fatal Plus (150 mg/kg; intra-cardiac) while still under anesthesia. Following VML surgery all mice recovered promptly and displayed only slight limitations in mobility. No unexpected deaths or adverse outcomes were noted in any group across the 4 months evaluated.

Volumetric muscle loss (VML) surgery

While anesthetized (isoflurane 1.5–2.0%) a surgical VML was created on the middle third of the posterior compartment using a surgical approach modified from previous work [22]. All mice received a pre-surgical (~ 30 min prior) administration of buprenorphine-SR (1.2 mg/kg; s.c.) for pain management. Briefly, a posterior-lateral incision was made through the skin to reveal the gastrocnemius muscle. Blunt and specific dissection of the skin, fascia, and hamstring muscle was used to reveal the posterior aspect of the gastrocnemius muscle. Blunt dissection was used to isolate the muscle compartment off the dorsal aspect of the tibia and a small metal plate was inserted below the deep soleus muscle but above the tibia and a punch biopsy (4 mm, approximately 20% volume loss of muscle; *see* Table 1) was performed through the middle third of the muscle compartment. Any bleeding was stopped with light pressure. Following the surgical injury the skin incision was closed with simple interrupted suture (6–0 Silk). In all cases the left limb underwent the VML injury and the contralateral was used as an injured intra-animal control for biochemical and gene expression analysis.

Rehabilitation

All rehabilitation sessions were conducted while the mouse was anesthetized (isoflurane 1.5–2.0%) and body temperature was maintained. At each bout the knee and foot of the left limb was stabilized at 90° (neutral position) and the foot was secured to a foot plate attached to a servomotor (300B-LR, Aurora Scientific, Aurora, Ontario, Canada). Under computer control, the servomotor passively rotated the ankle 40° through dorsi- and plantar-flexion, specifically 20° from neutral for both directions. Continuous range of motion was conducted for 30 min with each set taking 5 s, followed by a 5 s rest period at neutral for the range of motion alone groups. For groups that received combined range of motion and intermittent electrical stimulation, stimulation occurred during rest phases of the range of motion protocol. Stimulation was elicited using platinum-iridium (Pt-Ir) needle electrodes positioned percutaneously on either side of the sciatic nerve (S48 and SIU5, Grass Technologies, West Warwick, RI, USA). Progressive stimulation parameters were utilized to promote continuous adaptation and were as follows: 30 Hz, 50% duty cycle (immediate post-injury to 1 month); 45 Hz, 25% duty cycle (1 month to 2 months); and 80 Hz, 12.5% duty cycle (2 months to 4 months). These parameters were selected based on the following rationale: 1) 30, 45, and 80 Hz represent the linear phase of the torque-frequency relationship and reflect ~ 25, 50, and 75% peak-isometric torques in uninjured muscle [23, 24]; and 2) a reduced duty cycle for higher-frequencies contractions minimized potential for fatigue. All rehabilitation occurred twice per week throughout the study period, specifically for the acute study on days 2, 6, 9, and 13 days post-surgery. During rehabilitation sessions, ideal electrode placement and current (mAmps) were validate by a series of sub-maximal 20 Hz stimulations. These sub-maximal active torque (ROM-E group only), as well as passive torques (both ROM and ROM-E groups) about the ankle joint was evaluated post-hoc as an assessment of ongoing adaptation to the rehabilitation strategy (*see* Fig. 1).

Table 1 Multi-muscle volumetric muscle loss injury

	n	VML defect mass (mg)	Injured: uninjured gastrocnemius muscle mass	Force deficit from control (%)
3 days	4	18.6 ± 1.3	0.94 ± 0.09	–
7 days	4	18.8 ± 1.0	0.88 ± 0.08	–
14 days	4	19.1 ± 1.3	0.66 ± 0.02*	–
1 month	6	20.2 ± 0.5	0.77 ± 0.05	- 62.5 ± 3.2†
2 months	6	18.2 ± 0.9	0.88 ± 0.06	- 61.8 ± 4.7
4 months	6	19.8 ± 0.8	0.90 ± 0.02	- 51.0 ± 2.7
P-value		0.592	0.029	0.043

Mean ± SE; Significantly different than *3 days or †4 months post-VML

Muscle function

In vivo maximal isometric torque of the ankle plantarflexors (gastrocnemius, soleus, and plantaris muscle) was assessed as previously described [23–25] and was determined at the terminal time point. Briefly, mice were anesthetized using 2% isoflurane in oxygen, and then the left hindlimb was depilated and aseptically prepared, the foot placed in a foot-plate attached to a servomotor (Model 300C-LR; Aurora Scientific, Aurora, Ontario, Canada), and Pt-Ir needle electrodes (Grass Technologies, West Warwick, RI, USA) were inserted percutaneously on either side of the nerve. To avoid recruitment of the anterior crural muscles responsible for dorsiflexion, the common perineal nerve was severed [26]. Peak isometric torque was achieved by varying the current delivered to the sciatic nerve which branches to the tibial nerve thus innervating the ankle plantarflexor muscles. To account for differences

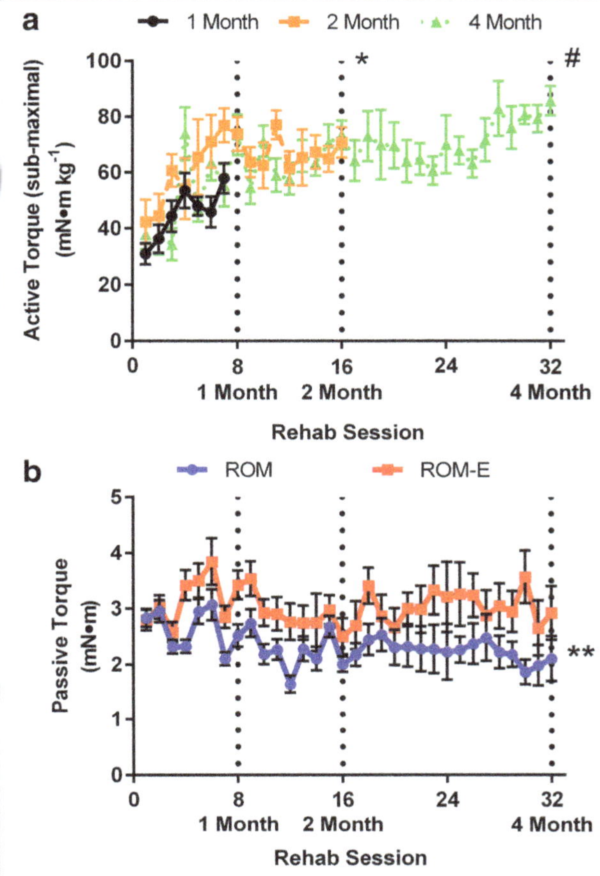

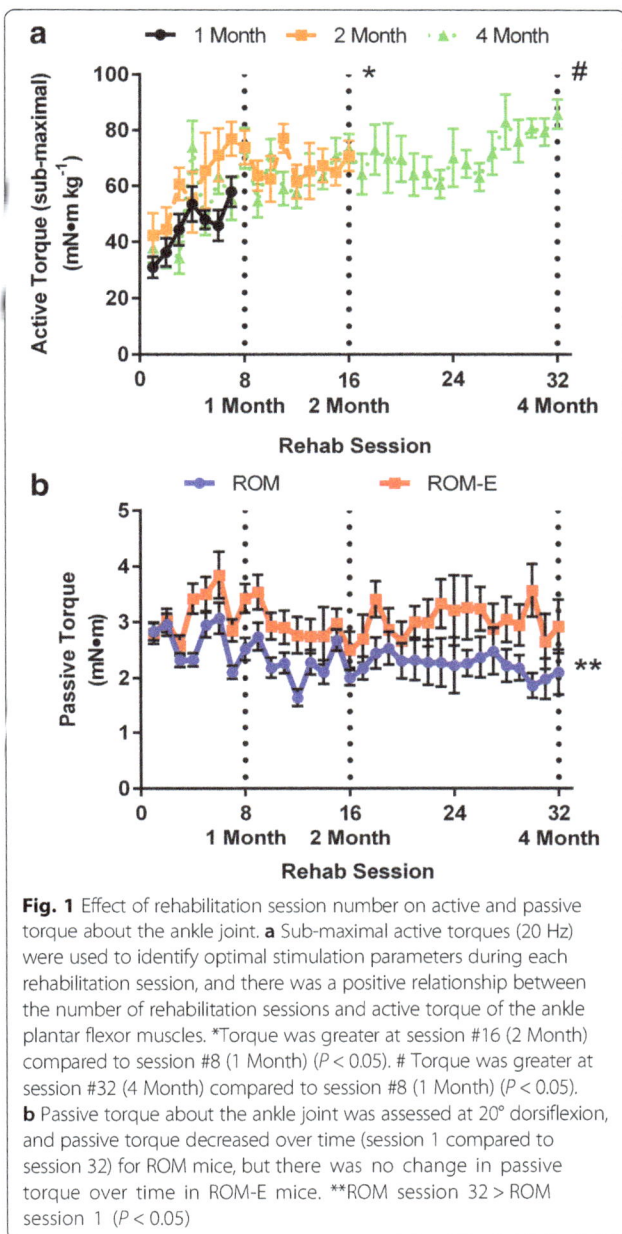

Fig. 1 Effect of rehabilitation session number on active and passive torque about the ankle joint. **a** Sub-maximal active torques (20 Hz) were used to identify optimal stimulation parameters during each rehabilitation session, and there was a positive relationship between the number of rehabilitation sessions and active torque of the ankle plantar flexor muscles. *Torque was greater at session #16 (2 Month) compared to session #8 (1 Month) ($P < 0.05$). # Torque was greater at session #32 (4 Month) compared to session #8 (1 Month) ($P < 0.05$). **b** Passive torque about the ankle joint was assessed at 20° dorsiflexion, and passive torque decreased over time (session 1 compared to session 32) for ROM mice, but there was no change in passive torque over time in ROM-E mice. **ROM session 32 > ROM session 1 ($P < 0.05$)

in body size among mice, torques (mN•m) was normalized by body mass (kg).

Hydroxyproline

Content of hyrdoxyproline in the muscle was used to determine collagen content following injury. Content was determined biochemically as previously described [27, 28].

Gene expression

At the time of tissue harvest the gastrocnemius were excised and placed in TRIzol and snap frozen in liquid nitrogen and stored at -80 °C until analysis. RNA was isolated and gene expression was analyzed using a custom designed gene array (RT^2 Profiler PCR Array; Qiagen) with genes related to myogenic, metabolic, fibrotic, inflammatory, and neural (Additional file 1: Table S1) response to injury per manufacture's instruction. Data was processed with GAPDH as the endogenous control and expression was calculated relative to contralateral control muscle or the non-repaired VML injured muscle at the same time point, as appropriate and noted. Differentially expressed genes were analyzed with iPathway using a fold change of 0.6 and adjusted *P*-value of 0.05 thresholds.

Mitochondrial

Immediately following dissection, portions of the medial and lateral gastrocnemius muscles from uninjured and injured limbs were dissected on a chilled aluminum block in 4 °C buffer X (7.23 mM K_2EGTA, 2.77 mM Ca K_2EGTA, 20 mM imidazole, 20 mM taurine, 5.7 mM ATP, 14.3 mM PCr, 6.56 mM $MgCl_2$-$6H_2O$, 50 mM k-MES) into thin muscle fiber bundles as reported previously [29]. Permeabilization of muscle fibers was achieved by transferring fibers to a vial containing buffer X and saponin (50 µg/ml) and incubating (i.e., gentle rocking) at 4 °C for 30 min. Muscle fiber bundles were rinsed for 15 min in buffer Z (105 mM k-MES, 30 mM KCl, 10 mM KH_2PO_4, 5 mM $MgCl_2$, 0.5 mg/ml BSA, 1 mM EGTA) at 4 °C. All measurements were performed using a Clark-type electrode (Oxygraph Plus System, Hansatech Instruments, UK) at 25 °C. Prior to each experiment, the electrode was calibrated according to the manufacturer's instructions and 1 ml of O_2 infused buffer Z was added to the chamber. Muscle fiber bundles were weighed (~ 2.5 mg for all samples) and added to the chamber. State 4 respiration (leak respiration in the absence of ADP) was initiated by the addition of glutamate (10 mM) and malate (5 mM). State 3 respiration (respiration coupled to ATP synthesis) was initiated by the addition of ADP (2.5 mM) and succinate (10 mM). Cytochrome c (10 µM) was added to measure the integrity of the outer mitochondrial membrane. State 3 uncoupled respiration (respiration uncoupled from ATP synthesis) was initiated by the addition of FCCP (0.5 µM). Mitochondrial respiration was terminated by the addition of cyanide (250 mM).

Statistical analysis

All data was analyzed using JMP (version 10.0 SAS Institute, Inc., NC). Data was analyzed separately using a variety of ANOVAs, when appropriate Tukey HSD post-hoc analysis was performed. Data are reported as mean ± SE, unless otherwise specified and significance was accepted at $P < 0.05$.

Results

Multi-muscle volumetric muscle loss (VML) injury

VML injury in military [30, 31] and civilian [32] populations commonly involve 2 or more muscles. To date most VML injury models have been to an isolated muscle, with only a limited number to multiple muscles within the quadriceps [33, 34]. Therefore, our first goal was to establish a murine multi-muscle VML injury model. Because the plantarflexor muscles within the posterior compartment of the rodent hind leg are highly recruited during normal ambulation and are weight bearing [35], this muscle group is ideal for rehabilitation studies. A full-thickness VML injury was created through the plantarflexor gastrocnemius, plantaris, and soleus muscles (Table 1) at the tibia mid-diaphyseal level, resulting in the removal of ~ 19 mg of tissue or ~ 20% of the combined plantarflexor muscle wet weight. The partial tissue resection caused an ~ 50% maximal isometric force loss and ~ 2 fold increase in passive torque (muscle stiffness) about the ankle through 4 months post-injury, indicating successful creation of a model that recapitulates pathophysiological aspects of VML injury in patients [2, 9].

Early rehabilitation

To validate early rehabilitation approaches, 2 days post-VML injury, mice were randomly assigned to one of the following groups: VML alone (VML), passive range of motion (ROM), or ROM plus intermittent electrical stimulation (ROM-E). Range of motion rehabilitation involved passively moving the ankle joint through 40° of motion and the intent was to reduce muscle stiffness associated with the deposition of collagens in and around the VML injury site. Intermittent electrical stimulation rehabilitation involved recruitment of the ankle plantar flexor muscles via sciatic nerve stimulation with Pt-Ir needle electrodes. The intent was to enhance strength by activating the remaining muscle after VML injury, during a time in which significant motoneuron axotomy is present following injury [36]. Rehabilitation strategies (twice weekly for 30 min) were continued in different cohorts of mice for 1, 2, or 4 months post-VML ($n = 6$ mice/group/time). A small cohort of completely uninjured mice was included to observe deficits associated with the VML injury and the relative recovery with early rehabilitation therapy ($n = 8$ mice).

Functional response to early rehabilitation

To determine if early rehabilitation approaches were beneficial, functional responses were analyzed at each rehabilitation bout. First, in both the ROM and ROM-E groups, passive torque about the ankle joint was recorded and analyzed during each therapy session. Additionally at each session, sub-maximal active torque about the ankle joint was evaluated in the ROM-E group only. There was a positive association between the number of rehabilitation sessions and sub-maximal plantar flexor muscle torque about the ankle (Main Effect Time, $P < 0.001$, Fig. 1), and overall torque was ~ 125% greater at the last compared to the first session. There was a significant interaction between group and time for passive torque about the ankle joint ($P = 0.034$), as passive torque decreased 25% with range of motion rehabilitation but was not changed over time with combined range of motion and electrical stimulation (Fig. 1). Collectively, these inter-rehabilitation session analyses demonstrated on-going functional remodeling of the injured limb.

Injured and contralateral uninjured gastrocnemius muscle masses were recorded to determine the long-term effect of injury and early rehabilitation on muscle atrophy and possible hypertrophy. There was no effect of early rehabilitation on injured gastrocnemius muscle mass relative to uninjured across time; however, independent of group, the relative mass was 18% greater at 4 months compared to 1 month (Main Effect Time, $P = 0.025$, Additional file 2: Figure S1). Body mass was not affected by early rehabilitation (Additional file 2: Figure S1).

At 1, 2 or 4 months post-VML injury, peak isometric torque of the ankle plantar flexor muscles was assessed to determine contractile function. Independent of time, peak isometric plantar flexor muscle torque was greater in ROM-E mice compared to VML and ROM mice (32 and 21%, respectively; Main Effect Group, $P < 0.001$, Fig. 2 and Additional file 3: Figure S2). At 4 months, VML injury represented a 51% deficit in torque (Control: 768 ± 34 mN•m kg^{-1} vs. VML: 376 ± 21 mN•m kg^{-1}; *see* Table 1), and while ROM-E mice were stronger than VML mice, a 35% deficit remained (Control: 768 ± 34 mN•m kg^{-1} vs. ROM-E: 496 ± 118 mN•m kg^{-1}). Collectively, rehabilitation using ROM-E gave rise to functional improvements but was not able to completely mitigate VML-related functional deficits.

Passive torque at 20° dorsiflexion (i.e., when plantar flexor muscles are passively resisting the stretch) was assessed to determine muscle stiffness. There was a strong trend for a significant interaction ($P = 0.056$). At 4 months, VML injury resulted in over a 3-fold increase in passive stiffness (Control: 1.5 ± 0.2 mN•m vs. VML: 4.9 ± 0.4 mN•m), but early ROM rehabilitation attenuated this effect. Independent of time, passive torque of the plantar flexor muscles following ROM and ROM-E rehabilitation were less compared to VML mice (– 52% and – 32%, respectively), and ROM resulted in 29% less passive torque compared to ROM-E (Main Effect Time, $P < 0.001$, Fig. 2).

Collagen content of the gastrocnemius muscles was measured since passive stiffness was greater with VML injury. There was a significant effect of injury, independent of time, as total collagen content was ~ 2-fold greater in injured limbs of VML, ROM, & ROM-E mice

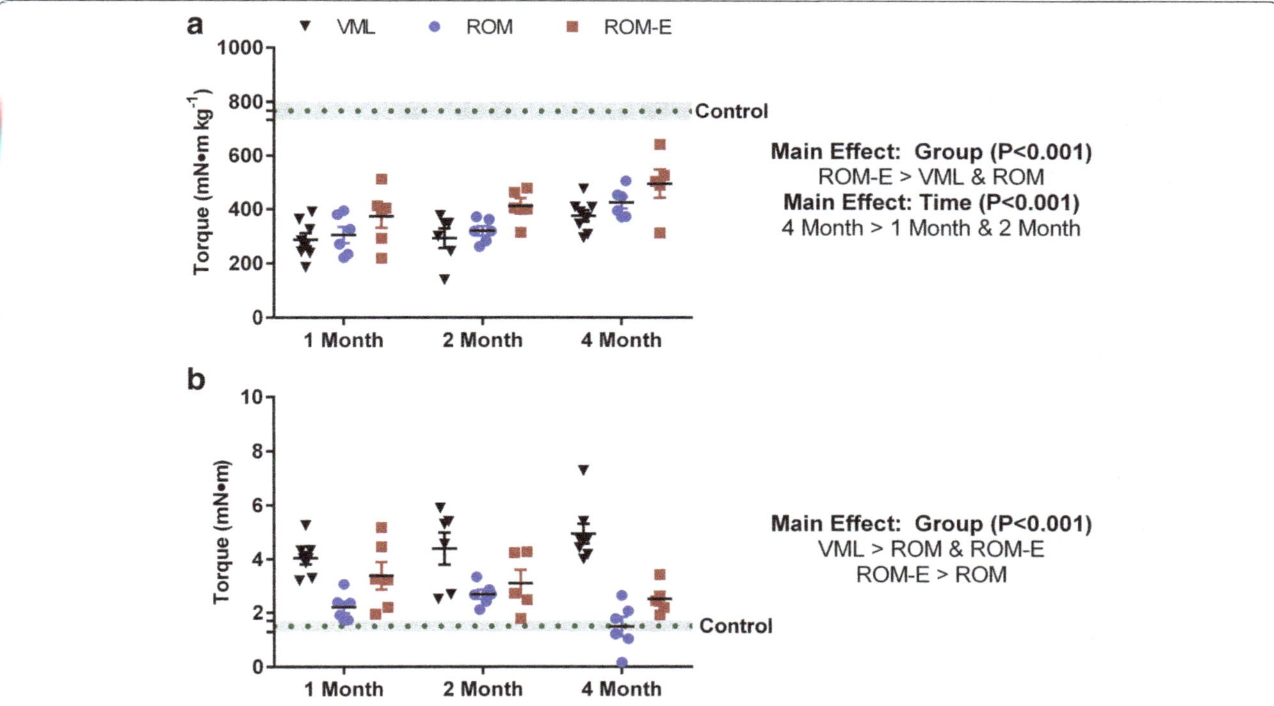

Fig. 2 Effect of VML injury and rehabilitation on study endpoint active and passive torque about the ankle joint. **a** Peak isometric torque of the ankle plantar flexor muscles was greater following ROM-E rehabilitation compared to VML-alone and ROM rehabilitation, independent of time. Control = 768 ± 34 mN•m kg $^{-1}$. **b** Passive torque of the ankle plantar flexor muscles at 20° dorsiflexion was greatest in VML-along compared to ROM and ROM-E rehabilitation, and lowest following ROM rehabilitation. Control = 1.5 ± 0.2 mN•m

compared to uninjured limbs ($P < 0.001$, Fig. 3). While there were noted improvements in passive torque about the ankle within the muscle following ROM rehabilitation the collagen deposition and expected fibrotic deposition remained unchanged.

Oxidative response to early rehabilitation

To determine the metabolic function of the remaining muscle tissue after VML injury, oxygen consumption rates for permeabilized fibers isolated adjacent to the injury site were compared to fibers from the contralateral uninjured limb. There was no significant interaction or main effects ($P \geq 0.112$, Fig. 4). However, independent of time and group, oxygen consumption rates were 25% greater in fibers from completely uninjured mice compared to mice that had a unilateral VML injury (Control: 5054 ± 233 nmol/min/g vs. VML-Injured: 4225 ± 87.39 nmol/min/g, $P < 0.001$, Fig. 4). This signals a previously

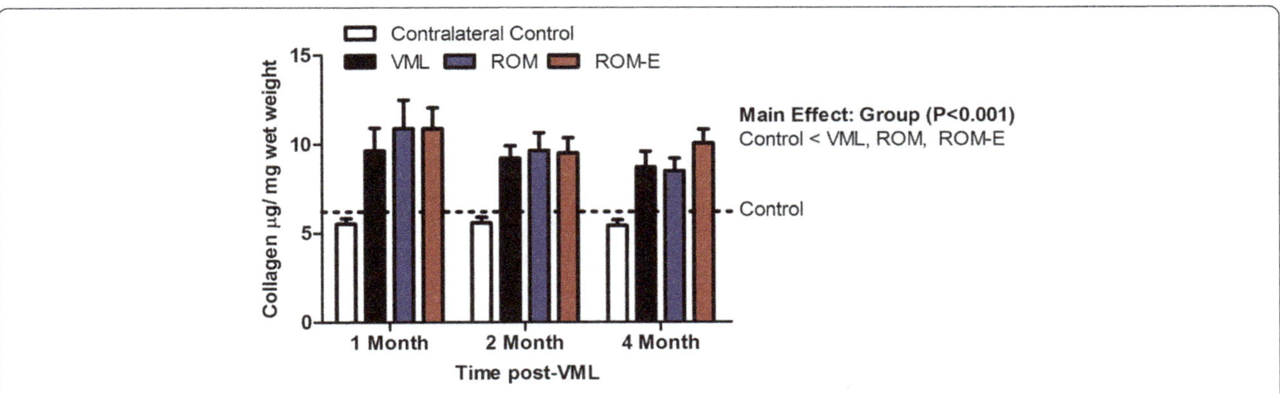

Fig. 3 Effect of VML injury and rehabilitation on gastrocnemius muscle collagen content. Gastrocnemius muscle collagen content was greater in uninjured compared to contralateral uninjured control limbs, independent of time and rehabilitation group ($P < 0.001$). Control = 6.21 ± 0.59 µg collagen per mg muscle wet weight

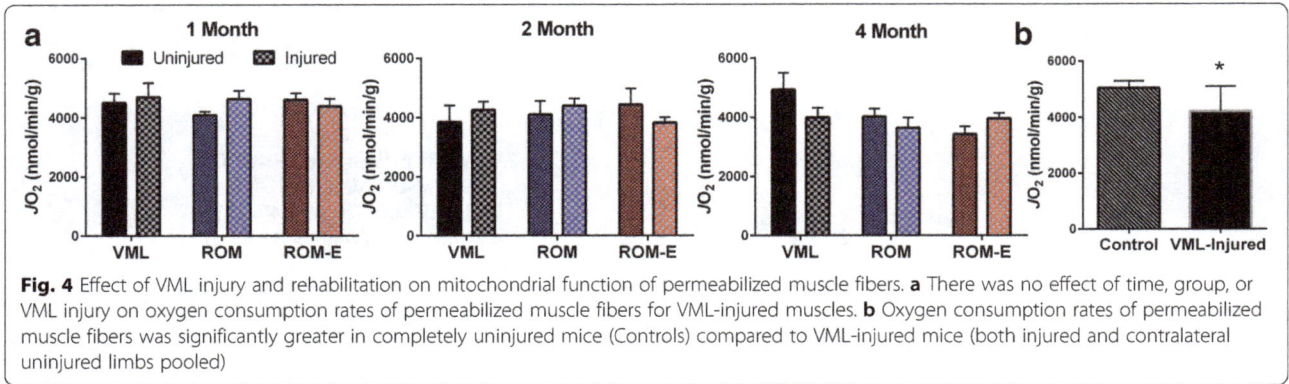

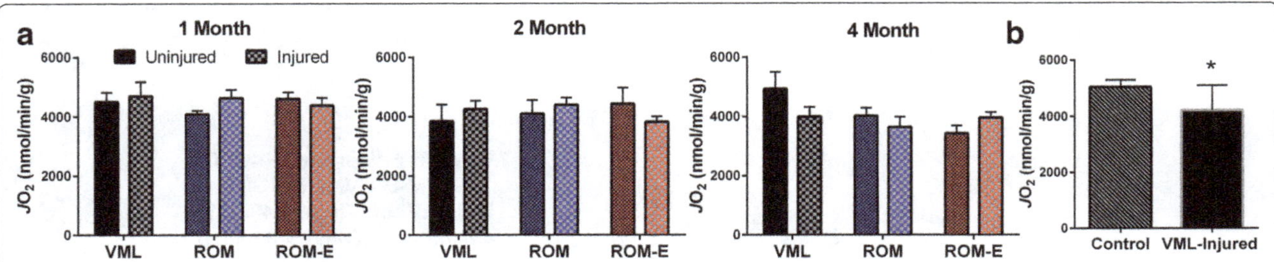

Fig. 4 Effect of VML injury and rehabilitation on mitochondrial function of permeabilized muscle fibers. **a** There was no effect of time, group, or VML injury on oxygen consumption rates of permeabilized muscle fibers for VML-injured muscles. **b** Oxygen consumption rates of permeabilized muscle fibers was significantly greater in completely uninjured mice (Controls) compared to VML-injured mice (both injured and contralateral uninjured limbs pooled)

undescribed impairment with VML injury, which may reflect metabolic maladaptation to changes in muscle recruitment that was resistant to rehabilitative approaches explored in this study.

Acute genetic response to volumetric muscle loss injury

To investigate cellular mechanisms of the VML injury pathophysiology, additional cohorts of injured mice were allocated to VML with no repair or early rehabilitation (ROM or ROM-E) for 3, 7, or 14 days following injury and transcriptional changes in inflammatory, neurogenic, fibrotic, myogenic, and metabolic genes were assessed (Additional file 1: Table S1). In the VML only group, there were 30 genes differentially regulated in the injured limb compared to the uninjured limb, independent of time (i.e., 3, 7, 14 days). Most all genes probed were significantly up-regulated over control tissue, notably only Mstn, Slc2a4, and Ppargc1a displayed down-regulation (Fig. 5 and Additional file 4: Table S2). Several of these genes demonstrated transient changes in differential regulation, as many myogenic, metabolic, and inflammatory genes were significantly up-regulated at 3 in comparison to both 7 and 14 days post-injury. A small number of fibrotic and neurogenic genes (Mmp9, Col3a1, Fbxo32, Tgfbr3, and Nrg1) were significantly up-regulated at 3 in comparison to only14 days. This supports a VML-related regulation of inflammatory genes which had at least a 4-fold increase at 3 days compared to both the 7 and 14 day time points, although notably inflammation was still significantly elevated at the later time points.

Acute genetic response to rehabilitation

To determine how early rehabilitation approaches may alter the gene expression pattern associated with VML injury, gene expression of the gastrocnemius muscle (24 h following the final rehabilitation bout) from mice that underwent rehabilitation (ROM & ROM-E) were compared to non-repaired VML muscle at the same time points (3, 7, or 14 days post-VML). Both the ROM and ROM-E groups were collapsed into 'early rehabilitation' (Fig. 5). Significant differences in gene expression were observed at 3 days post-injury between VML only and early rehabilitation groups (ROM & ROM-E). There was a significant down-regulation in mostly inflammatory gene expression with rehabilitation at 3 days post-injury compared to other time points. In particular, inflammatory (Il33, Tnf, Il4, CxCr3, CxC1, Ccl5, Ccl2) and metabolic (Akt2, Prkaal, Pparfcla, Sk2a4) genes were down-regulated at 3 days post-injury. This suggests that early rehabilitation may mitigate the acute maladaptive response to VML injury, which may be related to the chronic improvements in muscle function and passive stiffness.

Discussion

Current regenerative medicine and rehabilitation techniques for VML injured patients have not shown significant restoration of muscle strength or limb function [6]. A major limiting factor to rehabilitation is the remaining muscle tissue following injury, and its adaptability and/ or capacity to recover from injury. Unfortunately, in VML-injured patients, rehabilitation often begins after significant fibrosis has occurred in the muscle unit, contributing to low functional improvements [37]. To overcome this timing limitation we investigated techniques (i.e., passive range of motion and electrical stimulation) that can begin early after VML injury. The most salient findings were that 1) early initiation of passive range of motion therapy attenuated injury-induced elevations of muscle stiffness, but did not improve active muscle function (Fig. 2), early co-delivery of neural electrical stimulation with passive range of motion therapy 2) improved active muscle function, but did not attenuate rising muscle stiffness (Fig. 2), and 3) abrogated the capacity of passive range of motion therapy to prevent injury induced elevations of muscle stiffness.

Skeletal muscle fibrosis is known to impede muscle healing and regeneration, alter the microenvironment of the muscle, and causes destruction of muscle

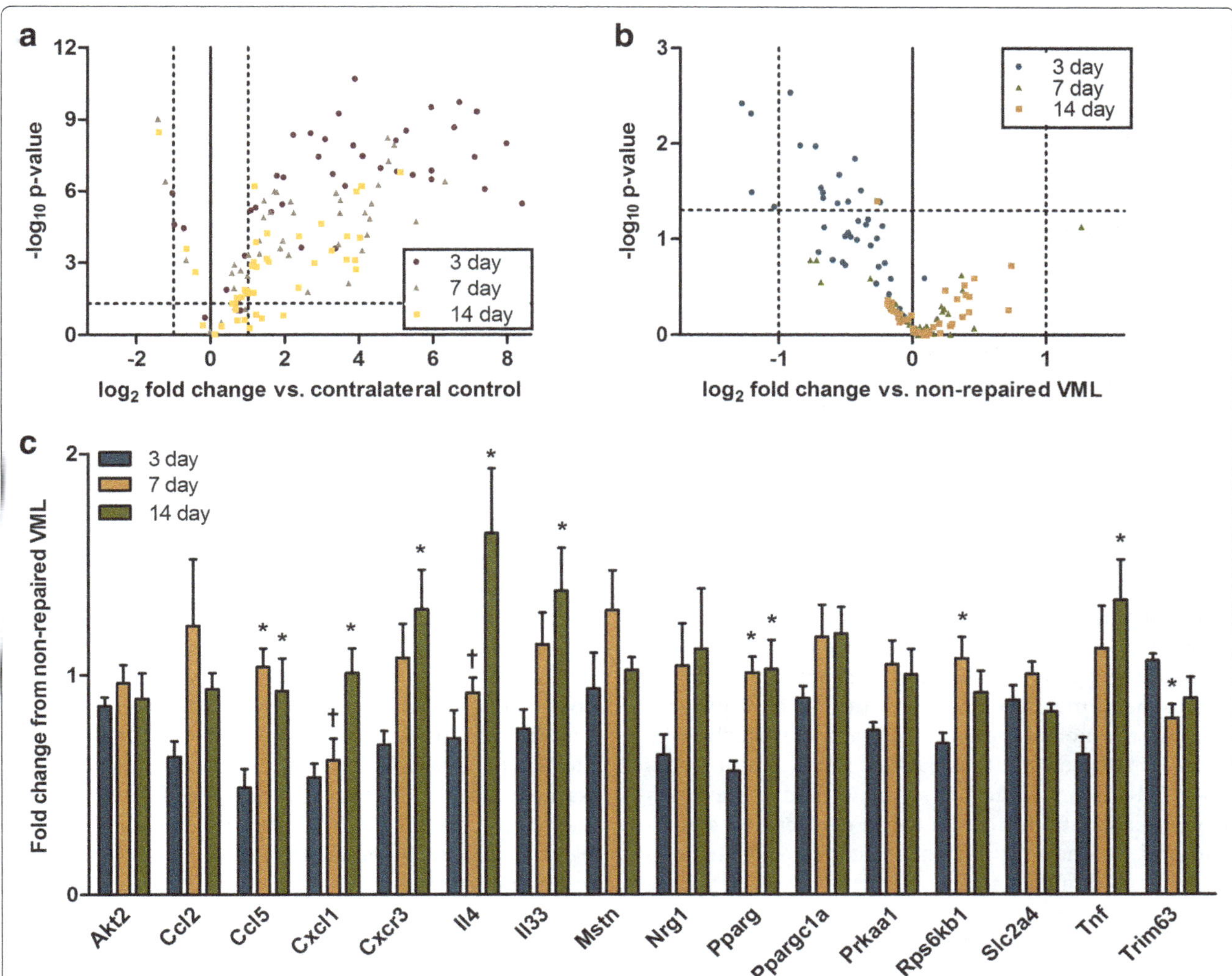

Fig. 5 Custom designed (inflammatory, neurogenic, fibrotic, myogenic, and metabolic, see Additional file 1: Table S1) PCR array analysis presents a significant change in regulation following VML injury and early rehabilitation. **a** The response to VML injury was assessed at 3, 7 and 14 days post-VML compared to contralateral control muscle. **b** The response to early rehabilitation was compared to non-repaired VML at the same time point (3, 7, or 14 days post-VML), treatment groups were collapsed. The dotted horizontal and longitudinal axes indicate the lower thresholds for statistical ($P < 0.05$) and biological significance (2 fold change) of expression, respectively. **c** Specific fold changes for genes that were significantly regulated due to rehabilitation are presented. (One way ANOVA; significantly different than *3 days or †14 days post-VML)

architecture [38]. It is possible that the overwhelming fibrotic response after injury may be limiting rehabilitation and/or further impacting the remaining muscle as it is left to follow the natural sequela of injury. In pathologies such as Duchenne muscular dystrophy and cerebral palsy it has been proposed that the organization and structure of the fibrotic deposition may have a greater role in functional impairments than the total amount of collagen [39]. Because fibrotic tissue fills the void left by VML injury [4, 37], we initially hypothesized that early range of motion therapy, alone or in combination with electrical stimulation, would attenuated fibrotic tissue deposition and stiffness. The observation of reduced stiffness after range of motion therapy partially supports this hypothesis; however, we did not detect predictable differences among rehabilitation groups in terms of total collagen content in the injured limb (Fig. 4). This discrepancy is similar to prior observations of disconnect between collagen crosslinking characteristics with tissue stiffness [40] and supports further investigation of range of motion therapy impact on collagen type, organization, or structure of collagen. The notable positive impact of reduced passive muscle stiffness with range of motion therapy alone does stand to have translatable benefits for this patient population, in which even modest improvements to daily activities may have significant impact on patient quality of life.

Skeletal muscle metabolic capacity is highly plastic and under most conditions has the capability to regenerate after injury. Specifically, during the normal regenerative processes, such as occurring after traumatic myotoxic injury, mitochondrial biogenesis accompanies muscle recovery from injury and is likely necessary to meet the energy demands of muscle repair [41, 42]. Injuries such as VML present a non-recoverable injury, in which the muscle has limited regenerative potential and loses the ability to recover [7]. Mitochondrial function was less in VML-injured mice compared to completely uninjured (i.e., naïve) control mice, however there was no detectable differences in mitochondrial function between injured and contralateral uninjured muscles paired across the same animal. This finding raises several intriguing questions regarding the systemic and chronic effects of VML injury and possibility of low-grade systemic inflammation. Large-scale traumatic injuries such as burn traumas have been associated with low-grade, systemic inflammation that is reported to negatively influence mitochondrial function [43, 44]. Furthermore, following various neuromusculoskeletal injuries such as hip fracture there is noted systemic inflammation which is hypothesized to contribute to lack of muscle regeneration [45]. VML injury induction of acute and chronic systemic inflammation presents a potential pivotal component of the pathogenic response that when left untreated may worsen disability and may impede rehabilitative and regenerative treatment efficacy.

To date only a few studies have examined fibrotic and myogenic responses at 1 to 2 weeks following VML injury. Previous work has indicated that connective tissue growth mediated regulation through TGF-1β family gene expression is greater at 1 week following VML and at 2 weeks there is induction of myogenic and inflammatory genes [13, 46]. Unique to VML injury however is the duration of inflammatory gene induction, which appears to be both heightened and prolonged following injury [34, 47] compared to common endogenously healing injuries [48]. This work investigated the early genetic response to VML injury inflammatory, neurogenic, fibrotic, myogenic, and metabolic genes over the first 2 weeks post-VML. Few selected genes were down-regulated following VML injury alone; specifically Mstn, Slc2a4, and Ppargc1a downregulation occurred at all time points through 2 weeks post-injury. Primarily there was a substantial up-regulation of probed genes following VML injury. In particular inflammatory genes probed appear to most up-regulated at 3 days over 7 and 14 days post-VML. Notably the expression at both 7 and 14 days was still greatly up-regulated from uninjured muscle. Early rehabilitation appears to dampen this inflammatory response, especially at 3 days post-injury and future work should investigate how early rehabilitation may impact any systemic inflammation related to VML injury.

It stands to reason that VML-injured animals are expected to be less physically active compared to uninjured controls, which could produce a lower basal metabolic capacity. A current limitation for the field is an understanding of the physical or metabolic activity of patients with VML injury. Importantly though, VML-injured rodents are able to elevate physical activity as evidenced by increased voluntary wheel running distance [11–14], but the ability of the VML-injured limb or uninjured limb to positively adapt to the elevated physical activity in terms of metabolic capacity, balance in protein synthesis/degradation, and fiber type distributions is unknown and future work should begin to understand this complex relationship. Additionally, future work is needed to continue to understand the pathophysiologic state of the muscle remaining after VML injury with or without additional rehabilitation, as there is a significant need to understand potential therapeutic targets that could benefit the loss of function following VML injury. Collectively, limited and/or lost mobility, poor metabolic function, and/or low-grade systemic inflammation after VML injury may all contribute to development and/or exacerbation of metabolic syndrome and cardiovascular disease in patients with VML injury. Therefore, identifying therapeutic interventions that promote muscle health and physical activity may lessen the health burden and medical costs of VML injury.

Conclusions

Many existing patients with a VML injury could benefit from more readily translatable strategies directed toward improving the remaining tissue, allowing them to engage in more daily actives, and improving quality of life. Strategies to improve the quality of the remaining muscle may also better prepare the individual to take advantage of advanced regenerative engineering approaches to regenerate tissue as they become available in the future. This work developed and evaluated early rehabilitation paradigms to understand the metabolic, genetic, and functional response of the remaining tissue after a multi-muscle VML injury, in efforts to improve the muscle remaining following injury. We expect that identifying genetic and functional plasticity in the remaining skeletal muscle with early rehabilitation approaches may facilitate evidenced-based practice at the clinical level following further translation. Herein we suggest that the remaining tissue following VML injury beneficially adapts to early rehabilitation, but that limitations in the metabolic plasticity of the muscle still exist.

Additional files

Additional file 1: Table S1. Genes probed following VML injury and early rehabilitation. (DOCX 22 kb)

Additional file 2: Figure S1. Effect of VML injury and rehabilitation on study endpoint body mass and gastrocnemius muscle mass. **a** There was a main effect of time, independent group, for body mass indicating mice at 4 Month post-VML injury weighed significantly more (~ 6%) than mice at 1 Month and 2 Month post-VML injury. **b** There was a main effect of time, independent of group, for injured gastrocnemius muscle mass as a fraction of the contralateral uninjured control indicating mice at 4 Month post-VML injury had significantly more (~ 13%) proportional injured gastrocnemius muscle mass than mice at 1 Month. (JPG 839 kb)

Additional file 3: Figure S2. Representative torque-time waveforms during peak isometric contraction from 4 Month VML, ROM, and ROM-E groups compared to completely uninjured controls. The rate of relaxation for all terminal peak isometric contractions was evaluated. The rate of relaxation was greater following ROM-E rehabilitation compared to VML-alone and ROM rehabilitation, independent of time. Control = 576 ± 34 mN•m sec − 1. (JPG 99 kb)

Additional file 4: Table S2. Fold change in gene expression (vs. control) following VML injury. (DOCX 30 kb)

Abbreviations
E: Intermittent electrical stimulation; Pt-Ir: Platinum-iridium; ROM: Range of motion; VML: Volumetric muscle loss

Acknowledgements
We thank Ms. Monica Jalomo, Mr. Javier Chapa, and Mr. Zach Agan for technical assistance in the completion of these studies.

Funding
This research received funding from the Alliance for Regenerative Rehabilitation Research & Training (AR^{3}T) awarded to SMG and JAC, which is supported by the Eunice Kennedy Shriver National Institute of Child Health and Human Development (NICHD), National Institute of Neurological Disorders and Stroke (NINDS), and National Institute of Biomedical Imaging and Bioengineering (NIBIB) of the National Institutes of Health under Award Number P2CHD086843. The content is solely the responsibility of the authors and does not necessarily represent the official views of the National Institutes of Health.

Declarations
The opinions or assertions contained here are the private views of the authors and are not to be construed as official or as reflecting the views of the Department of the Army, the Department of Defense, or the United States Government.

Authors' contributions
JAC and SMG designed the study. JAC, GLW, WMS, ASN, AMQ, and SMG performed experiments and collected data. JAC, BTC, and SMG analyzed and interpreted the data. JAC and SMG wrote the manuscript. All authors have read and approved the final version of this manuscript.

Competing interest
The authors declare that they have no competing interests.

Author details
[1]Extremity Trauma and Regenerative Medicine, United States Army Institute of Surgical Research, Fort Sam Houston, Texas 78234, USA. [2]Department of Physical Therapy, Byrdine F. Lewis School of Nursing and Health Professions, Georgia State University, Atlanta, GA 30302, USA. [3]Department of Kinesiology, University of Georgia, Athens, GA 30602, USA. [4]Regenerative Bioscience Center, University of Georgia, Athens, GA 30602, USA.

References
1. Corona BT, Rivera JC, Owens JG, Wenke JC, Rathbone CR. Volumetric muscle loss leads to permanent disability following extremity trauma. J Rehabil Res Dev. 2015;52(7):785–92.
2. Garg K, Ward CL, Hurtgen BJ, Wilken JM, Stinner DJ, Wenke JC, Owens JG, Corona BT. Volumetric muscle loss: persistent functional deficits beyond frank loss of tissue. J Orthop Res. 2015;33(1):40–6.
3. Grogan BF, Hsu JR. Skeletal trauma research C. Volumetric muscle loss J Am Acad Orthop Surg. 2011;19(Suppl 1):S35–7.
4. Corona BT, Rivera JC, Greising SM. Inflammatory and Physiological consequences of debridement of fibrous tissue after volumetric muscle loss injury. Clin Transl Sci. 2017;
5. Rivera JC, Corona BT. Muscle-related disability following combat injury increases with time. US Army Med Dep J. 2016:30–4.
6. Greising SM, Dearth CL, Regenerative CBT. Rehabilitative medicine: a necessary synergy for functional recovery from volumetric muscle loss injury. Cells Tissues Organs. 2016;202(3–4):237–49.
7. Corona BT, Wenke JC, Ward CL. Pathophysiology of volumetric muscle loss injury. Cells Tissues Organs. 2016;202(3–4):180–8.
8. Gentile NE, Stearns KM, Brown EH, Rubin JP, Boninger ML, Dearth CL, Ambrosio F, Badylak SF. Targeted rehabilitation after extracellular matrix scaffold transplantation for the treatment of volumetric muscle loss. Am J Phys Med Rehabil. 2014;93(11 Suppl 3):S79–87.
9. Mase VJ Jr, Hsu JR, Wolf SE, Wenke JC, Baer DG, Owens J, Badylak SF, Walters TJ. Clinical application of an acellular biologic scaffold for surgical repair of a large, traumatic quadriceps femoris muscle defect. Orthopedics. 2010;33(7):511.
10. Sicari BM, Rubin JP, Dearth CL, Wolf MT, Ambrosio F, Boninger M, Turner NJ, Weber DJ, Simpson TW, Wyse A *et al.* An acellular biologic scaffold promotes skeletal muscle formation in mice and humans with volumetric muscle loss. Sci Transl Med 2014; 6(234):234ra258.
11. Aurora A, Garg K, Corona BT, Walters TJ. Physical rehabilitation improves muscle function following volumetric muscle loss injury. BMC Sports Sci Med Rehabil. 2014;6(1):41.
12. Aurora A, Roe JL, Corona BT, Walters TJ. An acellular biologic scaffold does not regenerate appreciable de novo muscle tissue in rat models of volumetric muscle loss injury. Biomaterials. 2015;67:393–407.
13. Corona BT, Garg K, Ward CL, McDaniel JS, Walters TJ, Rathbone CR. Autologous minced muscle grafts: a tissue engineering therapy for the volumetric loss of skeletal muscle. Am J Physiol Cell Physiol. 2013; 305(7):C761–75.
14. Quarta M, Cromie M, Chacon R, Blonigan J, Garcia V, Akimenko I, Hamer M, Paine P, Stok M, Shrager JB, et al. Bioengineered constructs combined with exercise enhance stem cell-mediated treatment of volumetric muscle loss. Nat Commun. 2017;8:15613.
15. Corcoran JR, Herbsman JM, Bushnik T, Van Lew S, Stolfi A, Parkin K, McKenzie A, Hall GW, Joseph W, Whiteson J, et al. Early rehabilitation in the medical and surgical intensive care units for patients with and without mechanical ventilation: an Interprofessional performance improvement project. PM R. 2017;9(2):113–9.
16. Matsuo S, Suzuki S, Iwata M, Hatano G, Nosaka K. Changes in force and stiffness after static stretching of eccentrically-damaged hamstrings. Eur J Appl Physiol. 2015;115(5):981–91.
17. Chang KV, Hung CY, Han DS, Chen WS, Wang TG, Chien KL. Early versus delayed passive range of motion exercise for arthroscopic rotator cuff repair: a meta-analysis of randomized controlled trials. Am J Sports Med. 2015;43(5):1265–73.
18. Alemdaroglu I, Karaduman A, Yilmaz OT, Topaloglu H. Different types of upper extremity exercise training in Duchenne muscular dystrophy: effects on functional performance, strength, endurance, and ambulation. Muscle Nerve. 2015;51(5):697–705.
19. English AW, Wilhelm JC, Ward PJ. Exercise, Neurotrophins, and axon regeneration in the PNS. Physiology (Bethesda). 2014;29(6):437–45.
20. Baar K, Esser K. Phosphorylation of p70(S6k) correlates with increased skeletal muscle mass following resistance exercise. Am J Phys. 1999; 276(1 Pt 1):C120–7.
21. Hamilton DL, Philp A, MacKenzie MG, Baar KA. Limited role for PI(3,4,5)P3 regulation in controlling skeletal muscle mass in response to resistance exercise. PLoS One. 2010;5(7):e11624.
22. Pollot BE, Corona BT. Volumetric Muscle Loss. Methods Mol Biol. 2016; 1460:19–31.

23. Baltgalvis KA, Call JA, Cochrane GD, Laker RC, Yan Z, Lowe DA. Exercise training improves plantar flexor muscle function in mdx mice. Med Sci Sports Exerc. 2012;44(9):1671–9.
24. Call JA, Warren GL, Verma M, Lowe DA. Acute failure of action potential conduction in mdx muscle reveals new mechanism of contraction-induced force loss. J Physiol. 2013;591(Pt 15):3765–76.
25. Southern WM, Nichenko AS, Shill DD, Spencer CC, Jenkins NT, McCully KK, Call JA. Skeletal muscle metabolic adaptations to endurance exercise training are attainable in mice with simvastatin treatment. PLoS One. 2017; 12(2):e0172551.
26. Call JA, Ervasti JM, Lowe DA. TAT-muUtrophin mitigates the pathophysiology of dystrophin and utrophin double-knockout mice. J Appl Physiol (1985). 2011; 111(1):200–5.
27. Garlich MW, Baltgalvis KA, Call JA, Dorsey LL, Lowe DA. Plantarflexion contracture in the mdx mouse. Am J Phys Med Rehabil. 2010;89(12):976–85.
28. Greising SM, Call JA, Lund TC, Blazar BR, Tolar J, Lowe DA. Skeletal muscle contractile function and neuromuscular performance in Zmpste24 (–/–) mice, a murine model of human progeria. Age (Dordr). 2012;34(4):805–19.
29. Kuznetsov AV, Veksler V, Gellerich FN, Saks V, Margreiter R, Kunz WS. Analysis of mitochondrial function in situ in permeabilized muscle fibers, tissues and cells. Nat Protoc. 2008;3(6):965–76.
30. Owens BD, Kragh JF Jr, Macaitis J, Svoboda SJ, Wenke JC. Characterization of extremity wounds in operation Iraqi freedom and operation enduring freedom. J Orthop Trauma. 2007;21(4):254–7.
31. Owens BD, Kragh JF Jr, Wenke JC, Macaitis J, Wade CE, Holcomb JB. Combat wounds in operation Iraqi freedom and operation enduring freedom. J Trauma. 2008;64(2):295–9.
32. Bosse MJ, MacKenzie EJ, Kellam JF, Burgess AR, Webb LX, Swiontkowski MF, Sanders RW, Jones AL, McAndrew MP, Patterson BM, et al. An analysis of outcomes of reconstruction or amputation after leg-threatening injuries. N Engl J Med. 2002;347(24):1924–31.
33. Li MT, Willett NJ, Uhrig BA, Guldberg RE, Warren GL. Functional analysis of limb recovery following autograft treatment of volumetric muscle loss in the quadriceps femoris. J Biomech. 2014;47(9):2013–21.
34. Sadtler K, Estrellas K, Allen BW, Wolf MT, Fan H, Tam AJ, Patel CH, Luber BS, Wang H, Wagner KR, et al. Developing a pro-regenerative biomaterial scaffold microenvironment requires T helper 2 cells. Science. 2016;352(6283):366–70.
35. Roy RR, Hutchison DL, Pierotti DJ, Hodgson JA, Edgerton VREMG. Patterns of rat ankle extensors and flexors during treadmill locomotion and swimming. J Appl Physiol (1985). 1991;70(6):2522–9.
36. Corona BT, Flanagan KE, Brininger CM, Goldman SM, Call JA, Greising SM. Impact of volumetric muscle loss injury on persistent motoneuron axotomy. Muscle Nerve. 2017;
37. Garg K, Corona BT, Walters TJ. Losartan administration reduces fibrosis but hinders functional recovery after volumetric muscle loss injury. J Appl Physiol (1985). 2014;117(10):1120–31.
38. Lieber RL, Ward SR. Cellular mechanisms of tissue fibrosis. 4. Structural and functional consequences of skeletal muscle fibrosis. Am J Physiol Cell Physiol. 2013;305(3):C241–52.
39. Smith LR, Hammers DW, Sweeney HL, Barton ER. Increased collagen cross-linking is a signature of dystrophin-deficient muscle. Muscle Nerve. 2016;54(1):71–8.
40. Chapman MA, Pichika R, Lieber RL. Collagen crosslinking does not dictate stiffness in a transgenic mouse model of skeletal muscle fibrosis. J Biomech. 2015;48(2):375–8.
41. Duguez S, Feasson L, Denis C, Freyssenet D. Mitochondrial biogenesis during skeletal muscle regeneration. Am J Physiol Endocrinol Metab. 2002; 282(4):E802–9.
42. Wagatsuma A, Kotake N, Yamada S. Muscle regeneration occurs to coincide with mitochondrial biogenesis. Mol Cell Biochem. 2011;349(1–2):139–47.
43. Yasuhara S, Perez ME, Kanakubo E, Yasuhara Y, Shin YS, Kaneki M, Fujita T, Martyn JA. Skeletal muscle apoptosis after burns is associated with activation of proapoptotic signals. Am J Physiol Endocrinol Metab. 2000; 279(5):E1114–21.
44. Porter C, Herndon DN, Borsheim E, Bhattarai N, Chao T, Reidy PT, Rasmussen BB, Andersen CR, Suman OE, Sidossis LS. Long-term skeletal muscle mitochondrial dysfunction is associated with Hypermetabolism in severely burned children. J Burn Care Res. 2016;37(1):53–63.
45. Bamman MM, Ferrando AA, Evans RP, Stec MJ, Kelly NA, Gruenwald JM, Corrick KL, Trump JR, Singh JA. Muscle inflammation susceptibility: a prognostic index of recovery potential after hip arthroplasty? Am J Physiol Endocrinol Metab. 2015;308(8):E670–9.
46. Garg K, Ward CL, Rathbone CR, Corona BT. Transplantation of devitalized muscle scaffolds is insufficient for appreciable de novo muscle fiber regeneration after volumetric muscle loss injury. Cell Tissue Res. 2014;358(3):857–73.
47. Hurtgen BJ, Ward CL, Garg K, Pollot BE, Goldman SM, McKinley TO, Wenke JC, Corona BT. Severe muscle trauma triggers heightened and prolonged local musculoskeletal inflammation and impairs adjacent tibia fracture healing. J Musculoskelet Neuronal Interact. 2016;16(2):122–34.
48. Warren GL, Summan M, Gao X, Chapman R, Hulderman T, Simeonova PP. Mechanisms of skeletal muscle injury and repair revealed by gene expression studies in mouse models. J Physiol. 2007;582(Pt 2):825–41.

16

A comparison of the stem cell characteristics of murine tenocytes and tendon-derived stem cells

Katie Joanna Lee[1*], Peter David Clegg[1,2,3], Eithne Josephine Comerford[1,2] and Elizabeth Gail Canty-Laird[1,3]

Abstract

Tendon is a commonly injured soft musculoskeletal tissue, however, poor healing potential and ineffective treatment strategies result in persistent injuries and tissue that is unable to perform its normal physiological function. The identification of a stem cell population within tendon tissue holds therapeutic potential for treatment of tendon injuries. This study aimed, for the first time, to characterise and compare tenocyte and tendon-derived stem cell (TDSC) populations in murine tendon. Tenocytes and TDSCs were isolated from murine tail tendon. The cells were characterised for morphology, clonogenicity, proliferation, stem cell and tenogenic marker expression and multipotency. TDSCs demonstrated a rounded morphology, compared with a more fibroblastic morphology for tenocytes. Tenocytes had greater clonogenic potential and a smaller population doubling time compared with TDSCs. Stem cell and early tenogenic markers were more highly expressed in TDSCs, whereas late tenogenic markers were more highly expressed in tenocytes. Multipotency was increased in TDSCs with the presence of adipogenic differentiation which was absent in tenocytes. The differences in morphology, clonogenicity, stem cell marker expression and multipotency observed between tenocytes and TDSCs indicate that at least two cell populations are present in murine tail tendon. Determination of the most effective cell population for tendon repair is required in future studies, which in turn may aid in tendon repair strategies.

Keywords: Tendon, Tendon-derived stem cell, Tenocyte, Murine

Background

Tendon is prone to injury and degeneration, and this is most often seen in occupational and sporting environments [1–3]. The healing process for tendon is poorly understood, however it is well documented that tendon tissue is unable to heal effectively resulting in painful and debilitating scar tissue, which is unable to perform its normal physiological function [1, 4]. The current treatment options for damaged or degenerated tendon vary depending on the severity and location of the tendinopathy [5–8] and include physiotherapy; pharmacotherapies, such as anti-inflammatories; corticosteroid injections; or surgery [5, 6, 9]. However, these treatment strategies are largely ineffective [5]; therefore, an alternative approach for the management and treatment of tendinopathies is currently being sought.

Tenocytes are tendon-specific fibroblasts and traditionally were thought to be the only cell type present in tendon, however it is now thought that tenocytes account for approximately 95% of the cellular content of tendon, with progenitor cells, endothelial cells and chondrocytes comprising the remaining 5% [10]. Tenocytes are located between collagen fibrils and in the interfascicular matrix and they are responsible for the production of the ECM as well as the repair and maintenance of tendon tissue [10, 11]. The identification of a stem cell population within tendon tissue [12] holds therapeutic potential for treatment of tendon injuries. Tendon-derived stem cells (TDSCs) have been shown to be clonogenic, multipotent and express stem cell and tenogenic markers [12–15].

A number of tissue engineering strategies have utilised TDSCs for tendon repair with some successful outcomes

* Correspondence: leekj@liverpool.ac.uk
[1]Department of Musculoskeletal Biology, Institute of Ageing and Chronic Disease, University of Liverpool, William Henry Duncan Building, 6 West Derby Street, Liverpool L7 8TX, UK
Full list of author information is available at the end of the article

[16–20]. These studies highlight the potential use of TDSCs in tendon repair strategies, however further characterisation of TDSCs is necessary; particularly, the identification and characterisation of different cell populations within tendon tissue. Comparisons of tendon cell populations are lacking in the literature with only two studies comparing tenocytes and TDSC properties in the rabbit [14] and the horse [15]. These two studies reported conflicting results with large differences found between tenocyte and TDSC populations in the rabbit [14], but few differences observed in the horse [15]. No studies, to date, have compared tendon cell populations in rodents, despite the plethora of research on TDSCs in rats and mice.

This study aimed to isolate, characterise and compare tenocytes and TDSCs from murine tail tendon. We hypothesised that tenocytes would demonstrate phenotypic differences when compared with TDSCs, particularly differences in stem cell properties.

Methods

Isolation of murine tenocytes and TDSCs

HuR floxed embryos were obtained from Dimitris Kontoyiannis, Alexander Fleming Research Centre, Greece [21] and crossed with Aggrecan A1 Cre mice obtained from George Bou-Gharios, University of Liverpool, UK [22]. Tendon tissue was extracted from the tails of 6–8 week old C57BL/6 mice ($HuR^{fl/fl}$*Acan*-$Cre^{+/-}$) which were euthanased for reasons unrelated to this study, and digested for 3 h at 37 °C in 20 ml 375 U/ml collagenase type I and 0.05% trypsin. The resulting cell suspension was strained and then centrifuged at 1200 g for 10 min and the supernatant discarded. The cells were resuspended in complete DMEM (DMEM supplemented with 20% foetal calf serum, 100 U/ml penicillin, 100 µg/ml streptomycin and 2 µg/ml amphotericin B) and counted using a haemocytometer. For tenocyte isolation the cells were seeded at 1×10^5 cells in T25 culture flasks (4×10^3 cells/cm^2) [23, 24] and for TDSC isolation the cells were seeded at 100 cells per well of a 6-well plate (10 cells/cm^2) [13, 15, 16, 25–28]. All cells were cultured in complete DMEM at 37 °C, 5% CO_2 and 21% O_2. TDSCs were cultured for 6–8 days before passaging, whereas tenocytes were cultured for 2–3 days, cells were split 2:1 for subsequent passages. For TDSCs colonies were isolated using cloning cylinders and local application of 0.05% trypsin. All cells were analysed at passage 2–3 [15].

Cell proliferation assay

Cells at passage 2 were seeded at 10,000 cells in T25 culture flasks at day 0. At 80% confluency the cells were counted and the doubling time calculated using the formula below:

(LOG_{10}(cell number after proliferation)-LOG_{10}(initial seeding density))/$LOG_{10}(2)$ [29].

Colony formation assay

Cells at passage 2 were seeded at 100 cells/cm^2 in 6-well cell culture plates. After 7 days in culture the cells were washed and then fixed with 6% gluteraldehyde and stained with 0.5% crystal violet solution [30]. The cells were washed again and imaged using a biomolecular imager (Typhoon FLA 7000, GE Healthcare) and analysed using ImageQuant software (GE Healthcare) for colony number and size.

Tri-lineage differentiation assays

Cell monolayers were cultured for 21 days in osteogenic (complete DMEM containing 100 nM dexamethasone, 10 mM β-glycerophosphate and 50 mM ascorbic acid) [31] and adipogenic (complete DMEM containing 1 µM dexamethasone, 100 µM indomethacin, 10 µg/ml insulin and 500 µM IBMX) [32] induction media. Cell pellets (containing 5×10^5 cells) were cultured for 21 days in chondrogenic (complete DMEM containing 100 nM dexamethasone, 25 µg/ml ascorbic acid, 10 ng/ml TGF-β3 and ITS+ 3 supplement) [33] induction media. Control cells for all treatments were cultured in complete DMEM. After culturing, the cells were stained with alizarin red and alkaline phosphatase to assess osteogenic differentiation, Oil Red O to assess adipogenic differentiation, or alcian blue for chondrogenic differentiation, as described in the PromoCell MSC application notes (http://www.promocell.com/downloads/application-notes/). Chondrogenic pellets were also paraffin embedded and 4 µm sections taken which were rehydrated and further stained with 1% Alcian blue solution and 0.1% Safranin O solution. In addition, separate cell pellets were digested in 10 U/ml papain solution for 3 h at 60 °C before the total sulphated glycosaminoglycan (sGAG) content was quantified. Dimethylmethylene blue dye was added to each sample and the absorbance read immediately at 570 nm. The sGAG content was calculated from a standard curve produced using chondroitin sulphate standards [34]. RNA was extracted from all assays to analyse lineage-specific gene expression.

RNA extraction and quantitative real time-polymerase chain reaction (qRT-PCR)

RNA was extracted from all cell types by firstly applying Trizol to cell monolayers and using a cell scraper for cell detachment. After vortexing and centrifugation, 50 µg/ml glycoblue and 100% isopropanol were added to the aqueous phase for RNA precipitation. After centrifugation, the pellets were washed in 75% ethanol and resuspended in Tris-EDTA buffer. The quantity and quality of

RNA was assessed using a NanoDrop spectrophotometer (Thermo Fisher). 4 U DNase was then added to the samples to remove DNA, after which time an equal volume of phenol:chloroform:IAA was added to each sample. The RNA was then precipitated, centrifuged, washed in ethanol and the RNA quality assessed. cDNA was synthesised in a 25 μl reaction from 1 to 2 μg of total RNA. The conditions for cDNA synthesis were: incubation at 5 min at 70 °C, 60 min at 37 °C and 5 min at 93 °C with M-MLV reverse transcriptase and random-hexamer oligonucleotides (Promega) [35, 36].

qRT-PCR was conducted using a GoTaq(R) qPCR Master Mix (Promega), and in a 25 μl reaction 10 ng of cDNA was amplified in an AB 7300 Real Time PCR System (Applied Biosystems). After an initial denaturation for 10 min at 95 °C, 40 PCR cycles were performed consisting of 15 s at 95 °C and 1 min at 60 °C. Relative gene expression was calculated according to the comparative C_t method [35–37]. Murine specific primers were used (Table 1) and GAPDH was used as an internal control. Primers were designed using Primer-BLAST (NCBI), and the quality of each primer was tested using NetPrimer (Premier Biosoft). In addition, each primer was subjected to a BLAST (NCBI) search to ensure specificity. The best housekeeping gene was determined using the geNorm algorithm [38] and all primers were tested for efficiency; efficiencies between 90 and 110% were deemed to be acceptable.

Statistical analysis

Statistical analysis was performed using SPSS (IBM) and SigmaPlot (Systat Software Inc). To ensure data was normally distributed Shapiro Wilk tests were performed. For normally distributed data parametric tests were used for pairwise comparisons. For data which was not normally distributed Log_{10} data transformations were performed resulting in normally distributed data. For pairwise comparisons paired or independent Student's t-tests were used. *P*-values ≤0.05 were taken to be significant.

Results

Tenocyte and TDSC morphology and colony formation

Tenocytes and TDSCs demonstrated varying cell morphologies; tenocytes were large, flat and fibroblastic, whereas TDSCs were smaller and more rounded (Fig. 1a).

Both cell types were able to form colonies, however these colonies were not homogeneous. Tenocytes generally formed large sparse colonies, whereas TDSCs formed more compact, dense colonies. When quantified

Table 1 Primer sequences for murine genes

Gene	Forward Primer	Reverse Primer
GAPDH	GAGAGGCCCTATCCCAACTC	GTGGGTGCAGCGAACTTTAT
CD90	GGATGAGGGCGACTACTTTTGT	TTGGAGCTCATGGGATTCG
CD73	TGGTTCACCGTTTACAAAGG	CGCTCAGAATTGGAAATTTAAC
TNC	AGGCGATCCCAGCCAGTCAGT	ATGGACGGGGCACCTCCTGTC
SCX	AAGTTGAGCAAAGACCGTGACA	TGTGGACCCTCCTCCTTCTAAC
MKX	AGTAAAGACAGTCAAGCTGCCACTG	TCCTGGCCACTCTAGAAGCG
Sca-1	GTTTGCTGATTCTTCTTGTGGCCC	ACTGCTGCCTCCTGAGTAACAC
NANOG	AGGGTCTGCTACTGAGATGCTCTG	CAACCACTGGTTTTTCTGCCACCG
TNMD	AACTCCACCTCAGCAGTAGTCC	TTTCTTGGATACCTCGGGCCAGAA
THBS4	TCCTCCGCTACCTGAAGAATGATGG	TTCAATGGACTCTGGGTTCTGGGTG
CD45	AGTTAGTGAATGGAGACCAGGAA	TCCATAAGTCTGCTTTCCTTCG
RUNX2	ATGCGTATTCCTGTAGATCCG	TTGGGGAGGATTTGTGAAGAC
OC	CTCTGTCTCTCTGACCTCACA	CAGGTCCTAAA AGTGATACC
OSX	GAAAGGAGGCACAAAGAAG	CACCAAGGAGTAGGTGTGTT
OPN	CATGAGATTGGCAGTGATTTGC	TGCAGGCTGTAAAGCTTCTCCT
FABP4	GAAGCTTGTCTCCAGTCAAAA	AGTCACGCCTTTCATAACACAT
PPARγ	CTCCGTGATGGAAGACCACTC	AGACTCGGAACTCAATGGC
LEPTIN	CTTCACCCCATTCTGAGTTTGT	TTCTCCAGGTCATTGGCTATCT
SOX9	TGGCAGACCAGTACCCGCATCT	TCTTTCTTGTGCTGCACGCGC
COL2A1	GGTTTGGAGAGACCATGAAC	TGGGTTCGCAATGGATTGTG
AGG	TTGCCAGGGGGAGTTGTATTC	GACAGTTCTCACGCCAGGTTTG

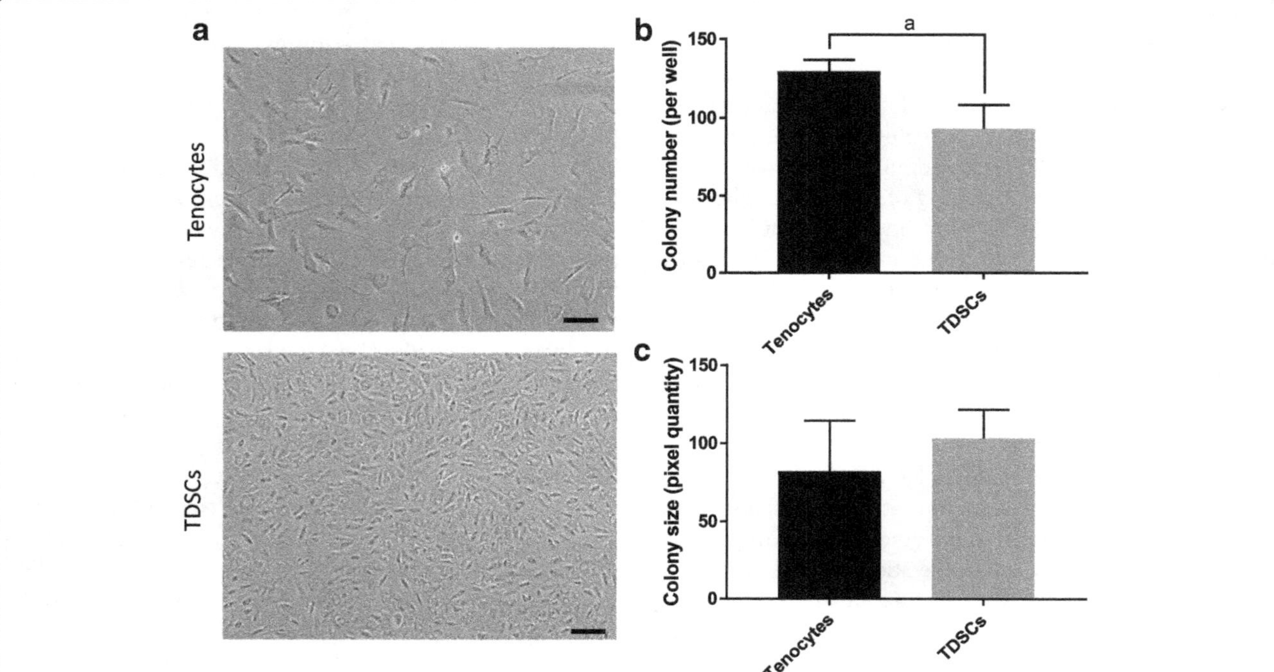

Fig. 1 Tenocyte and TDSC morphology and colony formation. Representative images of cell morphology are shown, bars = 100 μm (**a**). Colonies were counted (**b**) and measured (**c**) using ImageQuantTL software. Error bars shown represent SD. Pairwise comparisons were performed using a Student's independent t-test. [a]$p = 0.01$. $n = 4$ biological replicates

tenocytes produced significantly more colonies than TDSCs (Fig. 1b), however colony size was similar between cell types (Fig. 1c).

Tenocyte and TDSC proliferation

Both tenocytes and TDSCs proliferated very slowly and demonstrated very long population doubling times (PDT) with a mean (± SD) of 354 (±140) and 508 (±49) hours respectively (Fig. 2).

Tenocyte and TDSC marker expression

The gene expression of stem cell and tenogenic markers was assessed by qRT-PCR (Fig. 3). The majority of stem cell (Nanog and CD73) and early tenogenic markers (scleraxis and Mohawk) were more highly expressed in TDSCs when compared with tenocytes, whereas markers found in developed tendon (tenascin C, thrombospondin-4 and tenomodulin) exhibited higher expression in tenocytes compared to TDSCs. Expression of Nanog, scleraxis and Mohawk was significantly increased in TDSCs compared with tenocytes. Tenomodulin expression was significantly increased in tenocytes compared with TDSCs. The stem cell markers Sca-1 and CD90 were similarly expressed in both cell types. The haematopoietic stem cell marker CD45 demonstrated low expression with significantly higher levels observed for tenocytes compared with TDSCs.

Tenocyte and TDSC tri-lineage differentiation capacity

The ability of tenocytes and TDSCs to differentiate into different cell lineages was analysed by staining, glycosaminoglycan (GAG) assays and qRT-PCR for gene expression analysis.

Both cell types demonstrated osteogenic differentiation as assessed by alkaline phosphatase levels and alizarin

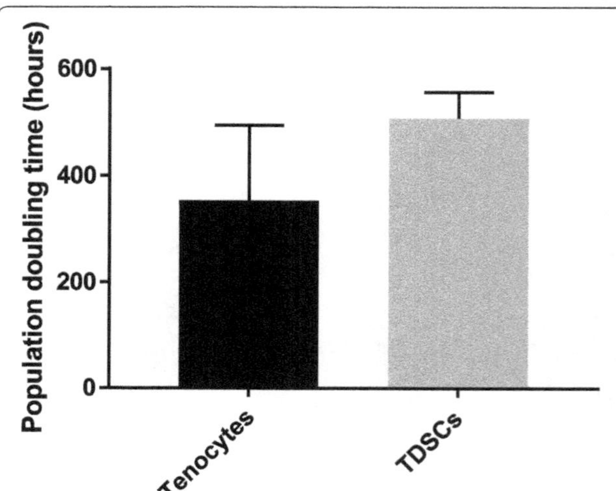

Fig. 2 Population doubling time for tenocytes and TDSCs. Error bars shown represent SD. Pairwise comparisons were performed using a Student's independent t-test. $n = 4$ biological replicates

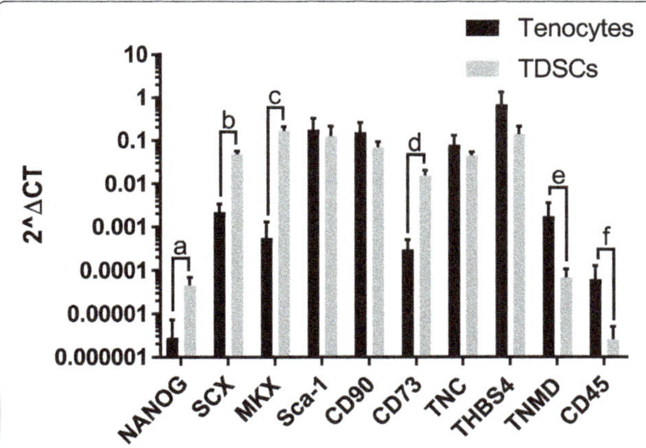

Fig. 3 Gene expression analysis of stem cell markers in tenocytes and TDSCs. Values are shown on a logarithmic scale and normalised to GAPDH. Error bars shown represent SD. Pairwise comparisons were performed using independent Student's t-tests after Log_{10} transformation of data. $^{a}p = 0.009$, $^{b}p = 0.011$, $^{c}p = 0.001$, $^{d}p = 0.011$, $^{e}p = 0.011$, $^{f}p = 0.011$. $n = 6$ biological replicates

red staining (Fig. 4). No adipogenic differentiation was observed for tenocytes, however oil red O staining was seen in differentiated TDSCs (Fig. 4). Tenocytes demonstrated some chondrogenic differentiation, with an increase in pellet size and intensity of safranin O staining in positive samples (chondrogenic induction media) compared with negative samples (control media). Due to low cell numbers, it was not possible to undertake chondrogenic differentiation assays on TDSCs (Fig. 4).

There was an increase in mean sGAG formation for tenocytes from 0.25 (±0.3) μg in negative samples to 0.5 (±0.54) μg in positive samples, however this was not significant. sGAG content was not analysed in TDSCs due to low cell numbers (Fig. 5).

Gene expression analysis of lineage specific genes showed a significant increase in the expression of osteogenic markers RUNX2 (runt-related transcription factor 2) and OPN (osteopontin) for TDSCs, however expression in tenocytes was similar between negative and positive samples (Fig. 6). There were small increases in all adipogenic

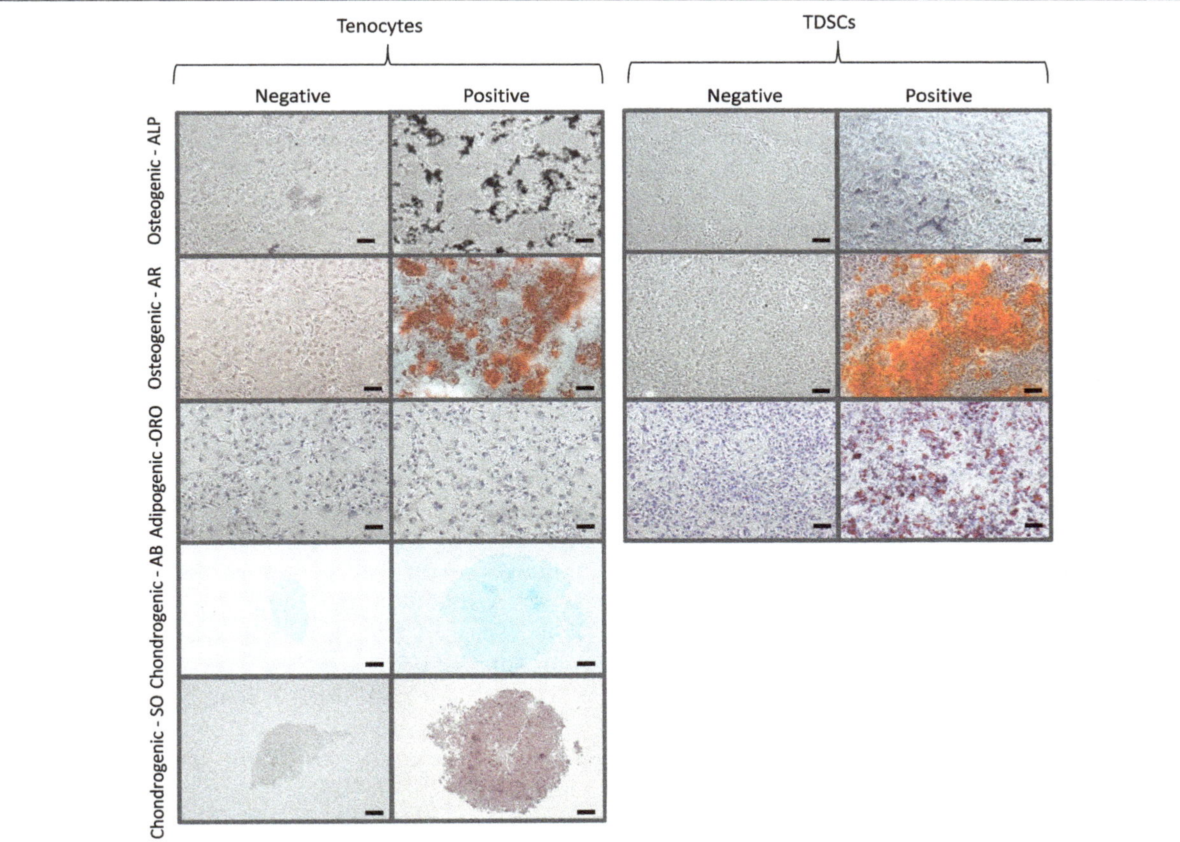

Fig. 4 Histological analysis of tri-lineage differentiation potential of tenocytes and TDSCs. Representative images are shown for both cell types after induction of osteogenic, adipogenic and chondrogenic differentiation (positive) and also for control samples (negative), after appropriate staining. Cells subjected to osteogenic differentiation media were stained for both alkaline phosphatase (ALP) activity and calcium deposits using alizarin red (AR). Cells subjected to adipogenic differentiation media were stained for oil droplet formation using oil red O (ORO), and cell pellets exposed to chondrogenic differentiation media, for GAG formation using alcian blue (AB) and safranin O (SO). Bar = 100 μm. Chondrogenic staining was not performed on TDSCs due to low cell numbers. $n = 6$ biological replicates

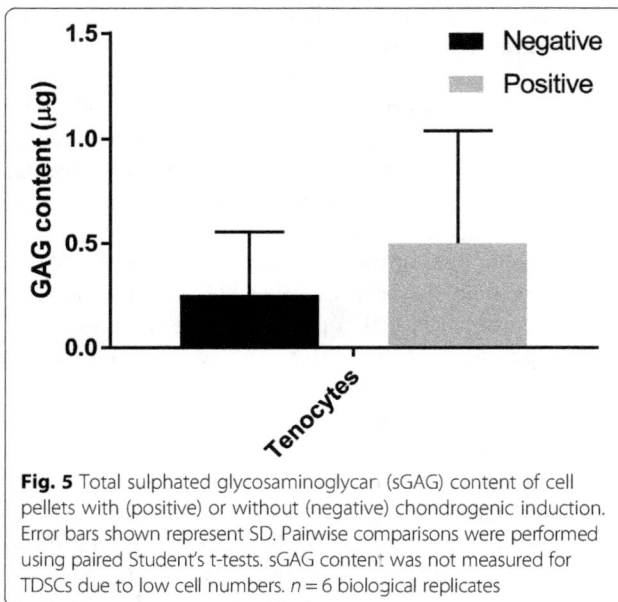

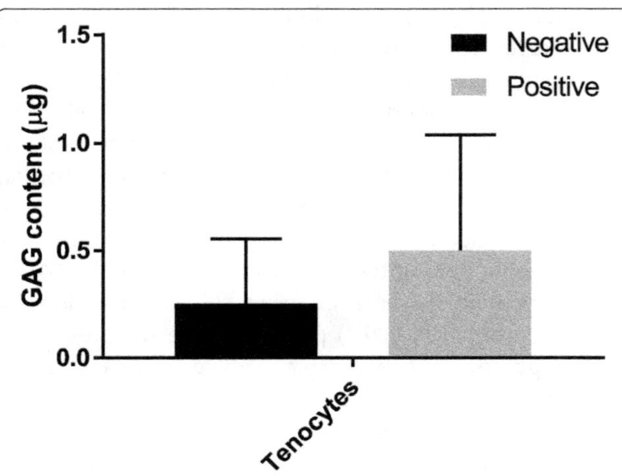

Fig. 5 Total sulphated glycosaminoglycan (sGAG) content of cell pellets with (positive) or without (negative) chondrogenic induction. Error bars shown represent SD. Pairwise comparisons were performed using paired Student's t-tests. sGAG content was not measured for TDSCs due to low cell numbers. $n = 6$ biological replicates

marker genes, such as LEPTIN, FABP4 (fatty acid binding protein 4) and PPARγ (peroxisome proliferator-activated receptor gamma), for tenocytes, and much larger significant increases for TDSCs in positive samples compared to negative samples (Fig. 6). Similarly, there was an increase in the majority of chondrogenic markers, such as AGG (aggrecan) and COL2 (collagen type II) in positive samples compared with negative samples for tenocytes although these were not significant. Chondrogenic markers were not analysed in TDSCs due to low cell numbers (Fig. 6).

Discussion

In this study we have isolated a population of cells in murine tendon that possess some of the traditional hallmarks of a stem cell: the ability to form colonies, the expression of stem cell markers and multipotency [39]. These findings are consistent with the published literature on murine TDSCs [12, 40–42]. The only discrepancy is the extended population doubling time observed in this study compared with previous reports. This could be explained by variations in cell isolation procedures. In this study we selected a low cell seeding density based on previous work in our group [15] and other studies [13, 16, 25–28], however some previous studies have used higher seeding densities. Alternatively, these differences may be due to mouse strain variation as research on murine mesenchymal stem cells (MSCs) has noted considerable variation in stem cell properties, including proliferation, between different strains of mice [43]. In addition, phenotypic differences of MSCs have been observed within certain strains of mice [44], highlighting the biological variation in murine stem cell populations. The TDSCs isolated in this study also stopped expanding at early passages which made certain assays impossible to perform due to low cell numbers. This may be due to stem cell quiescence, senescence or terminal differentiation and could indicate that these cells are not in fact stem cells but a progenitor cell population. For this reason we were unable to perform chondrogenic differentiation assays on TDSCs. We observed only moderate levels of chondrogenic differentiation for tenocytes which were low compared to reports in human tendon cells [45] and murine tendon tissue [46]. It is likely that the chondrogenic differentiation potential of TDSCs would be increased compared to tenocytes, as seen for osteogenic and adipogenic differentiation.

To our knowledge, no studies have compared the phenotype of murine tenocytes and TDSCs and we observed a number of phenotypic differences between these two cell populations. Tenocytes and TDSCs demonstrated different cell morphologies and colony forming ability as well as differences in the expression of certain stem cell markers, and some differences in multipotency. TDSCs generally conformed to the criteria of MSCs, as specified by the International Society for Cellular Therapy [39] (although chondrogenic potential could not be confirmed), whereas tenocytes did not due to a lack of adipogenic differentiation. The primary similarity between tenocytes and TDSCs was the expression of tenogenic markers such as tenascin C and thrombospondin 4, which was expected given that both cell populations were derived from tendon tissue. No studies have previously compared murine tenocytes and TDSCs, however such a comparison has been performed in other species [14, 15]. Our previous work demonstrated no discernible differences between tenocyte and TDSC populations in equine superficial digital flexor tendon, however a restricted differentiation potential was observed for equine TDSCs [15]. In contrast, a comparison of tenocytes and TDSCs in rabbit Achilles and patellar tendon demonstrated considerable differences in stemness between the two cell populations [14], which are more consistent with our study. The phenotypic differences observed in this study between tenocytes and TDSCs suggest that these cells are distinct populations with differing properties.

TDSCs have been used in a number of tissue engineering strategies to promote tendon healing with some encouraging results in human and animal models [16–20, 47, 48]. However, many of these studies do not state the exact TDSC isolation method used, or use varying cell seeding densities; in addition, many studies have not fully characterised the cells used for tendon repair. Therefore, it is possible that different tendon cell populations have been used across studies, which were not always defined as TDSCs. It is necessary to determine which tendon

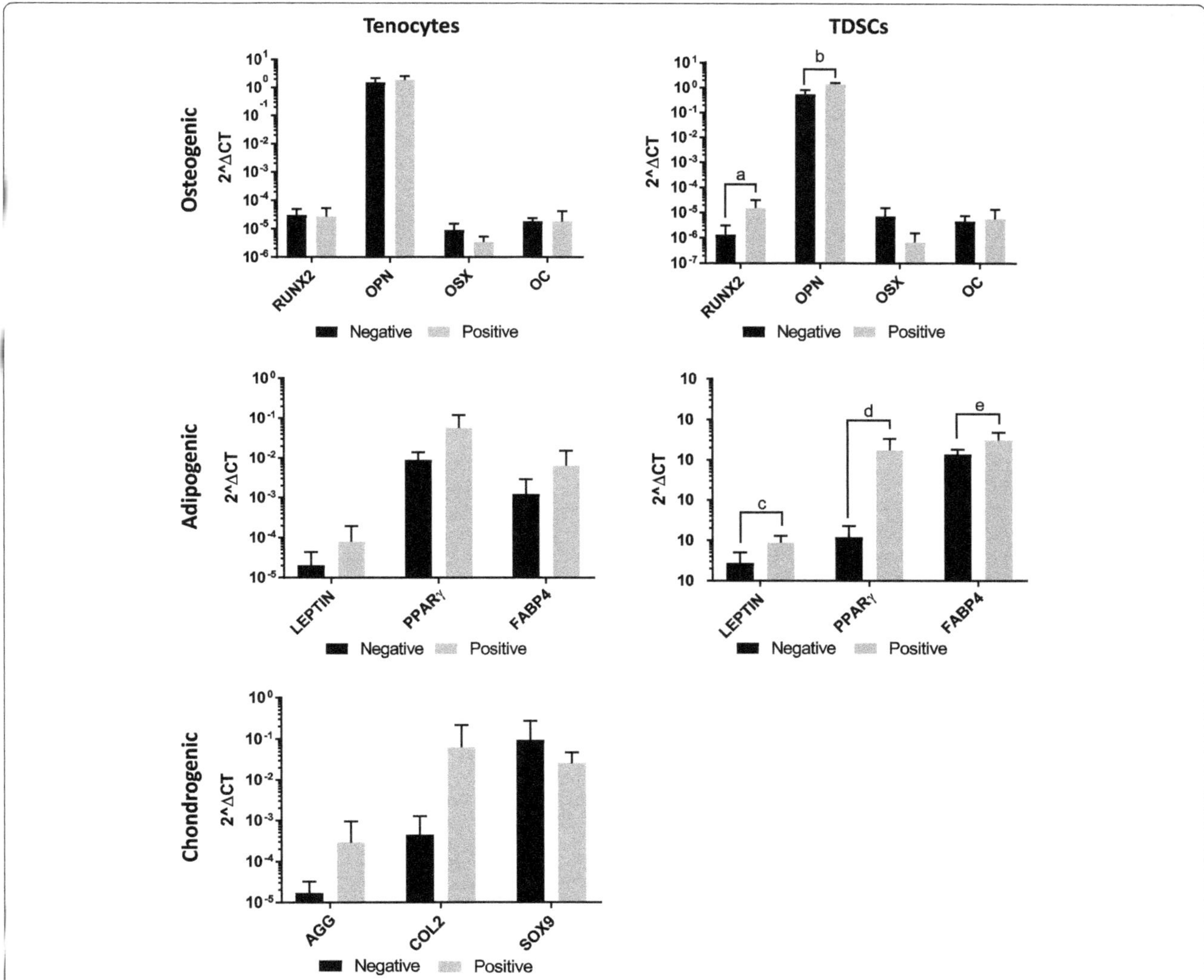

Fig. 6 Gene expression analysis of lineage specific markers for murine tenocytes and TDSCs. Values are shown on a logarithmic scale and normalised to GAPDH. Error bars shown represent SD. Pairwise comparisons were performed using paired Student's t-tests after Log_{10} transformation of data. [a]$p = 0.021$, [b]$p = 0.02$, [c]$p = 0.021$, [d]$p = 0.021$, [e]$p = 0.021$. Chondrogenic marker genes are not shown for TDSCs due to low cell numbers. $n = 6$ biological replicates

cell population is most effective for tendon repair. The increased stemness of murine TDSCs may promote tendon repair, however the poor proliferative potential of these cells is not conducive to tendon regeneration. Alternatively, murine tenocytes which demonstrated improved proliferative potential may provide a more suitable cell population for tendon regeneration. It is possible that the restricted differentiation potential of tenocytes may actually provide a therapeutic benefit during tendon healing by avoiding aberrant differentiation. Analysis of different tendon cell populations in human tendon has not yet been performed, however the presence of multiple tendon cell populations in several species [14, 15] would suggest the presence of more than one tendon cell population in human tendon. A comparison of tendon cell populations in humans is warranted, as well as investigation of the therapeutic potential of different tendon cell populations in vivo, which may highlight alternative, more effective tendon cell populations for human tendon repair strategies.

Conclusion

In conclusion, we have isolated and characterised two distinct tendon cell populations from murine tail tendon with differential properties. These tendon cell populations may provide therapeutic benefit for tendon injury and determination of the most effective cell population for tendon regeneration strategies in both humans and animals requires further investigation.

Abbreviations

AB: alcian blue; AGG: aggrecan; ALP: alkaline phosphatase; AR: alizarin red; CD: cluster of differentiation; cDNA: complementary deoxyribonucleic acid; COL2A1: collagen type II alpha 1; DMEM: Dulbecco's modified Eagle's medium; EDTA: ethylenediaminetetraacetic acid; FABP4: fatty acid binding protein 4; GAPDH: glyceraldehyde 3-phosphate dehydrogenase; IBMX: 3-isobutyl-1-methylxanthine; ITS: insulin transferrin selenium; MSC: mesenchymal stem cell; MKX: mohawk; OC: osteocalcin; OPN: osteopontin; ORO: oil red O; OSX: osterix; PDT: population doubling time; PPARγ: peroxisome proliferator-activated receptor gamma; qRT-PCR: quantitative real time-polymerase chain reaction; RNA: ribonucleic acid; RUNX2: runt-related transcription factor 2; Sca-1: stem cell antigen 1; SCX: scleraxis; SD: standard deviation; sGAG: sulphated glycosaminoglycan; SO: safranin O; TDSC: tendon-derived stem cell; TGFβ: transforming growth factor β; THBS4: thrombospondin 4; TNC: tenascin C; TNMD: tenomodulin

Acknowledgements

The authors would like to thank Dr. Simon Tew and Ms. Kirsty Johnson from the University of Liverpool for donation of murine tissue.

Funding

This project was funded by the Marjorie Forrest Bequest and by the Institute of Ageing and Chronic Disease at the University of Liverpool, UK. The funding source had no involvement in study design; collection, analysis and interpretation of data; in writing the report; or in the decision to submit the article for publication.

Authors' contributions

KJL acquired, analysed and interpreted data. PDC, EJC and EGC-L designed the study. KJL drafted the paper. All authors critically revised the manuscript and read and approved the final submitted version.

Consent for publication

Not applicable.

Competing interests

The authors declare that they have no competing interests.

Author details

[1]Department of Musculoskeletal Biology, Institute of Ageing and Chronic Disease, University of Liverpool, William Henry Duncan Building, 6 West Derby Street, Liverpool L7 8TX, UK. [2]School of Veterinary Science, Leahurst Campus, University of Liverpoo, Chester High Road, Neston CH64 7TE, UK. [3]The MRC-Arthritis Research UK Centre for Integrated research into Musculoskeletal Ageing (CIMA), Liverpool, UK.

References

1. Maffulli N, Wong J, Almekinders LC. Types and epidemiology of tendinopathy. Clinical Sports Medicine. 2003;22:675–92.
2. Kujala UM, Sarna S, Kapprio J. Cumulative incidence of Achilles tendon rupture and tendinopathy in male former elite athletes. Clin J Sport Med. 2005;15:133–5.
3. O'Neil BA, Forsythe ME, Stanish WD. Chronic occupational repetitive strain injury. Can Fam Physician. 2001;47:311–6.
4. Sharma P, Maffulli N. Biology of tendon injury: healing, modeling and remodeling. J Musculoskelet Neuronal Interact. 2006;6:181–90.
5. Mayor RB. Treatment of athletic tendonopathy. Conn Med. 2012;76:471–5.
6. Schwartz A, Watson JN, Hutchinson MR. Patellar tendinopathy. Sports Health. 2015;7:415–20.
7. Lempainen L, Johansson K, Banke IJ, Ranne J, Mäkelä K, Sarimo J, Niemi P, Orava S. Expert opinion: diagnosis and treatment of proximal hamstring tendinopathy. Muscles, Ligaments and Tendons Journal. 2015;5:23–8.
8. Goldin M, Malanga GA. Tendinopathy: a review of the pathophysiology and evidence for treatment. Phys Sportsmed. 2013;41:36–49.
9. Coleman BD, Khan KM, Maffulli N, Cook JL, Wark JD. Studies of surgical outcome after patellar tendinopathy: clinical significance of methodological deficiencies and guidelines for future studies. Scand J Med Sci Sports. 2000; 10:2–11.
10. Franchi M, Trire A, Quaranta M, Orsini E, Ottani V. Collagen structure of tendon relates to function. TheScientificWorldJOURNAL. 2007;7:404–20.
11. Kannus P. Structure of the tendon connective tissue. Scand J Med Sci Sports. 2000;10:312–20.
12. Bi Y, Ehirchiou D, Kilts TM, Inkson CA, Embree MC, Sonoyama W, Li L, Leet AI, Seo BM, Zhang L, et al. Identification of tendon stem/progenitor cells and the role of the extracellular matrix in their niche. Nat Med. 2007;13:1219–27.
13. Rui YF, Lui PP, Li G, Fu SC, Lee YW, Chan KM. Isolation and characterization of multipotent rat tendon-derived stem cells. Tissue Eng Part A. 2010;16:1549–58.
14. Zhang J, Wang JH. Characterization of differential properties of rabbit tendon stem cells and tenocytes. BMC Musculoskelet Disord. 2010;11:10.
15. Williamson KA, Lee KJ, Humphreys WJE, Comerford EJV, Clegg PD, Canty-Laird EG. Restricted differentiation potential of progenitor cell populations obtained from the equine superficial digital flexor tendon (SDFT). J Orthop Res. 2015;33:849–58.
16. Ni M, Lui PPY, Rui YF, Lee YW, Lee YW, Tan Q, Wong YM, Kong SK, Lau PM, Li G, Chan KM. Tendon-derived stem cells (TDSCs) promote tendon repair in a rat patellar tendon window defect model. J Orthop Res. 2012;30:613–9.
17. Ni M, Rui YF, Tan Q, Liu Y, Xu LL, Chan KM, Wang Y, Li G. Engineered scaffold-free tendon tissue produced by tendon-derived stem cells. Biomaterials. 2013;34:2024–37.
18. Zhang J, Li B, Wang JH. The role of engineered tendon matrix in the stemness of tendon stem cells in vitro and the promotion of tendon-like tissue formation in vivo. Biomaterials. 2011;32:6972–81.
19. Jiang D, Xu B, Yang M, Zhao Z, Zhang Y, Li Z. Efficacy of tendon stem cells in fibroblast-derived matrix for tendon tissue engineering. Cytotherapy. 2013;16:662–73.
20. Yin Z, Chen X, Chen JL, Shen WL, Hieu Nguyen TM, Gao L, Ouyang HW. The regulation of tendon stem cell differentiation by the alignment of nanofibers. Biomaterials. 2010;31:2163–75.
21. Katsanou V, Milatos S, Yiakouvaki A, Sgantzis N, Kotsoni A, Alexiou M, Harokopos V, Aidinis V, Hemberger M, Kontoyiannis DL. The RNA-binding protein Elavl1/HuR is essential for placental branching morphogenesis and embryonic development. Mol Cell Biol. 2009;29:2762–76.
22. Cascio LL, Liu K, Nakamura H, Chu G, Lim NH, Chanalaris A, Saklatvala J, Nagase H, Bou-Gharios G. Generation of a mouse line harboring a bi-transgene expressing luciferase and tamoxifen-activatable creERT2 recombinase in cartilage. Genesis. 2014;52:110–9.
23. Güngörmüş C, Kolankaya D. Characterization of type I, III and V collagens in high-density cultured tenocytes by triple-immunofluorescence technique. Cytotechnology. 2008;58:145–52.
24. Schulze-Tanzil G, Mobasheri A, Clegg PD, Sendzik J, John T, Shakibaei M. Cultivation of human tenocytes in high-density culture. Histochem Cell Biol. 2004;122:219–28.
25. Cheng B, Ge H, Zhou J, Zhang Q. TSG-6 mediates the effect of tendon derived stem cells for rotator cuff healing. European Rev for Medical and Pharmacol Sci. 2014;18:247–51.
26. Lee WY, Lui PP, Rui YF. Hypoxia-mediated efficient expansion of human tendon-derived stem cells in vitro. Tissue Eng Part A. 2012;18:484–98.
27. Mienaltowski M, Adams S, Birk D. Tendon proper- and peritenon-derived progenitor cells have unique tenogenic properties. Stem Cell Research and Therapy. 2014;5:86.
28. Tsai RYL, McKay RDG. Cell contact regulates fate choice by cortical stem cells. J Neurosci. 2000;20:3725–35.
29. Nagura I, Kokubu T, Mifune Y, Inui A, Takase F, Ueda Y, Kataoka T, Kurosaka M. Characterization of progenitor cells derived from torn human rotator cuff tendons by gene expression patterns of chondrogenesis, osteogenesis, and adipogenesis. J Orthop Surg Res. 2016;11:40.
30. Franken NAP, Rodermond HM, Stap J, Haveman J, van Bree C. Clonogenic assay of cells in vitro. Nat Protocols. 2006;1:2315–9.
31. Jaiswal N, Haynesworth SE, Caplan AI, Bruder SP. Osteogenic differentiation of purified, culture-expanded human mesenchymal stem cells in vitro. J Cell Biochem. 1997;64:295–312.

32. Cheng MT, Yang HW, Chen TH, Lee OKS. Isolation and characterization of multipotent stem cells from human cruciate ligaments. Cell Prolif. 2009;42:448–60.
33. Murdoch AD, Grady LM, Ablett MP, Katopodi T, Meadows RS, Hardingham TE. Chondrogenic differentiation of human bone marrow stem cells in Transwell cultures: generation of scaffold-free cartilage. Stem Cells. 2007;25:2786–96.
34. Farndale RW, Buttle DJ, Barrett AJ. Improved quantitation and discrimination of sulphated glycosaminoglycans by use of dimethylmethylene blue. Biochim Biophys Acta Gen Subj. 1986;883:173–7.
35. McDermott BT, Ellis S, Bou-Gharios G, Clegg PD, Tew SR. RNA binding proteins regulate anabolic and catabolic gene expression in chondrocytes. Osteoarthr Cartil. 2016;24:1263–73.
36. Reynolds JA, Haque S, Williamson K, Ray DW, Alexander MY, Bruce IN. Vitamin D improves endothelial dysfunction and restores myeloid angiogenic cell function via reduced CXCL-10 expression in systemic lupus erythematosus. Sci Rep. 2016;6:22341.
37. Peffers MJ, Fang Y, Cheung K, Wei TKJ, Clegg PD, Birch HL. Transcriptome analysis of ageing in uninjured human Achilles tendon. Arthritis Research & Therapy. 2015;17:33.
38. Vandesompele J, De Preter K, Pattyn F, Poppe B, Van Roy N, De Paepe A, Speleman F. Accurate normalization of real-time quantitative RT-PCR data by geometric averaging of multiple internal control genes. Genome Biology. 2002;3:research0034.0031–11.
39. Dominici M, Le Blanc K, Mueller I, Slaper-Cortenbach I, Marini F, Krause D, Deans R, Keating A, Prockop D, Horwitz E. Minimal criteria for defining multipotent mesenchymal stromal cells. The International Society for Cellular Therapy position statement. Cytotherapy. 2006;8:315–7.
40 Alberton P, Dex S, Popov C, Shukunami C, Schieker M, Docheva D. Loss of Tenomodulin results in reduced self-renewal and augmented senescence of tendon stem/progenitor cells. Stem Cells Dev. 2014;24:597–609.
41. Mienaltowski MJ, Adams SM, Birk DE. Regional differences in stem cell/ progenitor cell populations from the mouse achilles tendon. Tissue Eng Part A. 2013;19:199–210.
42. Zhang J, Wang JHC. The effects of mechanical loading on tendons - an in vivo and in vitro model study. PLoS One. 2013;8:e71740.
43. Peister A, Mellad JA, Larson BL, Hall BM, Gibson LF, Prockop DJ. Adult stem cells from bone marrow (MSCs) isolated from different strains of inbred mice vary in surface epitopes, rates of proliferation, and differentiation potential. Blood. 2004;103:1662–8.
44. Lei J, Hui D, Huang W, Liao Y, Yang L, Liu L, Zhang Q, Qi G, Song W, Zhang Y, et al. Heterogeneity of the biological properties and gene expression profiles of murine bone marrow stromal cells. Int J Biochem Cell Biol. 2013;45:2431–43.
45. Stanco D, ViganÒ M, Perucca Orfei C, Di Giancamillo A, Thiebat G, Peretti G, de Girolamo L. In vitro characterization of stem/progenitor cells from semitendinosus and gracilis tendons as a possible new tool for cell-based therapy for tendon disorders. Joints. 2014;2:159–68.
46. Mikic B, Rossmeier K, Bierwert L. Sexual dimorphism in the effect of GDF6 deficiency on murine tendon. Journal of orthopaedic research : official publ of the Orthopaedic Res Soc. 2009;27:1603–11.
47. Lui PPY, Wong OT, Lee YW. Transplantation of tendon-derived stem cells pre-treated with connective tissue growth factor and ascorbic acid in vitro promoted better tendon repair in a patellar tendon window injury rat model. Cytotherapy. 2016;18:99–112.
48. Chen L, Liu JP, Tang KL, Wang Q, Wang GD, Cai XH, Liu XM. Tendon derived stem cells promote platelet-rich plasma healing in collagenase-induced rat Achilles tendinopathy. Cell Physiol Biochem. 2014;34:2153–68.

17

Comparison of single-dose radial extracorporeal shock wave and local corticosteroid injection for treatment of carpal tunnel syndrome including mid-term efficacy

Pichitchai Atthakomol[1*], Worapaka Manosroi[2], Areerak Phanphaisarn[1], Sureeporn Phrompaet[1], Sawan Iammatavee[3] and Siam Tongprasert[4]

Abstract

Background: Recent studies have reported that radial extracorporeal shock wave therapy (rESWT) reduces pain and improves function in patients with mild to moderately severe carpal tunnel syndrome (CTS) compared to a placebo. However, most of those studies used multi-session rESWT combined with wrist support and evaluation of efficacy was limited to a maximum of 14 weeks.

Methods: The prospective randomized controlled trial compared efficacy in relieving pain and improving clinical function between single-dose rESWT and local corticosteroid injection (LCsI) over the mid-term (24 weeks). Twenty-five patients with mild to moderately severe CTS were randomized to receive either single-dose rESWT ($n = 13$) or LCsI ($n = 12$). Primary outcomes were evaluated using the Boston self-assessment questionnaire (BQ), while secondary outcomes used the Visual analogue scale (VAS) and electrodiagnostic parameters. Evaluations at baseline and at 1, 4, 12 and 24 weeks after treatment were performed.

Results: There was significantly greater improvement in symptom severity scores, functional scores and Boston questionnaire scores at weeks 12 to 24 in the rESWT group compared to the LCsI group. When compared to the baseline, there was significant reduction of VAS and functional score in the rESWT group at weeks 12 and 24. The LCsI group had no statistically significant differences in VAS reduction and functional score of the same period.

Conclusions: Treatment of CTS using single-dose rESWT has a carry-over effect lasting up to 24 weeks suggesting that single-dose rESWT is appropriate for treatment of mild to moderate CTS and provides longer-lasting benefits than LCsI.

Keywords: Extracorporeal shock wave, Steroid injection, Carpal tunnel syndrome, Randomized controlled trial, Treatment

* Correspondence: p.atthakomol@gmail.com
[1]Department of Orthopaedics, Faculty of Medicine, Chiang Mai University, Chiang Mai, Thailand
Full list of author information is available at the end of the article

Background

Carpal tunnel syndrome (CTS) is the most common entrapment neuropathy in the upper extremities [1]. Previous studies using varying based diagnostic criteria have reported population prevalence estimates from 2.7 to 14.4%, with a higher incidence in females than males among the elderly [2]. Specific causes of CTS are currently unknown, although evidence suggests that space occupying lesions can disturb blood circulation leading to demyelination of the median nerve and axonal loss [3–6]. Many risk factors are potentially associated with CTS including repetitive wrist motion, diabetes mellitus, hypothyroidism, rheumatism, obesity, arthritis, menopause and pregnancy [7–12].

Among the variety of optional treatments for CTS, local corticosteroid injection (LCsI) is widely used in mild to moderate cases and achieve improved symptom scores within 1 week [13]. A 2007 review by Cochrane reported greater symptom improvement 1 month after injection compared to placebo and significantly improved clinical outcomes compared to oral corticosteroids for up to 3 months [14]. Other publications have shown that LCsI provides benefits in terms of pain reduction and functional scores in patients with CTS. Those effects, however, were only reported to have occurred in the short term (up to 10 weeks) [15–17]. American Academy of Orthopaedic surgeons (AAOS) guidelines in 2008 and 2016 recommended LCsI or splinting for the treatment of CTS prior to considering a surgical option [18, 19].

There has been recent interest in extracorporeal shockwave therapy (ESWT) for CTS. Seok et al. demonstrated significant improvement in pain and symptom severity scores in CTS patients using focused ESWT (fESWT). At 3 months, however, symptom relief was not different from LCsI [20]. Several later studies have focused on the effect of radial ESWT (rESWT). CTS patients receiving 3 sessions of rESWT showed better clinical symptom improvement for 12–14 weeks compared to patients receiving sham ESWT [21, 22].

Patient compliance can affect the success of treatment [23, 24], so to reduce the period of time that a patient needs to repeat rESWT, we developed a single-dose rESWT for CTS and compared the efficacy of that treatment with LCsI up to the mid-term mark (week 24).

Methods

Design

This prospective, randomized, single-blind study was conducted at a tertiary level hospital. After receiving approval from our institutional review board, the Ethics Committee and registration at www.clinicaltrials.in.th (TCTR20150709001), we enrolled all new CTS patients who came to that hospital between January and June 2016 who gave their informed consent to participate in this study.

Participants

Only CTS patients older than 18 years were included. CTS diagnosis was based on guidelines of the American Academy of Neurology (AAN) for CTS. Diagnostic criteria consisted of standard symptoms, provocative factors, mitigating factors and standard physical examination results [25]. Practice parameter for electrodiagnostic studies in CTS of the American Association of Electrodiagnostic Medicine 2002 was used as the criteria for neurophysiologic diagnoses [26, 27]. We included only patients with mild or moderate severe CTS following the electrodiagnostic criteria as specified by Sucher [27]. Patients with underlying metabolic disorders such as diabetes mellitus, genetic disorders, upper limb surgery, peripheral polyneuropathy, traumatic nerve injury, blood coagulation disorder while using anticoagulants, pregnancy, thrombosis, cancer or previous surgical treatment for cancer, treatment with ultrasound, cryo-ultrasound, oral steroids or Nonsteroidal anti-inflammatory drugs (NSAIDs) within 7 days prior to enrollment or local injection of corticosteroid for CTS in the previous year were excluded. In patients with bilateral CTS, the hand with the more severe condition was selected for evaluation of treatment outcome.

Randomization and allocation

Patients who met the inclusion and exclusion criteria were randomly assigned to either the rESWT or the LCsI group in blocks of four (number of subjects per block = 4, number of block = 7) using a random number generator (free program from www.randomization.com). The notes in each treatment was prepared and put into envelopes according to the allocation orders.

The nurse assistant who did not take the responsibility in the allocation method would open the envelope and informed PA or SP to do the treatment.

In data collection process, research assistants who were blinded to the randomization and treatment methods evaluated VAS and the Thai version of BQ at baseline (before treatment) and at weeks 1, 4, 12 and 24 following treatment for both treatment methods [28]. Electrodiagnostic evaluation was performed at baseline (before treatment) and 12 weeks after treatment in both groups.

Patients whose CTS symptoms progressed to the point they could not be tolerated and those who asked for additional or alternative treatment were eliminated from this study.

Interventions

rESWT

Each patient in the rESWT group received shockwaves of continuous frequency and intensity (4 Bar, 15 Hz frequency, 5000 shocks, BTL-6000 SWT, radial shockwave mode). The probe was oriented perpendicular to the patient's palm between the distal wrist crease and Kaplan's cardinal line; ultrasound gel was used as a coupling agent. The duration of treatment was 3–7 min. A cold pack was applied for 15 min after rESWT.

LCsI

We used 1 ml. of triamcinolone (acetonide) 10 mg mixed with 1 ml of 1% lidocaine in a 3 ml disposable syringe. The injection was performed using a 25 gauge needle applied 1 cm proximal to the wrist flexion crease between the palmaris longus and flexor carpi radialis tendons. The angle of the needle was about 45 degrees distally and was advanced 1 cm, where it penetrated the flexor retinaculum. If paresthesia was provoked, we withdrew the needle and reinserted it 1 cm medial to the previous injection site. We advanced 1 cm at a time until the solution was injected. After injection, we instructed the patient to use their hand freely without splinting. Each patient was injected only once [29].

Outcome measures

Primary outcome

BQ [30], the most commonly used instrument to assess improvement of clinical symptoms and functional recovery of patients with CTS, consisted of 11 questions covering symptom severity and 8 questions to evaluate functional status (functional score) which rate the level of difficulty to perform activities in daily life. The rating scale ranged from 1 to 5, with 5 being the most difficult. In our study, we used the Thai version of the BQ [28].

Secondary outcomes

1) VAS was used to evaluate the intensity of pain at rest on a 10 cm VAS in cm. The patient marked the scale on which the start point represented no pain and the endpoint represented maximum or intolerable pain. 2) Electrodiagnostic evaluation was performed by a Rehabilitation Medicine board qualified senior staff member. Median peak sensory latency in millisecond (ms), distal motor latency in millisecond (ms), sensory nerve action potential (SNAP) amplitude in microvolt (uV) and compound muscle action potential (CMAP) amplitude in millivolt (mV) were the parameters used in this study.

Data analysis

Data were analyzed using Stata program (StataCorp. 2017. Stata Statistical Software: Release 15. College Station, TX: StataCorp LLC). For categorical variables, frequencies and percentages of were recorded; for continuous variables, means and standard deviations. Demographic data were analyzed using Fisher's exact test for categorical variables, the independent t-test for normally distributed continuous variables and the Mann-Whitney U test for non-normally distributed continuous variables. The paired t-test was used to evaluate the outcomes at each follow-up visit (weeks 1, 4, 12 and 24 after treatment) compared to the baseline. Differences between the two treatment groups at each follow-up visit were analyzed using mixed-model analysis of repeated measures including measurement of the effect of treatment, time, severity and interaction between treatment and time. Statistical significance was accepted at $p < 0.05$.

Estimated sample size for two-sample comparison of means with repeated measures. The preliminary data of BQ scores were used to calculate the sample size in each group [alpha = 0.05 (two-sided), power = 0.9. mean in population 1 = 22.33, mean in population 2 = 29, SD in population 1 = 2.51, SD in population 2 = 3]. Estimated required sample size in each group was 4.

Results

After screening for eligibility, a total of 25 patients were enrolled in the study and randomly assigned to receive one intervention (rESWT or LCsI). During the follow-up period, 3 patients rejected to provide electrodiagnostic measurement at week 12 after the treatment. At the final follow-up period (week 24), another 2 patients withdrew due to travel problems and additional 2 patients in the LCsI group developed severe symptom progression which required additional treatment (Fig. 1).

There were no statistically significant differences between the groups in terms of demographic characteristics (age, gender, body mass index) or in clinical characteristics (lesion site, baseline of pain, symptom and functional score and severity determined by electrodiagnostic measurement (Table 1).

There was a significant reduction of VAS and functional scores in the rESWT group at weeks 12 and 24 compared to baseline, while there was no significant change for the LCsI group. There were also significant reductions in symptom severity score and Boston questionnaire score at weeks 4, 12 and 24 in the rESWT group compared to baseline. In the LCsI group, there was significant reduction in terms of symptom severity score at weeks 1 and 4 as well as in the Boston questionnaire score at week 1 compared to the baseline. As to electrodiagnostic parameters, the rESWT group showed significant reduction in peak sensory distal latency at week 12 compared to the baseline as did the LCsI group. There were no significant changes from baseline in the

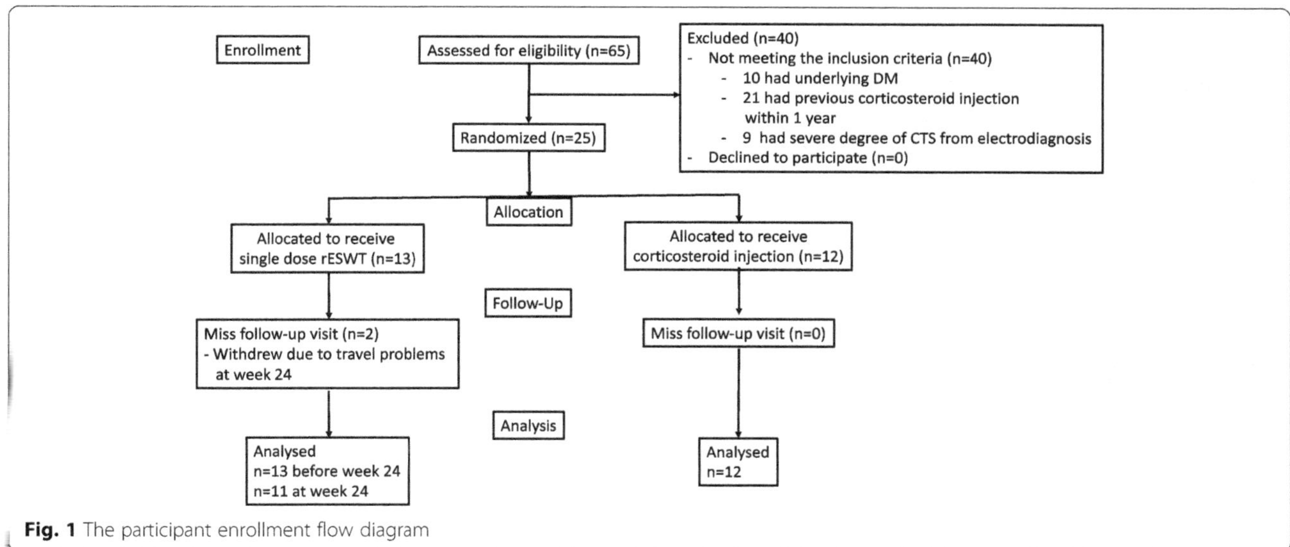

Fig. 1 The participant enrollment flow diagram

Table 1 Demographic and baseline characteristics of the groups

Characteristic	rESWT[a] (*n* = 13)	LCsI[b] (*n* = 12)	*p* value
Age, median (mean +/− SD), y	46 +/− 9	53 +/− 12	0.12
Gender, n (%)			0.16
Male	5 (62)	1 (8)	
Female	8 (38)	11 (92)	
Body mass index, (mean +/− SD)	28 (5)	24 (3)	0.09
Lesion site, n (%)			> 0.99
Right	9 (69)	8 (67)	
Left	4 (31)	4 (33)	
Unilateral	9 (69)	12 (100)	
Bilateral	4 (31)	0	
Severity, n (%)			> 0.99
Mild	5 (62)	4 (33)	
Moderate	8 (38)	8 (67)	
Baseline visual analogue scale, (mean +/− SD)	2.4 +/− 2.5	2.6 +/− 2.0	0.60
Baseline symptom severity score, (mean +/− SD)	21 +/− 6.4	22 +/− 5.1	0.63
Baseline functional score, (mean +/− SD)	14 +/− 3.2	12 +/− 4.1	0.16
Baseline Boston questionnaire score, (mean +/− SD)	35 +/− 8.5	34 +/− 8.5	0.77
Baseline peak sensory distal latency, (mean +/− SD)	4.5 +/− 0.72	3.7 +/− 1.3	0.057
Baseline SNAP[c] amplitude, (mean +/− SD)	17 +/− 6.9	18 +/− 10	0.72
Baseline motor distal latency, (mean +/− SD)	4.5 +/− 0.35	4.7 +/− 0.90	0.57
Baseline CMAP[d] amplitude, (mean +/− SD)	6.9 +/− 1.5	6.0 +/− 0.61	0.16

[a]rESWT = Radial extracorporeal shockwave therapy
[b]LCsI = Local corticosteroid injection
[c]SNAP = Sensory nerve action potential
[d]CMAP = Compound muscle action potential

other electrodiagnostic parameters in either group at week 12 (Table 2).

A comparison of post-treatment values of outcome variables between groups at each follow-up period is provided in Table 3. There was a significant declination in symptom severity score, functional score and Boston questionnaire score between week 12 and week 24 in the rESWT group compared to the LCsI group. While the VAS did not show the statistically significant difference between two groups in this period of time. There was a greater reduction in peak sensory distal latency between baseline and week 12 in the rESWT group than the LCsI group. Mixed-model analysis of repeated measures found that severity from electrodiagnostic measurement (mild or moderate) did not affect all outcome parameters ($p > 0.05$) with the exception of SNAP amplitude ($p < 0.05$).

Discussion

Session rESWT is becoming a popular treatment for patients with mild to moderate CTS. Published results of prospective, randomized control trials have shown regression in pain intensity and improvement of clinical symptoms compared to sham rESWT. However, session

Table 2 Comparison of pre-treatment and post-treatment values of outcome variables in each group

		rESWT[a] (*n* = 13)		LCsI[b] (*n* = 12)	
Outcome variable	Follow-up sessions	Mean +/− SD	*p* value	Mean +/− SD	*p* value
Visual analogue scale	Baseline	2.4 +/− 2.5		2.6 +/− 2.0	
	Week 1	1.3 +/− 2.0	0.18	1.6 +/− 1.7	0.08
	Week 4	1.3 +/− 1.9	0.15	1.4 +/− 1.5	0.08
	Week 12	0.65 +/− 1.2	0.022*	1.9 +/− 2.7	0.52
	Week 24	0.35 +/− 0.81[c]	0.0075*	1.7 +/− 2.1	0.19
Symptom severity score	Baseline	21 +/− 6.4		22 +/− 5.1	
	Week 1	19 +/− 7.4	0.33	17 +/− 4.5	0.0047*
	Week 4	17 +/− 4.3	0.031*	17 +/− 5.1	0.011*
	Week 12	15 +/− 4.5	0.0082*	18 +/− 5.5	0.13
	Week 24	13 +/− 2.9[c]	0.0059*	19 +/− 7.9	0.20
Functional score	Baseline	14 +/− 3.2		12 +/− 4.1	
	Week 1	13 +/− 4.2	0.27	11 +/− 3.2	0.31
	Week 4	13 +/− 3.5	0.12	11 +/− 3.3	0.39
	Week 12	11 +/− 3.0	0.0065*	10 +/− 3.4	0.19
	Week 24	11 +/− 2.2[c]	0.0073*	13 +/− 7.0	0.65
Boston questionnaire score	Baseline	35 +/− 8.5		34 +/− 8.5	
	Week 1	32 +/− 10	0.28	28 +/− 7.0	0.037*
	Week 4	30 +/− 7.1	0.032*	28 +/− 8.0	0.05
	Week 12	26 +/− 6.8	0.0040*	29 +/− 8.2	0.13
	Week 24	24 +/− 4.7[c]	0.0037*	32 +/− 14	0.47
Peak sensory distal latency	Baseline	4.5 +/− 0.72		3.7 +/− 1.3	
	Week 12	4.1 +/− 0.74[d]	0.0047*	3.6 +/− 1.3	0.026*
SNAP[e] amplitude	Baseline	17 +/− 6.9		18 +/− 11	
	Week 12	18 +/− 6.5[d]	0.66	21 +/− 12	0.28
Motor distal latency	Baseline	4.5 +/− 0.35		4.7 +/− 0.90	
	Week 12	4.2 +/− 0.42[d]	0.084	4.4 +/− 0.75	0.06
CMAP[f] amplitude	Baseline	6.9 +/− 1.5		6.0 +/− 0.61	
	Week 12	6.9 +/− 1.6[d]	0.91	6.5 +/− 1.2	0.20

*$p < 0.05$
[a]rESWT = Radial extracorporeal shockwave therapy
[b]LCsI = Local corticosteroid injection
[c]$n = 11$
[d]$n = 10$
[e]SNAP = Sensory nerve action potential
[f]CMAP = Compound muscle action potential

Table 3 Comparison of post-treatment values of outcome variables between both groups in each follow-up peroid

Outcome variable	Follow-up sessions	Coefficeint (rESWT[a] VS LCsI[b])	*p* value	95% CI
Visual analogue scale	Baseline to week 1	−0.10	0.90	−1.7 to 1.5
	Week 1 to week 4	0 .049	0.95	− 1.6 to 1.7
	Week 4 to week 12	−1.0	0.23	−2.7 to 0.63
	Week 12 to week 24	−1.2	0.17	− 2.9 to 0.49
Symptom severity score	Baseline to week 1	2.6	0.27	−2.0 to 7.2
	Week 1 to week 4	1.5	0.53	−3.2 to 6.1
	Week 4 to week 12	−1.9	0.43	−6.5 to 2.8
	Week 12 to week 24	−5.1	0.036*	−9.8 to −0.33
Functional score	Baseline to week 1	0.43	0.81	−3.1 to 3.9
	Week 1 to week 4	−0.20	0.91	−3.7 to 3.3
	Week 4 to week 12	−1.8	0.32	−5.3 to 1.7
	Week 12 to week 24	−4.5	0.015*	−8.1 to −0.87
Boston questionnaire score	Baseline to week 1	3.0	0.43	−4.5 to 11
	Week 1 to week 4	1.3	0.74	−6.2 to 8.8
	Week 4 to week 12	−3.7	0.34	−11 to 3.8
	Week 12 to week 24	−9.5	0.015*	−17 to − 1.9
Peak sensory distal latency	Baseline to week 12	−0.24	0.022*	− 0.44 to − 0.034
SNAP[c] amplitude	Baseline to week 12	−2.8	0.36	−8.9 to 3.2
Motor distal latency	Baseline to week 12	−0.038	0.84	−0.41 to 0.33
CMAP[d] amplitude	Baseline to week 12	−0.44	0.34	−1.4 to 0.46

*$p < 0.05$
[a]rESWT = Radial extracorporeal shockwave therapy
[b]LCsI = Local corticosteroid injection
[c]SNAP = Sensory nerve action potential
[d]CMAP = Compound muscle action potential

rESWT requires patients to return to a medical center to receive treatments for 3 to 4 consecutive weeks [21, 22, 31], a situation that is reflected in reports of compliance affecting the success of treatment [23, 24]. We theorized that if a single-dose rESWT provides a good functional outcome in mild and moderate CTS patients, it might resolve the compliance problem by eliminating the need for repeated interventions. The levels and duration of efficacy of a single-dose rESWT treatment of CTS are still controversial, including rESWT efficacy compared to LCsI, a CTS treatment frequently recommended prior considering surgical options [18, 19], i.e., the relative efficacy of single-dose rESWT treatment compared to LCsI was still an open question.

To the best our knowledge, this study examines a new dimension in the treatment of CTS. Single-dose rESWT, which has a carry-over effect lasting up to 24 weeks, showed significant improvement in terms of clinical symptoms and functional recovery compared to LCsI from weeks 12 to week 24. Most previous studies have conducted the final follow up at week 12 or week 14 [20–22, 32, 33]. The methodology evaluated in this study showed the efficacy of single-dose rESWT in the absence of any other confounding treatment, e.g., the wrist splints used in combination with rESWT in other studies [21, 22, 31, 32, 34]. This study used mixed-model analysis of repeated measures to analyze differences between treatments which can detect the effect of time on the results of treatment while other cohort studies have used the Mann-Whitney U test [20, 21] and the independent t-test [31, 32].

One limitation of our study is the relatively low number of patients compared to other studies [20–22, 31–34], although our sample did have enough statistical power to detect the significant difference between groups at weeks 12 and 24. A second limitation is that the different dose intensity of rESWT might affect the results of treatment. Finally, long- term results, beyond 24 weeks, were not measured. Future studies should include larger numbers of patients, different treatment protocols and longer follow-up periods.

In our study, the pain relief benefit of rESWT appeared to begin at week 12 and to continue through week 24 compared to baseline, while LCsI initially provided statistically insignificant pain reduction which disappeared entirely by week 24. Compared to previous studies, the effect of pain reduction from session rESWT seemed to begin earlier in our study [21, 31, 32]. In terms of symptom severity and functional outcomes, with single-dose rESWT significant improvement compared to the baseline began at week 4, while the LCsI group had significant improvement at only week 1. Conversely, symptom and functional improvement were not significant after that time. This differs from Wo et al. which reported an earlier effect of session rESWT for symptom and functional improvement beginning at week 1 [21]. The differences in pain, symptom and functional improvement of single dose rESWT in our study compared to session rESWT in others studies might be the result of differences in the method of rESWT (single vs. session) as well as the effect of wrist splinting in the other studies (single-dose rESWT vs. session rESWT +wrist splinting) [21, 31, 32].

Our study found a significant decrease in peak sensory distal latency in both groups at week 12 compared to the baseline while other electrodiagnostic parameters showed no significant difference between the baseline and week 12. The only significant difference in improvement of electrodiagnostic parameters between the groups was the greater reduction in peak sensory distal latency in the rESWT group. Two other studies reported a significant increase in sensory nerve conduction velocity between baseline and week 12 with rESWT [21, 32]. One of those studies detected no difference between the baseline and week 12 for all electrodiagnostic parameters in a fESWT group [20], while the other study reported a significant decrease in CMAP and SNAP distal latency between baseline and week 12 in an ESWT group [31]. Taken together, these results seem to indicate that the effect of electrodiagnostic changes seems to be inconclusive. The reason the results of electrodiagnostic changes varied might be a reflection of the fact that the other studies also found no significant relationship between symptom severity score and electrodiagnostic findings [35, 36]. Additionally, one study reported that the electrodiagnosis could access only large myelinated nerves functions. Small non-myelinated sensory nerve functions, which are commonly associated with CTS symptoms, could not be evaluated by electrodiagnostic measurement [37].

Our study demonstrated that single rESWT provided greater benefits in term of symptom severity reduction and functional improvement compared to LCsI during weeks 12 and 24, while other studies have reported on maintenance of benefits from LCsI for only short periods (up to 3 months) [13, 14, 17].

The mechanisms by which rESWT helps CTS patients remain inconclusive. One experimental study reported that ESWT down-regulated the inflammatory effect by inducing tyrosine dephosphorylation of endothelial nitric oxide synthase which increases the level of nitric oxide. After that the amount of the nitric oxide suppresses NF-kappa B activation which inhibits LPS/IFN-gamma-elicited expression of genes in the inflammatory process [38]. A study in rat glioma cell line C6 also reported an anti-inflammatory effect caused by the same mechanism [39]. Previous reports have also described effects of ESWT including enhancing elimination of injured axons, promoting Schwann cell proliferation and increasing axonal regeneration [40–42].

The efficacy of ESWT relies on the dose intensity, duration and number of attempts. A recent study reported a longer-lasting effect with multiple-session attempts compared to a single-dose [22]. Our single-dose rESWT protocol had a higher dose intensity than that study (3–7 min 4 Bar, frequency: 15 Hz, number of shocks: 5000 shocks VS 4 Bar, frequency: 5 Hz, number of shocks: 2000 shocks) [22]. Our rESWT protocol provided a long-lasting effect, up to 24 weeks, without multiple-session attempts.

No serious complications in terms of severe pain or progression of symptoms occurred with single-dose rESWT. A few patients mentioned minimal pain during treatment, but that pain was relieved within a minute following application of a cold pack. To date, there have been no severe complications reported from using fESWT or rESWT to treat CTS patients [20–22, 31–34]. The literature does mention that transient pain, skin redness or small hematoma might present after ESWT, but those are typically resolved spontaneously [43].

Conclusions

Based on the results of this study, single-dose rESWT provides longer-lasting benefits than LCsI in the treatment of mild to moderate CTS.

Abbreviations

AAN: American Academy of Neurology; AAOS: American Academy of Orthopaedic surgeons; BQ: The Boston self-assessment questionnaire; CMAP: Compound muscle action potential; CTS: Carpal tunnel syndrome; LCsI: Local corticosteroid injection; NSAIDs: Nonsteroidal anti-inflammatory drugs; rESWT: Radial extracorporeal shock wave therapy; SNAP: Sensory nerve action potential; VAS: Visual analogue scale

Acknowledgements

This study was supported by the Faculty of Medicine, Chiang Mai University. The authors are grateful to Thipphakorn Kanthawong, MA; Jirachart Kraisarin, MD for collecting the data and to G. Lamar Robert, PhD, for reviewing the manuscript.

Funding

Faculty of Medicine, Chiang Mai University.

Authors' contributions

PA initiated study conception and design. SP performed single-dose radial extracorporeal shock wave therapy. PA injected local corticosteroid injection. ST performed electrodiagnosis. SI performed data collection and acquisition of data. WM and AP performed analysis and interpretation of data. PA wrote and edited the manuscript. PA had role in critical revision. All authors have read and approved the manuscript.

Consent for publication
Not Applicable

Competing interests
The authors declare that they have no competing interests.

Author details
[1]Department of Orthopaedics, Faculty of Medicine, Chiang Mai University, Chiang Mai, Thailand. [2]Division of Endocrinology, Department of Internal Medicine, Bangkok Chiang Mai Hospital, Chiang Mai, Thailand. [3]Department of Orthopaedics, Nakornping Hospital, Chiang Mai, Thailand. [4]Department of Rehabilitation Medicine, Faculty of Medicine, Chiang Mai University, Chiang Mai, Thailand.

References

1. Olney RK. Carpal tunnel syndrome: complex issues with a "simple" condition. Neurology. 2001;56(11):1431–2.
2. Atroshi I, Gummesson C, Johnsson R, Ornstein E, Ranstam J, Rosen I. Prevalence of carpal tunnel syndrome in a general population. JAMA. 1999; 282(2):153–8.
3. Gelberman RH, Hergenroeder PT, Hargens AR, Lundborg GN, Akeson WH. The carpal tunnel syndrome. A study of carpal canal pressures. J Bone Joint Surg Am. 1981;63(3):380–3.
4. Gelberman RH, Szabo RM, Williamson RV, Hargens AR, Yaru NC, Minteer-Convery MA. Tissue pressure threshold for peripheral nerve viability. Clin Orthop Relat Res. 1983;178:285–91.
5. Lundborg G, Gelberman RH, Minteer-Convery M, Lee YF, Hargens AR. Median nerve compression in the carpal tunnel–functional response to experimentally induced controlled pressure. J Hand Surg Am. 1982;7(3):252–9.
6. Szabo RM, Gelberman RH, Williamson RV, Hargens AR. Effects of increased systemic blood pressure on the tissue fluid pressure threshold of peripheral nerve. J Orthop Res. 1983;1(2):172–8.
7. Werner RA, Andary M. Carpal tunnel syndrome: pathophysiology and clinical neurophysiology. Clin Neurophysiol. 2002;113(9):1373–81.
8. van Dijk MA, Reitsma JB, Fischer JC, Sanders GT. Indications for requesting laboratory tests for concurrent diseases in patients with carpal tunnel syndrome: a systematic review. Clin Chem. 2003;49(9):1437–44.
9. Shiri R. Hypothyroidism and carpal tunnel syndrome: a meta-analysis. Muscle Nerve. 2014;50(6):879–83.
10. Padua L, Di Pasquale A, Pazzaglia C, Liotta GA, Librante A, Mondelli M. Systematic review of pregnancy-related carpal tunnel syndrome. Muscle Nerve. 2010;42(5):697–702.
11. Pourmemari MH, Shiri R. Diabetes as a risk factor for carpal tunnel syndrome: a systematic review and meta-analysis. Diabet Med. 2016;33(1):10–6.
12. Shiri R, Pourmemari MH, Falah-Hassani K, Viikari-Juntura E. The effect of excess body mass on the risk of carpal tunnel syndrome: a meta-analysis of 58 studies. Obes Rev. 2015;16(12):1094–104.
13. Cartwright MS, White DL, Demar S, Wiesler ER, Sarlikiotis T, Chloros GD, Yoon JS, Won SJ, Molnar JA, Defranzo AJ, et al. Median nerve changes following steroid injection for carpal tunnel syndrome. Muscle Nerve. 2011;44(1):25–9.
14. Marshall S, Tardif G, Ashworth N. Local corticosteroid injection for carpal tunnel syndrome. Cochrane Database Syst Rev. 2007;2:CD001554.
15. Armstrong T, Devor W, Borschel L, Contreras R. Intracarpal steroid injection is safe and effective for short-term management of carpal tunnel syndrome. Muscle Nerve. 2004;29(1):82–8.
16. Carlson H, Colbert A, Frydl J, Arnall E, Elliot M, Carlson N. Current options for nonsurgical management of carpal tunnel syndrome. Int J Clin Rheumatol. 2010;5(1):129–42.
17. Atroshi I, Flondell M, Hofer M, Ranstam J. Methylprednisolone injections for the carpal tunnel syndrome: a randomized, placebo-controlled trial. Ann Intern Med. 2013;159(5):309–17.
18. Keith MW, Masear V, Amadio PC, Andary M, Barth RW, Graham B, Chung K, Maupin K, Watters WC 3rd, Haralson RH 3rd, et al. Treatment of carpal tunnel syndrome. J Am Acad Orthop Surg. 2009;17(6):397–405.
19. Graham B, Peljovich AE, Afra R, Cho MS, Gray R, Stephenson J, Gurman A, MacDermid J, Mlady G, Patel AT, et al. The American Academy of Orthopaedic Surgeons Evidence-Based Clinical Practice Guideline on: Management of Carpal Tunnel Syndrome. J Bone Joint Surg Am. 2016; 98(20):1750–4.
20. Seok H, Kim SH. The effectiveness of extracorporeal shock wave therapy vs. local steroid injection for management of carpal tunnel syndrome: a randomized controlled trial. Am J Phys Med Rehabil. 2013;92(4):327–34.
21. Wu YT, Ke MJ, Chou YC, Chang CY, Lin CY, Li TY, Shih FM, Chen LC. Effect of radial shock wave therapy for carpal tunnel syndrome: a prospective randomized, double-blind, placebo-controlled trial. J Orthop Res. 2016;34(6):977–84.
22. Ke MJ, Chen LC, Chou YC, Li TY, Chu HY, Tsai CK, Wu YT. The dose-dependent efficiency of radial shock wave therapy for patients with carpal tunnel syndrome: a prospective, randomized, single-blind, placebo-controlled trial. Sci Rep. 2016;6:38344.
23. Demonceau J, Ruppar T, Kristanto P, Hughes DA, Fargher E, Kardas P, De Geest S, Dobbels F, Lewek P, Urquhart J, et al. Identification and assessment of adherence-enhancing interventions in studies assessing medication adherence through electronically compiled drug dosing histories: a systematic literature review and meta-analysis. Drugs. 2013;73(6):545–62.
24. Corrao G, Parodi A, Nicotra F, Zambon A, Merlino L, Cesana G, Mancia G. Better compliance to antihypertensive medications reduces cardiovascular risk. J Hypertens. 2011;29(3):610–8.
25. American Academy of Neurology. Practice parameter for carpal tunnel syndrome (summary statement). Report of the quality standards subcommittee of the American Academy of Neurology. Neurol. 1993;43(11):2406–9.
26. American Association of Electrodiagnostic Medicine AAoN, American Academy of Physical M, Rehabilitation. Practice parameter for electrodiagnostic studies in carpal tunnel syndrome: summary statement. Muscle Nerve. 2002;25(6):918–22.
27. Sucher BM. Grading severity of carpal tunnel syndrome in electrodiagnostic reports: why grading is recommended. Muscle Nerve. 2013;48(3):331–3.
28. Upatham S, Kumnerddee W. Reliability of Thai version Boston questionnaire. J Med Assoc Thail. 2008;91(8):1250–6.
29. Gelberman RH, Aronson D, Weisman MH. Carpal-tunnel syndrome. Results of a prospective trial of steroid injection and splinting. J Bone Joint Surg Am. 1980;62(7):1181–4.
30. Levine DW, Simmons BP, Koris MJ, Daltroy LH, Hohl GG, Fossel AH, Katz JN. A self-administered questionnaire for the assessment of severity of symptoms and functional status in carpal tunnel syndrome. J Bone Joint Surg Am. 1993;75(11):1585–92.
31. Vahdatpour B, Kiyani A, Dehghan F. Effect of extracorporeal shock wave therapy on the treatment of patients with carpal tunnel syndrome. Adv Biomed Res. 2016;5:120.
32. Raissi GR, Ghazaei F, Forogh B, Madani SP, Daghaghzadeh A, Ahadi T. The effectiveness of radial extracorporeal shock waves for treatment of carpal tunnel syndrome: a randomized clinical trial. Ultrasound Med Biol. 2017; 43(2):453–60.
33. Paoloni M, Tavernese E, Cacchio A, D'Orazi V, Ioppolo F, Fini M, Santilli V, Mangone M. Extracorporeal shock wave therapy and ultrasound therapy improve pain and function in patients with carpal tunnel syndrome. A randomized controlled trial. Eur J Phys Rehabil Med. 2015;51(5):521–8.
34. Notarnicola A, Maccagnano G, Tafuri S, Fiore A, Pesce V, Moretti B. Comparison of shock wave therapy and nutraceutical composed of Echinacea angustifolia, alpha lipoic acid, conjugated linoleic acid and quercetin (perinerv) in patients with carpal tunnel syndrome. Int J Immunopathol Pharmacol. 2015;28(2):256–62.
35. Chan L, Turner JA, Comstock BA, Levenson LM, Hollingworth W, Heagerty PJ, Kliot M, Jarvik JG. The relationship between electrodiagnostic findings and patient symptoms and function in carpal tunnel syndrome. Arch Phys Med Rehabil. 2007;88(1):19–24.
36. Longstaff L, Milner RH, O'Sullivan S, Fawcett P. Carpal tunnel syndrome: the correlation between outcome, symptoms and nerve conduction study findings. J Hand Surg Br. 2001;26(5):475–80.

37. Gursoy AE, Kolukisa M, Yildiz GB, Kocaman G, Celebi A, Kocer A. Relationship between electrodiagnostic severity and neuropathic pain assessed by the LANSS pain scale in carpal tunnel syndrome. Neuropsychiatr Dis Treat. 2013;9:65–71.
38. Mariotto S, Cavalieri E, Amelio E, Ciampa AR, de Prati AC, Marlinghaus E, Russo S, Suzuki H. Extracorporeal shock waves: from lithotripsy to anti-inflammatory action by NO production. Nitric Oxide. 2005;12(2):89–96.
39. Ciampa AR, de Prati AC, Amelio E, Cavalieri E, Persichini T, Colasanti M, Musci G, Marlinghaus E, Suzuki H, Mariotto S. Nitric oxide mediates anti-inflammatory action of extracorporeal shock waves. FEBS Lett. 2005;579(30):6839–45.
40. Hausner T, Nogradi A. The use of shock waves in peripheral nerve regeneration: new perspectives? Int Rev Neurobiol. 2013;109:85–98.
41. Hausner T, Pajer K, Halat G, Hopf R, Schmidhammer R, Redl H, Nogradi A. Improved rate of peripheral nerve regeneration induced by extracorporeal shock wave treatment in the rat. Exp Neurol. 2012;236(2):363–70.
42. Lee JH, Cho SH. Effect of extracorporeal shock wave therapy on denervation atrophy and function caused by sciatic nerve injury. J Phys Ther Sci. 2013; 25(9):1067–9.
43. Wild C, Khene M, Wanke S. Extracorporeal shock wave therapy in orthopedics. Assessment of an emerging health technology. Int J Technol Assess Health Care. 2000;16(1):199–209.

Association between Fas/FasL gene polymorphism and musculoskeletal degenerative diseases

Donghua Huang[1†], Jinrong Xiao[2†], Xiangyu Deng[1], Kaige Ma[1], Hang Liang[1], Deyao Shi[1], Fashuai Wu[1] and Zengwu Shao[1*]

Abstract

Background: It was reported that Fas (rs1800682, rs2234767) and FasL (rs5030772, rs763110) gene polymorphism might be related to the risk of musculoskeletal degenerative diseases (MSDD), such as osteoarthritis (OA), intervertebral disc degeneration (IVDD) and rheumatoid arthritis (RA). However, data from different studies was inconsistent. Here we aim to elaborately summarize and explore the association between the Fas (rs1800682, rs2234767) and FasL (rs5030772, rs763110) and MSDD.

Methods: Literatures were selected from PubMed, Web of Science, Embase, Scopus and Medline in English and VIP, SinoMed, Wanfang and the China National Knowledge Infrastructure (CNKI) in Chinese up to August 21, 2017. All the researches included are case-control studies about human. We calculated the pooled odds ratios (ORs) with 95% confidence intervals (95% CI) to evaluate the strengths of the associations of Fas (rs1800682, rs2234767) and FasL (rs5030772, rs763110) polymorphisms with MSDD risk.

Results: Eleven eligible studies for rs1800682 with 1930 cases and 1720 controls, 6 eligible studies for rs2234767 with 1794 cases and 1909 controls, 3 eligible studies for rs5030772 with 367 cases and 313 controls and 8 eligible studies for rs763110 with 2010 cases and 2105 controls were included in this analysis. The results showed that the G allele of Fas (rs1800682) is associated with an increased risk of IVDD in homozygote and recessive models. The G allele of Fas (rs2234767) is linked to a decreased risk of RA but an enhanced risk of OA in allele and recessive models. In addition, the T allele of FasL (rs763110) is correlated with a reduced risk of IVDD in all of models. However, no relationship was found between FasL (rs5030772) and these three types of MSDD in any models.

Conclusions: Fas (rs1800682) and FasL (rs763110) polymorphism were associated with the risk of IVDD and Fas (rs2234767) was correlated to the susceptibility of OA and RA. Fas (rs1800682) and Fas (rs2234767) are more likely to be associated with MSDD for Chinese people. FasL (rs763110) is related to the progression of MSDD for both Caucasoid and Chinese race groups. But FasL (rs5030772) might not be associated with any types of MSDD or any race groups statistically.

Keywords: Fas/FasL polymorphism, Musculoskeletal degenerative diseases, Intervertebral disc degeneration, Osteoarthritis, Rheumatoid arthritis

* Correspondence: szwpro@163.com
[†]Equal contributors
[1]Department of Orthopaedics, Union Hospital, Tongji Medical College, Huazhong University of Science and Technology, 1277 JieFang Avenue, Wuhan 430022, China
Full list of author information is available at the end of the article

Background

Degenerative disease is the consequence of a successive process resulted from degenerative cell changes, influencing tissues or organs, which will gradually deteriorate over time. The most common degenerative diseases in musculoskeletal systems include intervertebral disc degeneration (IVDD), osteoarthritis (OA) and rheumatoid arthritis (RA). IVDD, which results from ageing, small injuries and natural daily compression on intervertebral disc (IVD), has been regarded as one of the main causes to low back pain and motor deficiency. OA, a common type of joint disease, is owing to the destruction of joint cartilage and subchondral bone and is traditionally considered to be associated with articular cartilage degeneration [1]. RA, a long term autoimmune dysfunction that primarily affects joints, is also considered to be a degenerative rheumatoid and arthritis [2, 3]. All of the three diseases are of high prevalence in the society and exert huge burdens to the global medical care [4]. And they were all have been found to be related to gene alternations or heredity by recent studies [5–8].

Apoptosis represents a physiological procedure in order to remove harmful, damaged, or unwanted cells [9]. Fas is a cell-surface receptor referring to apoptotic signaling in various cell types and interacts with the natural ligand Fas ligand (FasL) to start the death signal cascade, which can contribute to apoptotic cell death [10, 11]. Fas/FasL genetic polymorphisms have been reported to be related to the development or progression of several common diseases such as cancer, systemic lupus erythematosus [12–14]. Fas (- 670 G > A rs1800682, - 1377 G > A rs2234767) and FasL (IVS2nt-124 A > G rs5030772, - 844 T > C rs763110) are the most commonly studied sites in Fas/FasL gene recently.

Although the exact etiology of OA is still unclear, current researches have explored an association between chondrocyte apoptosis and the progression of OA [15, 16]. RA, which is characterized by synovial cells proliferation and T lymphocyte collection inside the synovial tissue, is partly due to the inhibition of T cell death by which Fas/FasL participated in [17, 18]. One of the main processes in the initiation and development of IVDD is the decrease in disc cells, leading to decline in ability of synthesizing and repairing extracellular matrix [19]. Recent studies have observed a significantly higher expression levels of Fas and FasL in disc cells of the herniated lumbar disc tissues, which may result in a rapid apoptosis of resident disc cells [20, 21]. From the evidences above, we hypothesize that there may be an association of Fas and FasL gene polymorphisms with musculoskeletal degenerative diseases (MSDD). A few previous researches have reported that Fas and FasL variations were associated with these MSDD risks but came to a contradictory published results [19, 22–32]. However, no meta-analysis has investigated the association between IVDD or OA and Fas/FasL polymorphism up to now. Two meta-analyses, Zhu et al. (published in 2016) [31] and Lee et al. [33] have analyzed the association between RA and Fas/FasL recently. For Zhu et al.(published in 2016) [31] it only included and analyzed Chinese patients for Fas (rs2234767) site. For Lee et al. [33], it only analyzed Fas polymorphism and there are some mistakes in data extractions for some studies included, such as, Huang et al. [26], Lee et al. [28] and Coakley et al. [25]

So we performed a comprehensive meta-analysis containing three MSDD (OA, RA and IVDD) and enrolling all races of populations besides Chinese. Also we corrected the mistakes of the previous meta-analysis, Lee et al. [33] and added a new study, Zhu et al. (published in 2016) [31] when analyzing. This meta-analysis is designed to explore the association of MSDD (OA, RA and IVDD) with Fas/FasL polymorphism, which could assist to forecast the susceptibility of MSDD for specific individuals or conduct the clinical treatment for 'high-risk' individuals.

Methods

Strategy for literature search

To identify all literatures that studied the association of Fas and FasL genes polymorphisms with MSDD, we searched nine electronic databases including PubMed, Web of Science (WOS), Embase, Scopus and Medline in English and VIP, SinoMed, Wanfang and the China National Knowledge Infrastructure (CNKI) in Chinese. The search period for all these nine databases was up to August 21, 2017. The search strategy to explore all potential studies involved the use of the following terms: "Intervertebral Disk Degeneration" or "IDD" or "Disc Degeneration" or "disc herniation" or "low back pain" or "IVDD", "Osteoarthritides" or "Osteoarthrosis" or "Arthritis, Degenerative" or "Degenerative Arthritis" or "Osteoarthrosis Deformans", "Rheumatoid Arthritis", "CD95 antigen, human" or "Fas" or "tumor necrosis factor receptor superfamily, member 6 protein, human" or "CD95L" or "Fas Ligand" or "FasL Protein" or "tumor necrosis factor ligand superfamily member 6" or "CD178 Antigens" or "CD95 Antigen Ligand" or "TNFRSF6 protein, human" or "Fas1 protein, human" or "rs1800682" or "rs2234767" or "rs5030772" or "rs763110", "polymorphism" and "SNP".

Inclusion and exclusion criteria

To be included in this meta-analysis, studies should satisfy the following inclusion criteria: (1) evaluated the association of Fas and FasL genes polymorphisms with IVDD, OA and RA; (2) case-control studies; (3) offered sufficient data to calculate an odds ratio (OR) with 95% confidence interval (CI). What's more, the following exclusion disciplines were also applied: (1) non–case-control studies; (2) repeated publications; (3) the study only concerned with a case group; (4) comment or review; and (5) not relevant to MSDD. Two investigators (Xiao and Huang) independently evaluated the articles in accord with the inclusion and exclusion criteria. Any inconsistency was solved by discussion. If these 2 authors could still not reach the uniformity, senior authors (Ma and Deng) were asked to resolve the disputes.

Data extraction

For each study, the following characteristics were collected: (1) name of the first author; (2) year of publication; (3) country of enrollment; (4) ethnicity, age range and gender of the study population; (5) diagnosis and diagnostic criteria for MSDD cases; (6) genotyping methods; (7) source of controls; (8) matching criteria. (9) number of subjects under MSDD cases and controls; and (10) the HWE among the controls. Data were extracted cautiously from all eligible articles independently by 2 authors (Xiao and Huang). For conflict resolution, the accordance was realized by discussion.

Methodological quality assessment

The qualities of all the included studies were assessed by two investigators (Xiao and Huang) separately using the Clark scores system, which includes 10 items [34]. Scores under 5 represent low quality; while 5–7 scores denote moderate quality and 8–10 scores indicate high quality [34].

Statistical analysis

The PRISMA checklists and their guidelines were carefully followed in the whole process of this study [35]. The HWE in control groups for all the studies were calculated by χ^2 test before statistical analysis and $P < 0.05$ was thought to indicate significant disequilibrium. We examined Fas (rs1800682, rs2234767) and FasL (rs5030772, rs763110) genotypes using the allele (G vs. A, C vs. T) model, homozygote (GG vs. AA, CC vs. TT) model, heterozygote (GA vs. AA, CT vs. TT) model, dominant (GG + GA vs. AA, CC + CT vs. TT) model, recessive (GG vs. GA + AA, CC vs. CT + TT) model. The strength of the association between Fas (rs1800682, rs2234767) and FasL (rs5030772, rs763110) polymorphism and MSDD was assessed by the pooled ORs and 95% CI. Subgroup analyses were conducted to find whether diagnosis of MSDD or race groups was also related to the value of the pooled ORs and 95% CI. The statistical heterogeneity was verified by I^2 statistics. Fixed-effects model was applied to estimate the ORs and 95% CI when heterogeneity was low ($I^2 < 50\%$); instead, the random-effects was used when heterogeneity was high ($I^2 > 50\%$) [36]. Sensitivity analyses were carried out by removing one study each time to test the stability of the results. Publication bias was evaluated by the Begg's test [37] and the Egger's test [38] ($P < 0.05$ was considered to be statistically significant). All statistical analyses were managed using STATA 14 (Stata, College Station, TX). All P-values were two-sided.

Results

Characteristics of the studies

A flow chart showing the exclusion/inclusion of literatures is presented as Fig. 1. The comprehensive publications search screened 1761 potentially relevant articles, of which 267 articles were excluded for duplication and 1469 articles were omitted after browsing the title and/or abstract due to obvious irrelevance to MSDD or Fas/FasL gene we studied. Eight articles were deleted because they did not study MSDD or single nucleotide polymorphisms (SNPs) unrelated to the object of our study; 1 article was excluded on account of no detailed data; and 4 articles were wiped off because they were reviews. Finally, 12 case-control studies [19, 22–32] were identified for meta-analysis based on the inclusion criteria. As shown in Table 1, 4 eligible studies for IVDD, 1 eligible study for OA, 7 eligible studies for RA. Also, 5 eligible studies for Chinese, 5 eligible studies for Caucasoid and 2 eligible studies for other race groups.

As shown in Table 2, 11 eligible studies for rs1800682 with 1930 cases and 1720 controls, 6 eligible studies for rs2234767 with 1794 cases and 1909 controls, 3 eligible studies for rs5030772 with 367 cases and 313 controls and 8 eligible studies for rs763110 with 2010 cases and 2105 controls were included in this analysis. The characteristics of all the included studies are also listed in the Table 1 and Table 2, including the year, country and continent of studies, the ethnicity, age and gender of subjects, the type of MSDD, the diagnosis methods, genotyping methods, source of controls, matching items of cases and controls, the number of subjects in control/case group and Hardy-Weinberg equilibrium (HWE) in each studies. The genotype distributions for all of the control groups were consistent with the HWE, except Sezgin et al. [22]. The quality assessment of study was listed in Table 3.

Association between Fas (rs1800682) polymorphism and MSDD risk

No significant heterogeneity was noted among the studies of rs1800682 in the overall analysis, subgroup analysis leveled by diagnosis or recessive model of subgroup analysis leveled by race groups. Thus, the fixed-effects model was used for analysis in these models mentioned above. And other models used the random-effects model. However, no significant associations were found in any models for overall analysis.

The results of subgroup analyses leveled by diagnosis were listed below: For OA subgroup, no significant

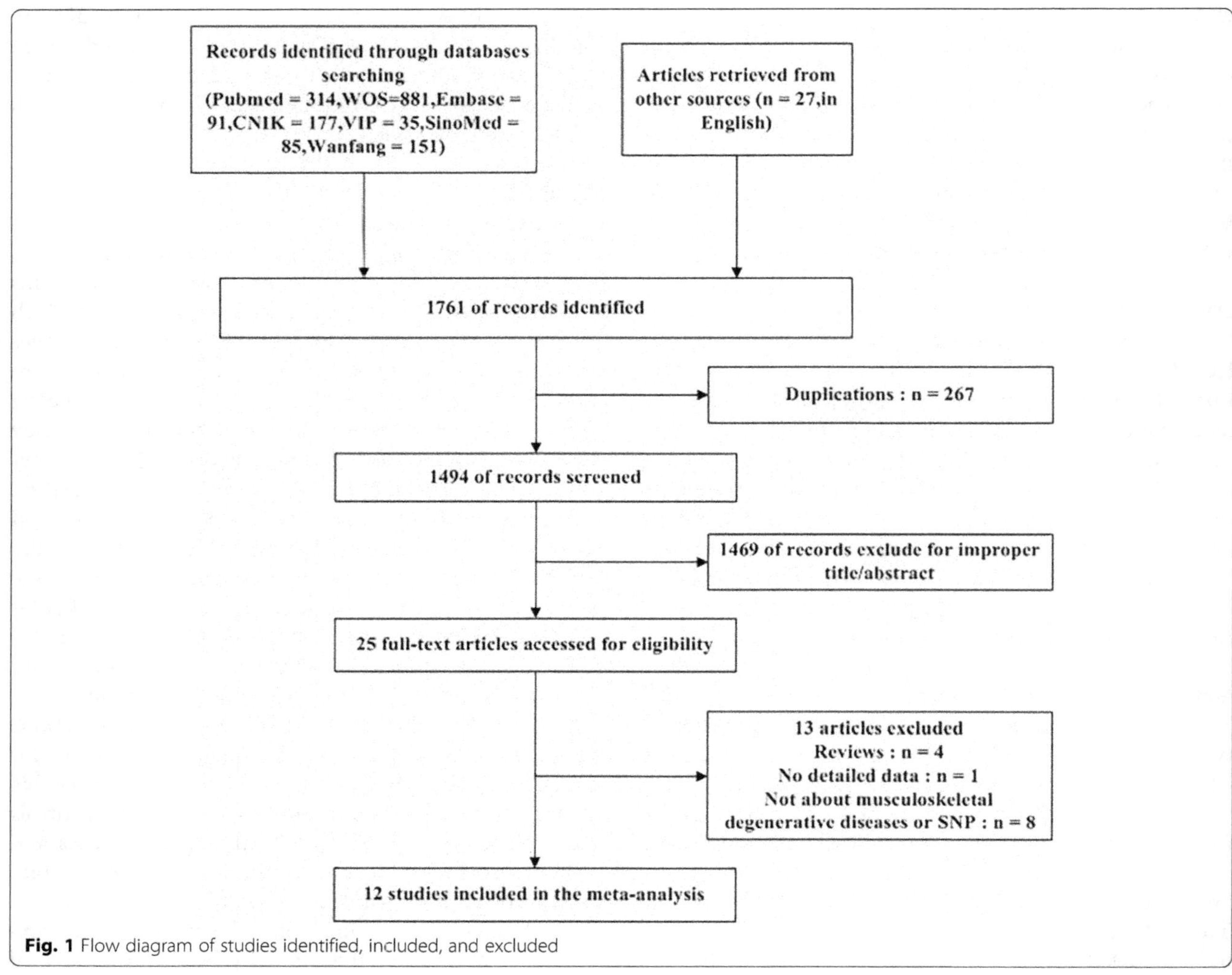

Fig. 1 Flow diagram of studies identified, included, and excluded

relationship was found in any models. For IVDD subgroup, significant associations were noted in GG vs. AA, OR = 1.388, 95% CI: 1.062–1.812, $P = 0.016$; in GG vs. GA + AA, OR = 1.357, 95% CI: 1.063–1.731, $P = 0.014$ (Fig. 2). However, no significant relationship was observed in other models. For RA subgroup, no significant relationship was found in any models. (Additional file 1: Table S1) The results of subgroup analyses leveled by race groups were listed below: For Caucasoid subgroup, no significant relationship was found in any models. For Chinese subgroup, significant associations were noted in GG vs. AA, OR = 1.388, 95% CI: 1.062–1.812, $P = 0.016$; in GG vs. GA + AA, OR = 1.357, 95% CI: 1.063–1.731, $P = 0.014$ (Fig. 3). However, no significant relationship was observed in other models. (Additional file 2: Table S2).

Association between Fas (rs2234767) polymorphism and MSDD risk

Significant heterogeneity was observed among the studies of rs2234767 in the allele and recessive models for overall analysis and subgroup analysis leveled by diagnosis and allele, heterozygote and recessive models of subgroup analysis leveled by race groups. Thus, the random-effects model was chosen to assess the connection between rs2234767 polymorphism and MSDD risk in these models mentioned above. And other models used the fixed-effects model. Significant associations were noted in GG vs. AA, OR = 0.771, 95% CI: 0.608–0.976, $P = 0.031$. However, no significant relationship was observed in other models.

The results of subgroup analyses leveled by diagnosis were showed below: For OA subgroup, significant associations were found in G vs. A, OR = 1.826, 95% CI: 1.199–2.779, $P = 0.005$; in GG vs. GA + AA, OR = 2.561, 95% CI: 1.525–4.299, $P = 0.000$ (Fig. 4). However, no significant relationship was observed in other models. For IVDD subgroup, no significant relationship was found in any models. For RA subgroup, significant associations were explored in G vs. A, OR = 0.855, 95% CI: 0.734–0.996, $P = 0.044$; in GG vs. GA + AA, OR = 0.785, 95% CI: 0.641–0.961, $P = 0.019$ (Fig. 4). However, no significant relationship was observed

Table 1 Main Characteristics of Studies Included in This Meta-analysis

Study ID	Year	Enrolled Country	Ethnicity	Age Range	Gender	Diagnosis	Diagnosis by	Genotyping Method	Control Source	Matching	Cases	Controls
Lv et al. [32]	2009	China	Chinese	N/D	N/D	IVDD	N/D	PCR-seq	N/D	N/D	223	124
Zhu et al. [24]	2011	China	Chinese	30–68	both	IVDD	MRI	PCR-seq	healthy subjects	age, sex, occupation, smoking	348	215
Sun et al. [19]	2013	China	Chinese	N/D&	both	IVDD	MRI	PCR-seq	participants with nonspine-related problems	age, sex, race	472	528
Zhang et al. [23]	2013	China	Chinese	33–61	both	IVDD	MRI	PCR-seq	patients or participants without back pain	race, sex, age, living areas	129	132
Sezgin et al. [22]	2013	Turkey	Caucasoid	43–70	both	OA	ACR	PCR-seq	patients without OA related disease	N/D	148	102
Coakley et al. [25]	1999	UK	Caucasoid	24–87	both	RA	ACR	PCR-seq	healthy subjects	age	18	128
Huang et al. [26]	1999	Australia	Caucasoid	23–65	both	RA	ARA	PCR-seq	healthy subjects	N/D	185	86
Lee et al. [28]	2001	Korea	Korean	16–75	both	RA	ACR	PCR-seq	healthy subjects	ethnically	87	87
Mohammad-zadeh et al. [29]	2012	Iran	Caucasoid	28–59	both	RA	N/D	PCR-seq	healthy subjects	N/D	120	112
Kobak et al. [27]	2012	Turkey	N/D	19–72	both	RA	ACR	PCR-seq	healthy subjects	age, sex	101	105
Seyfi et al. [30]	2013	Turkey	Caucasoid	20–80	both	RA	ACR	PCR-seq	patients without musculoskeletal diseases	age,sex, ethnically	100	101
Zhu et al. [31]	2016	China	Chinese	40–70	both	RA	ACR	N/D	patients without RA	age, sex	839	615

Abbreviations: *ACR* the American college of rheumatology diagnostic criteria for RA, *ARA* American rheumatology association 1987 criteria, *IVDD* Intervertebral disc degeneration, *OA* osteoarthritis, *RA* rheumatoid arthritis, *N/D* not described, *PCR-seq* restriction analysis polymerase chain reaction sequencing. &, the author only mentioned the mean ages of the case and control groups were 36.5 and 38.7 years, respectively

Table 2 Distribution of genotypes among cases and controls

	Study ID	Year	Diagnosis	Ethnicity	Case Group			Control Group			P_{HWE}
FAS (CD95) site											
-670 G > A rs1800682					GG	GA	AA	GG	GA	AA	
	Lv et al. [32]	2009	IVDD	Chinese	47	125	51	21	67	36	0.28
	Zhu et al. [24]	2011	IVDD	Chinese	57	162	129	30	96	89	0.62
	Sun et al. [19]	2013	IVDD	Chinese	74	217	181	61	265	202	0.06
	Zhang et al. [23]	2013	IVDD	Chinese	20	59	49	14	68	50	0.19
	Sezgin et al. [22]	2013	OA	Caucasoid	27	63	58	21	46	35	0.41
	Coakley et al. [25]	1999	RA	Caucasoid	4	8	6	31	61	36	0.61
	Huang et al. [26]	1999	RA	Caucasoid	32	105	48	22	44	20	0.83
	Lee et al. [28]	2001	RA	Korean	16	38	33	13	48	26	0.23
	Mohammadzadeh et al. [29]	2012	RA	Caucasoid	17	64	39	18	50	44	0.55
	Kobak et al. [27]	2012	RA	N/D	24	50	27	14	52	39	0.61
	Seyfi et al. [30]	2013	RA	Caucasoid	20	45	35	22	40	39	0.06
−1377 G > A rs2234767					GG	GA	AA	GG	GA	AA	
	Zhu et al. [24]	2011	IVDD	Chinese	121	172	55	99	92	24	0.71
	Sun et al. [19]	2013	IVDD	Chinese	218	209	45	236	248	44	0.06
	Zhang et al. [23]	2013	IVDD	Chinese	59	55	14	56	65	11	0.19
	Sezgin et al. [22]	2013	OA	Caucasoid	95	51	2	42	60	0	< 0.01
	Seyfi et al. [30]	2013	RA	Caucasoid	74	26	0	81	18	2	0.41
	Zhu et al. [31]	2016	RA	Chinese	246	284	68	389	357	85	0.82
FASL (CD178) site											
IVS2nt-124 A > G rs5030772					GG	GA	AA	GG	GA	AA	
	Sezgin et al. [22]	2013	OA	Caucasoid	4	37	107	4	30	68	0.76
	Mohammadzadeh et al. [29]	2012	RA	Caucasoid	8	35	77	6	31	75	0.25
	Seyfi et al. [30]	2013	RA	Caucasoid	6	25	68	10	29	60	0.03
−844 T > C rs763110					CC	CT	TT	CC	CT	TT	
	Zhu et al. [24]	2011	IVDD	Chinese	175	148	25	131	76	8	0.46
	Sun et al. [19]	2013	IVDD	Chinese	236	188	48	308	200	20	0.07
	Zhang et al. [23]	2013	IVDD	Chinese	64	51	13	77	50	5	0.37
	Sezgin et al. [22]	2013	OA	Caucasoid	45	80	23	37	47	18	0.65
	Mohammadzadeh et al. [29]	2012	RA	Caucasoid	33	63	24	43	49	20	0.36
	Kobak et al. [27]	2012	RA	N/D	30	40	31	33	40	23	0.12
	Seyfi et al. [30]	2013	RA	Caucasoid	20	55	25	31	54	14	0.22
	Zhu et al. [31]	2016	RA	Chinese	331	228	34	453	317	51	0.65

Abbreviations: HWE Hardy–Weinberg equilibrium

in other models. (Additional file 1: Table S1) The results of subgroup analyses leveled by race groups were showed below: For Caucasoid subgroup no significant relationship was observed in any models. For Chinese subgroup significant associations was explored in GG vs. AA, OR = 0.761, 95% CI: 0.599–0.966, $P = 0.025$ (Fig. 5). However, no significant relationship was observed in other models. (Additional file 2: Table S2).

Association between FasL (rs5030772) polymorphism and MSDD risk

Significant heterogeneity was explored among the studies of rs5030772 in the allele model of overall and subgroup leveled by diagnosis analysis. Thus, the random-effects model was used to evaluate the association between rs5030772 polymorphism and MSDD risk in allele model. The other models used the fixed-effects

Table 3 Quality assessment of the included articles

Study ID	year	A	B	C	D	E	F	G	H	I	J	Sum
Huang et al. [26]	1999	1	1	1	1	1	0	0	1	1	1	8
Coakley et al. [25]	1999	1	1	1	1	1	0	0	1	1	0	7
Lee et al. [28]	2001	1	1	1	1	1	0	0	1	1	0	7
Lv et al. [32]	2009	0	1	1	1	1	0	0	1	1	0	6
Zhu et al. [24]	2011	0	1	1	1	1	1	0	1	1	0	7
Mohammadzadeh et al. [29]	2011	0	1	1	1	1	0	0	1	1	0	6
Kobak et al. [27]	2012	1	1	1	1	1	0	0	1	1	0	7
Sun et al. [19]	2013	1	1	1	1	1	1	1	1	1	0	9
Zhang et al. [23]	2013	1	1	1	1	1	0	0	1	1	0	7
Sezgin et al. [22]	2013	0	0	1	1	1	1	0	1	1	0	6
Seyfi et al. [30]	2013	1	0	1	1	1	0	0	1	1	0	6
Zhu et al. [31]	2016	1	1	1	1	1	0	0	1	1	1	8

Abbreviations: *A* Control group, *B* Hardy–Weinberg equilibrium, *C* Case group, *D* Primer, *E* Reproducibility, *F* Blinding, *G* Power calculation, *H* Statistics, *I* Corrected statistics, *J* Independent replication, *Sum* sum of quality assessment score, *1* done, *0* undone or unclear

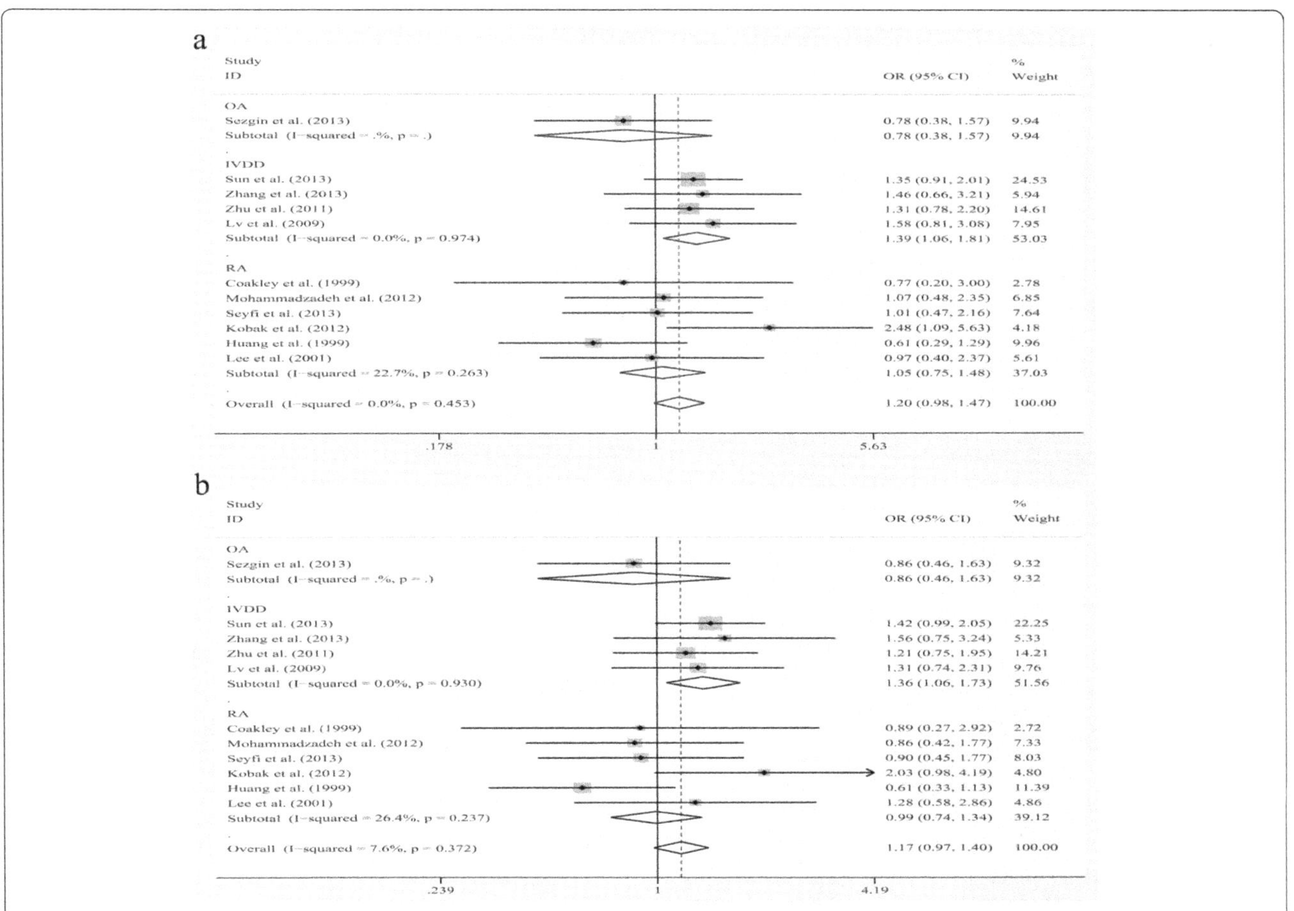

Fig. 2 The associations of Fas (rs1800682) with MSDD leveled by diagnosis in different genetic models. **a** Homozygote model (GG vs. AA). **b** Recessive model (GG vs. GA + AA)

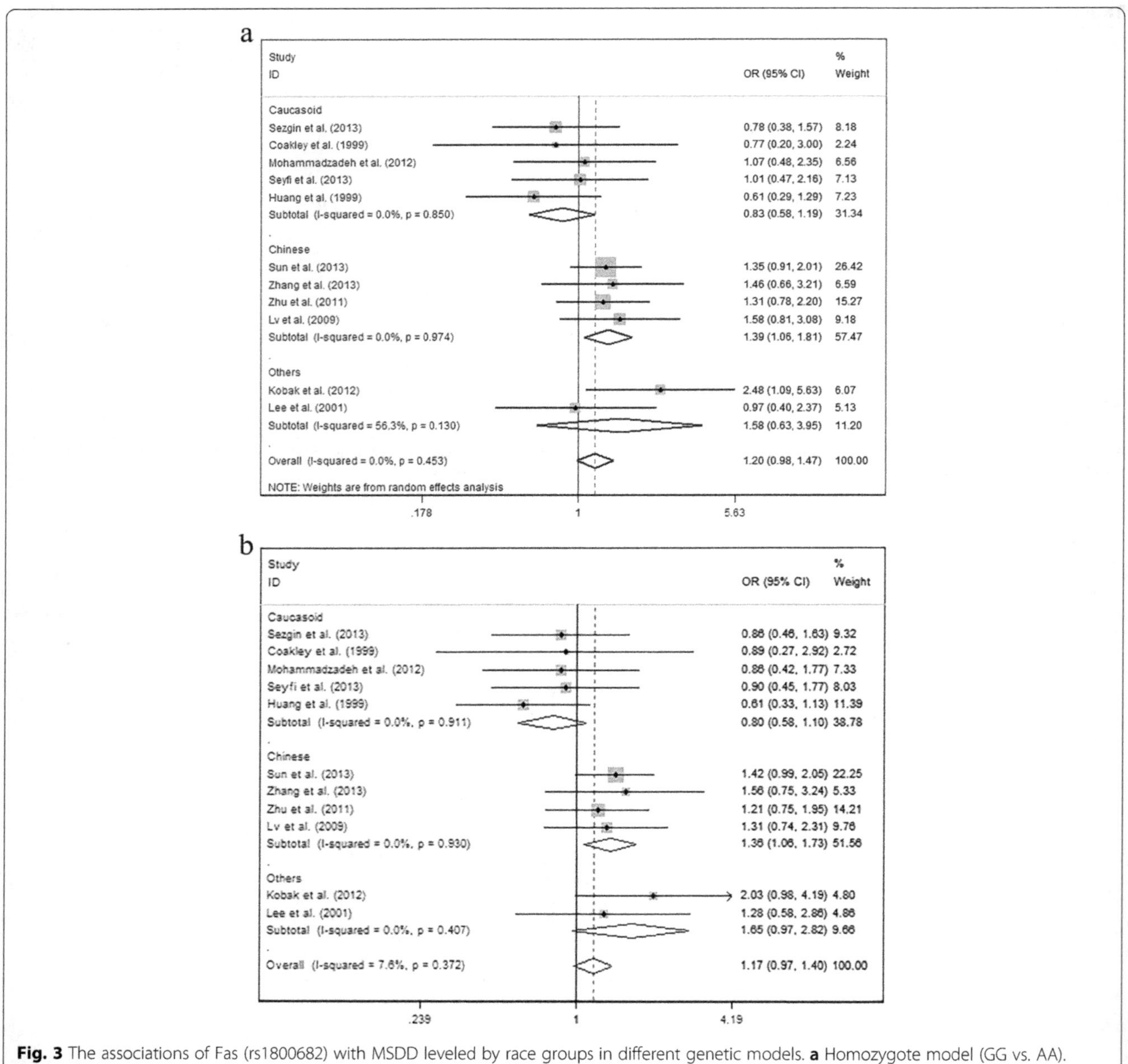

Fig. 3 The associations of Fas (rs1800682) with MSDD leveled by race groups in different genetic models. **a** Homozygote model (GG vs. AA). **b** Recessive model (GG vs. GA + AA)

model. However, no significant associations were observed in any models for overall analysis. The results of subgroup analyses leveled by diagnosis were listed below: For OA subgroup, no significant relationship was found in any models. For RA subgroup, no significant relationship was found in any models. (Additional file 3: Table S3) The results of subgroup analyses leveled by race groups were listed below: For Caucasoid subgroup, no significant relationship was found in any models. (Additional file 4: Table S4).

Association between FasL (rs763110) polymorphism and MSDD risk

Significant heterogeneity was observed among the studies of rs763110 in the allele, homozygote and dominant models for overall analysis and subgroup analyses stratified by diagnosis and all the models stratified by race groups. So the random-effects model was applied to assess the association between rs763110 polymorphism and MSDD risk in models mentioned above. Other models used the fixed-effects model. Significant associations were noted in all models: in the allele model, C vs.

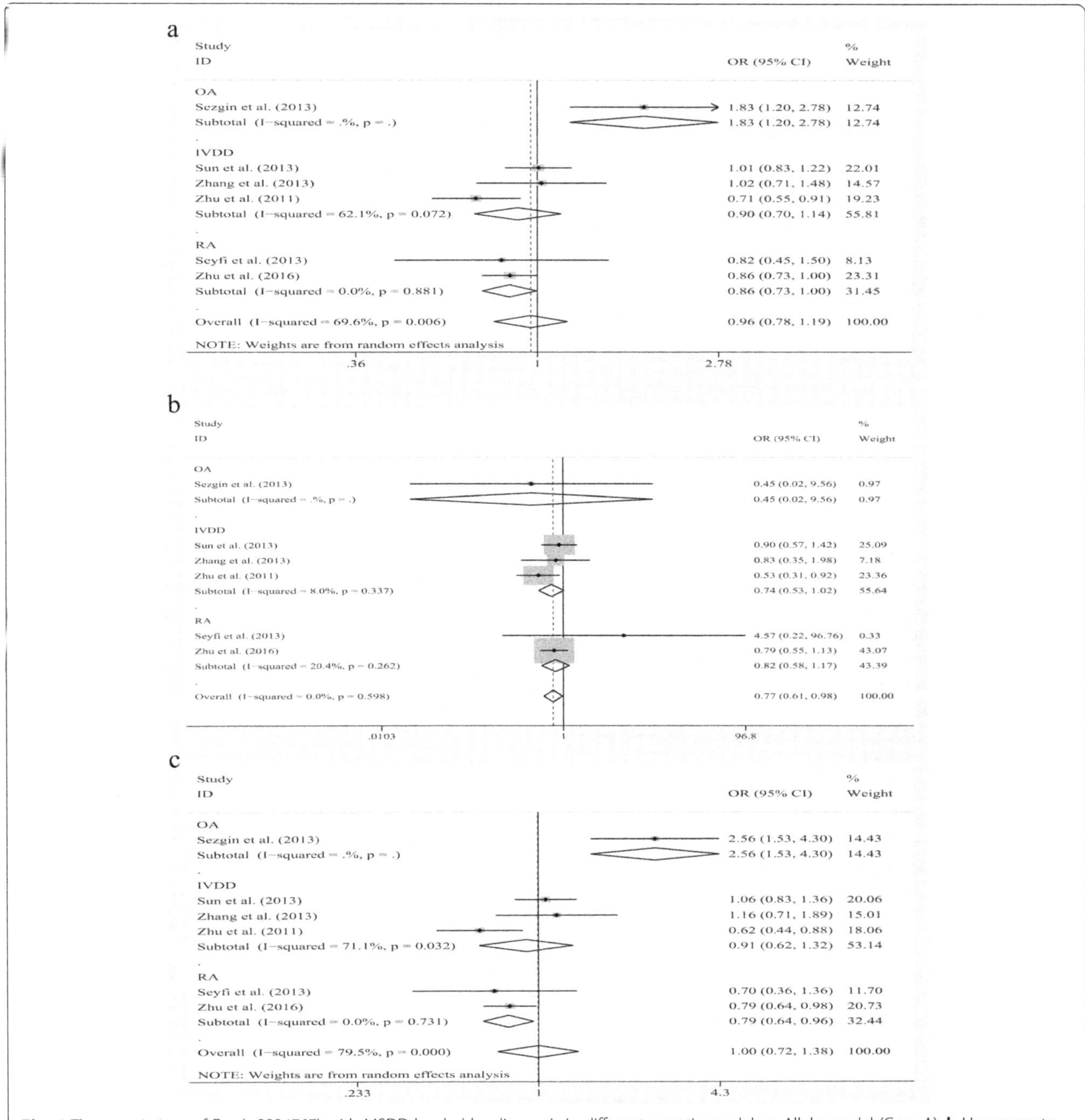

Fig. 4 The associations of Fas (rs2234767) with MSDD leveled by diagnosis in different genetic models. **a** Allele model (G vs. A). **b** Homozygote model (GG vs. AA). **c** Recessive model (GG vs. GA + AA)

T, OR = 0.780, 95% CI: 0.671–0.907, $P = 0.001$; in the homozygote model, CC vs. TT, OR = 0.565, 95% CI: 0.383–0.834, $P = 0.004$; in the heterozygote model, CT vs. TT, OR = 0.746, 95% CI: 0.591–0.946, $P = 0.013$; in the dominant model, CC + CT vs. TT, OR = 0.656, 95% CI: 0.461–0.934, $P = 0.019$; and in recessive model, CC vs. CT + TT, OR = 0.794, 95% CI: 0.700–0.901, $P = 0.000$ (Fig. 6).

The results of subgroup analyses leveled by diagnosis were showed below: For OA subgroup, no significant relationship was found in any models. For IVDD subgroup, significant associations were explored in C vs. T, OR = 0.684, 95% CI: 0.588–0.795, $P = 0.000$; in CC vs. TT, OR = 0.344, 95% CI: 0.226–0.525, $P = 0.000$; in CT vs. TT, OR = 0.442, 95% CI: 0.288–0.679, $P = 0.000$; in CC + CT vs. TT, OR = 0.382, 95% CI: 0.253–0.577, $P = 0.001$; in CC

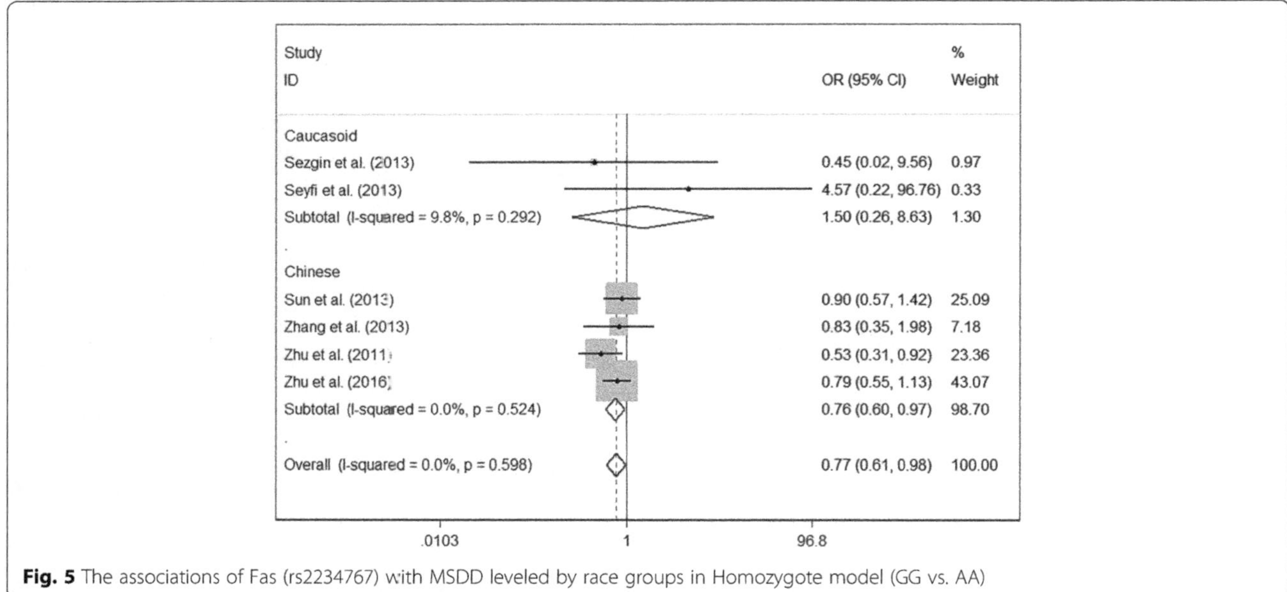

Fig. 5 The associations of Fas (rs2234767) with MSDD leveled by race groups in Homozygote model (GG vs. AA)

vs. CT + TT, OR = 0.694, 95% CI: 0.576–0.837, $P = 0.001$ (Fig. 6). For RA subgroup, no significant relationship was found in any models. (Additional file 3: Table S3) The results of subgroup analyses leveled by race groups were showed below: For Caucasoid subgroup, significant associations were explored in C vs. T, OR = 0.777, 95% CI: 0.626–0.964, $P = 0.022$; in CC vs. CT + TT, OR = 0.647, 95% CI: 0.465–0.901, $P = 0.010$ (Fig. 7). However, no significant relationship was observed in other models. For Chinese subgroup, significant associations were explored in C vs. T, OR = 0.772, 95% CI: 0.603–0.989, $P = 0.041$; in CC vs. CT + TT, OR = 0.786, 95% CI: 0.618–0.998, $P = 0.048$ (Fig. 7). However, no significant relationship was observed in other models. (Additional file 4: Table S4).

Sensitivity analysis

Sensitivity analysis was performed to assess the influence set by one study on the pooled ORs for Fas (rs1800682, rs2234767) and FasL (rs5030772, rs763110) polymorphism by deleting one study each turn in every genetic model.

We observed that the pooled ORs significantly differed when we deleted Huang et al. [26] in homozygote model (GG vs. AA, OR = 1.269, 95% CI: 1.030–1.565, $P = 0.025$) and in recessive model (GG vs. GA + AA, OR = 1.240, 95% CI: 1.026–1.499, $P = 0.026$) for Fas (rs1800682) site. We also noted that the overall ORs significantly changed when we deleted Zhu et al. (published in 2011) [24] in homozygote model (GG vs. AA, OR = 0.843, 95% CI: 0.647–1.098, $P = 0.204$) and Zhu et al. (published in 2016) [31] in homozygote model (GG vs. AA, OR = 0.755, 95% CI: 0.550–1.037, $P = 0.082$) for Fas (rs2234767) site. We found that the pooled ORs significantly differed when we deleted Sun et al. 19] in dominant model (GG + GA vs. AA, OR = 0.760, 95%CI: 0.560–1.031, $P = 0.078$) and Seyfi et al. [30] in dominant model (GG + GA vs. AA, OR = 0.679, 95% CI: 0.459–1.005, $P = 0.053$) for FasL (rs763110) site as well. However, there was no change in the significance of results in any models for FasL (rs5030772) site.

Publication bias

The Begg funnel plot (Fig. 8) and the Egger's test were conducted to evaluate the publication bias in selected literature. No evidence of publication bias was noted in this study for Fas rs1800682 (Begg's test: $P = 0.436$, Egger's test: $P = 0.576$ for allele model; Begg's test $P = 0.640$, Egger's test $P = 0.609$ for homozygote model; Begg's test $P = 0.876$, Egger's test $P = 0.694$ for heterozygote model; Begg's test: $P = 0.640$, Egger's test: $P = 0.965$ for dominant model; Begg's test: $P = 1.000$, Egger's test: $P = 0.508$ for recessive model).(Table 4) Because of the limited number (below 10) of studies included in Fas (rs2234767) and FasL (rs5030772, rs763110), publication bias was not evaluated in these sites.

Discussion

MSDD are common and one of the most clinically vital somatic disorders. A large number of genetic factors have been discovered among the crucial causes of IVDD [39], RA [40] and OA [41, 42] Several studies have reported the Fas/FasL genetic polymorphisms to be related to MSDD, but with conflicting results. In order to offer insight into the connection between Fas/FasL gene and diseases, large sample studies about predisposing gene polymorphisms are required. A meta-analysis, critically

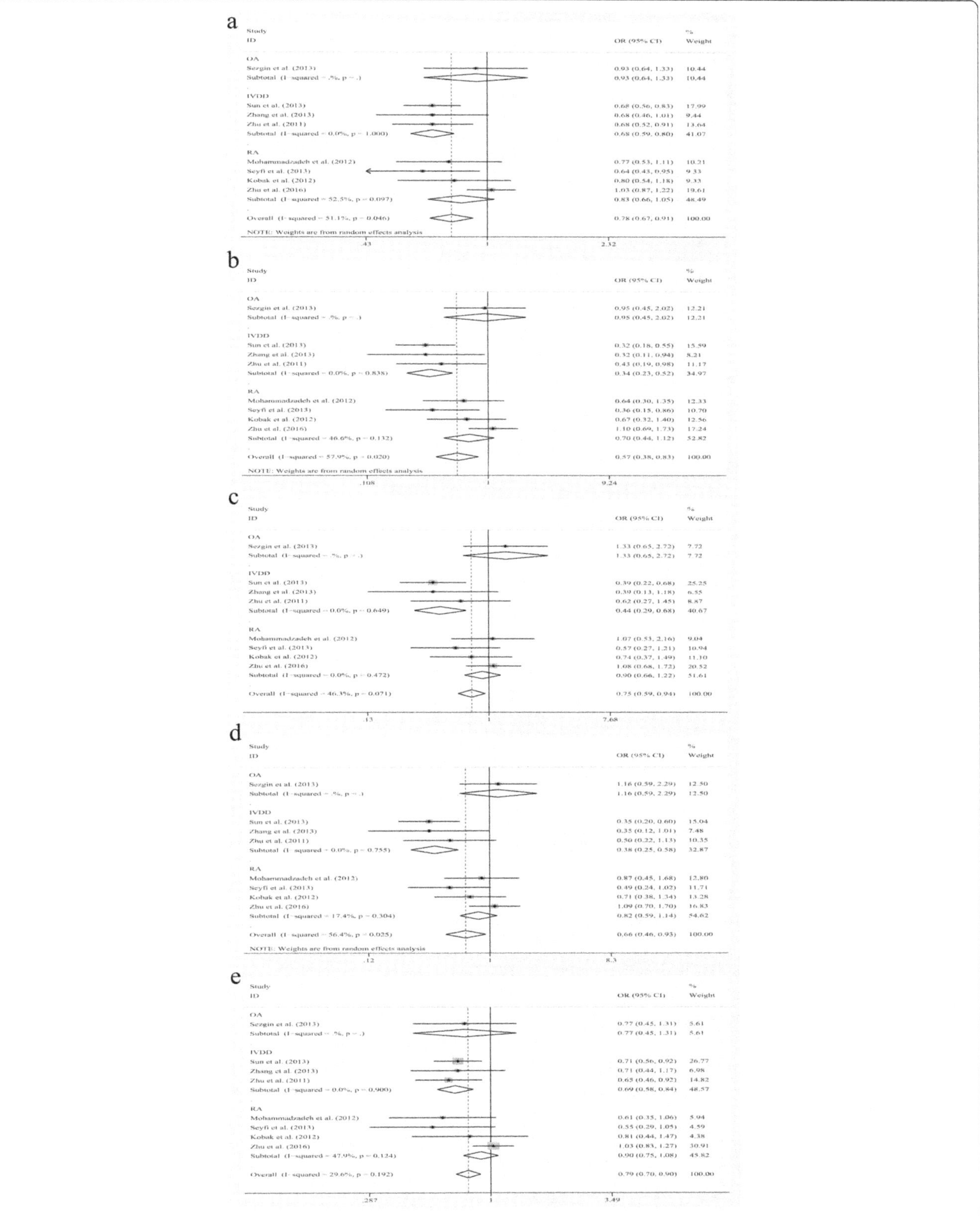

Fig. 6 The associations of FasL (rs763110) with MSDD leveled by diagnosis in different genetic models. **a** Allele model (C vs. T). **b** Homozygote model (CC vs. TT). **c** Heterozygote model (CT vs. TT). **d** Dominant model (CC + CT vs. TT). **e** Recessive model (CC vs. CT + TT)

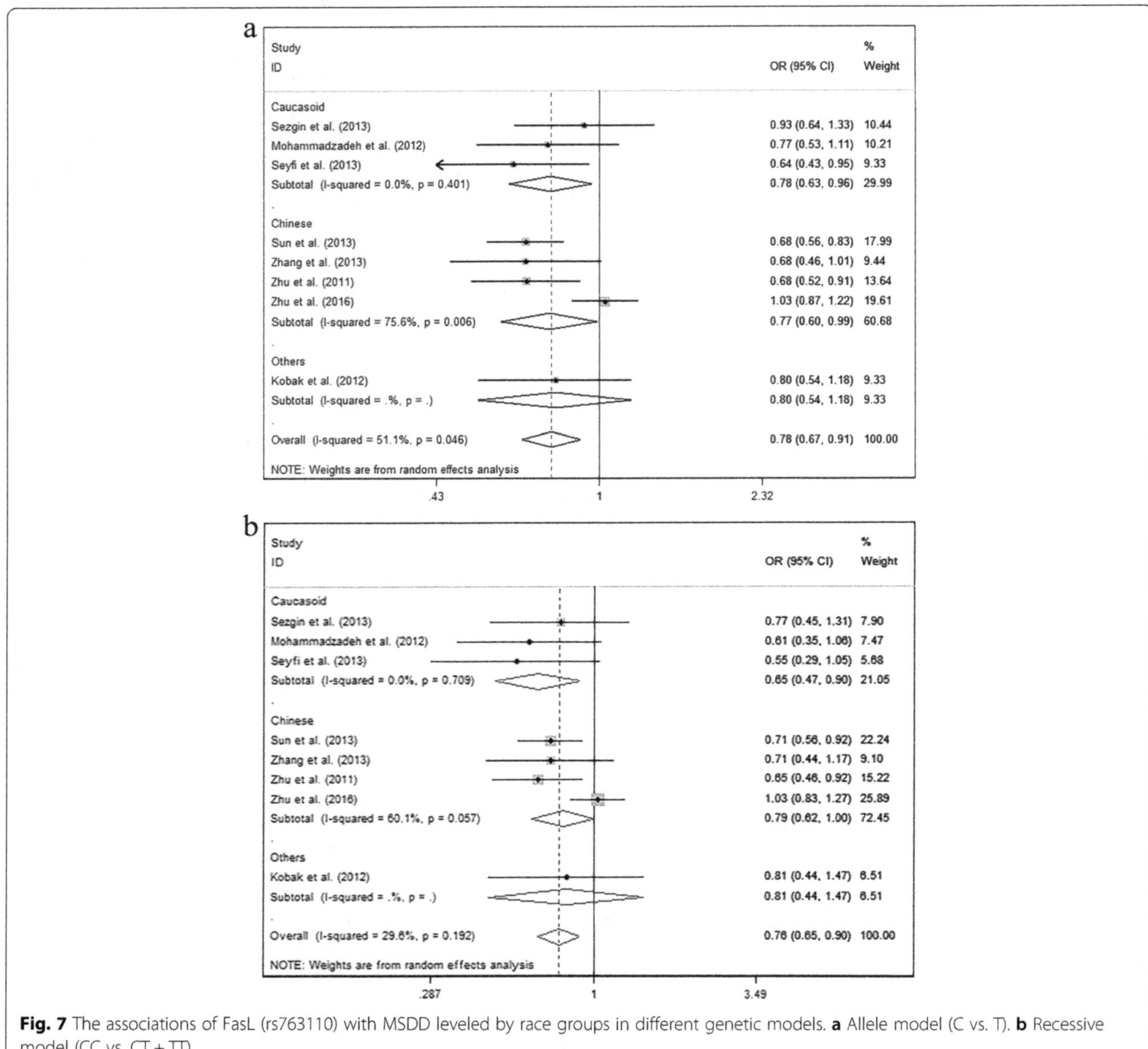

Fig. 7 The associations of FasL (rs763110) with MSDD leveled by race groups in different genetic models. **a** Allele model (C vs. T). **b** Recessive model (CC vs. CT + TT)

reviewing 11 studies on Fas (rs1800682), 6 studies on Fas (rs2234767), 3 studies on FasL (rs5030772) and 8 studies on FasL (rs763110), was performed to assess the association of Fas/FasL genetic polymorphisms with the risk of MSDD. Its strength came from the accumulation of published data, offering more information to evaluate significant differences.

In current meta-analysis, the main findings were that the G allele of Fas (rs2234767) was linked to a decreased risk of MSDD only in homozygote model and the T allele of FasL (rs763110) was associated with a reduced risk of MSDD in all of the comparison models. Besides that, subgroup analyses leveled by diagnosis suggested that the G allele of Fas (rs1800682) was associated with an increased risk of IVDD in homozygote and recessive models. The G allele of Fas (rs2234767) was linked to a decreased risk of RA but an enhanced risk of OA in allele and recessive models. In addition, the T allele of FasL (rs763110) was correlated with a reduced risk of IVDD in all of models. However, no relationship was found between FasL (rs5030772) and these three types of MSDD in any models. In addition, subgroup analyses leveled by race groups showed that the G allele of Fas (rs1800682) was associated with an increased risk of MSDD in homozygote and recessive models only in Chinese people. The G allele of Fas (rs2234767) was linked to a decreased risk of MSDD in homozygote model for Chinese people. What's more, the T allele of

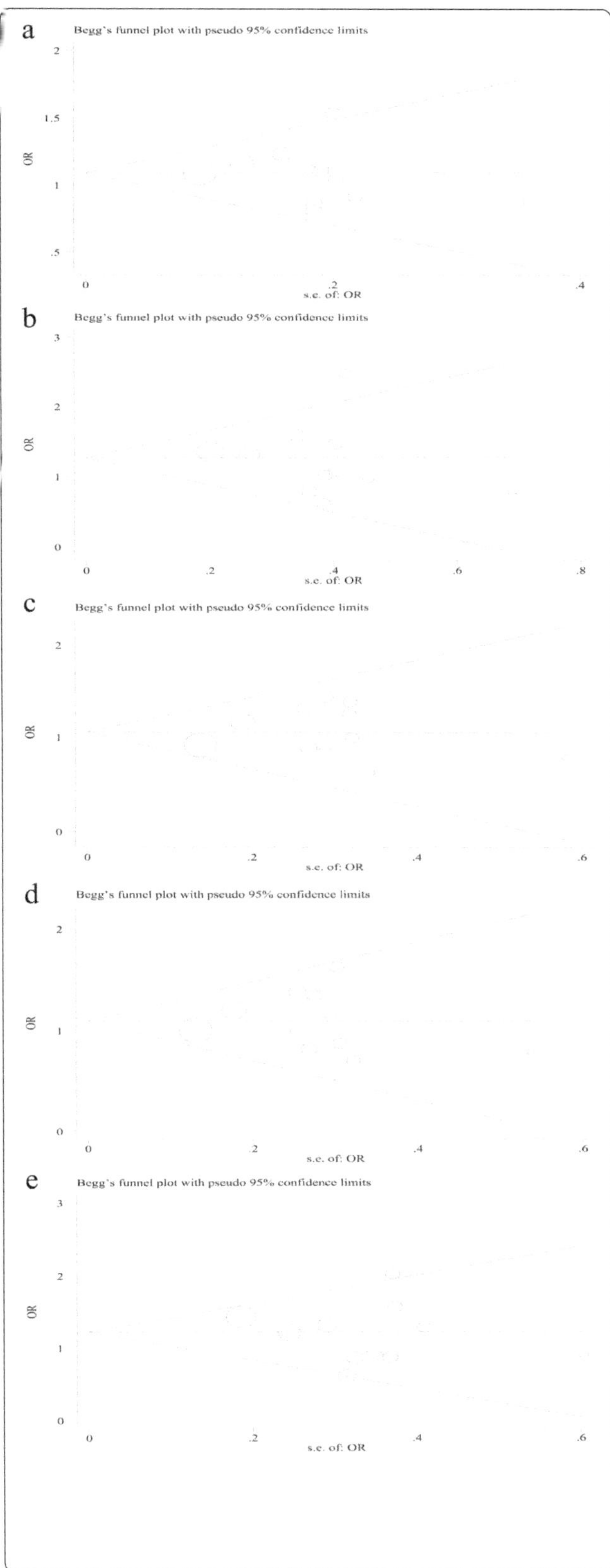

Fig. 8 Begg's funnel plot of publication bias for the association of FAS (rs1800682) polymorphism with MSDD in different genetic models. **a** Allele model (G vs. A). **b** Homozygote model (GG vs. AA). **c** Heterozygote model (GA vs. AA). **d** Dominant model (GG + GA vs. AA). **e** Recessive model (GG vs. GA + AA). Each point represents a separate study for the indicated association

FasL (rs763110) was correlated with a reduced risk of MSDD in allele and recessive models for both Caucasoid and Chinese race groups. However, no relationship was found between FasL (rs5030772) and these two race groups of MSDD in any models. Our results have several differences with the previous meta-analyses of RA recently published [31, 33]. Compared with Lee et al. 33], we observed no significance between FasL rs763110 and RA but it got an opposite result. A possible explanation for this phenomenon is that we include one more study with large participants, Zhu et al. (published in 2016) [31] Although Lee et al. [33] got the same result with us in Fas (rs1800682) site, it has some errors in data extraction of articles as mentioned above. We corrected the mistakes and analyzed again. Compared with Zhu et al. (published in 2016) [31], the small differences of result in Fas (rs2234767) for RA might be due to a new study [30] that we added in analysis. Furthermore, these Fas/FasL polymorphisms influencing the risk of MSDD can be explained partly by that these mutations can remarkably alter the percent of resident cells in tissues, such as disc cells in IVD and T-lymphocyte in synovial tissue, gradually causing occurrence of these MSDD [17, 19]. In addition, the same single nucleotide polymorphism exerted disproportionate levels of influence on different MSDD. These might be interpreted by various histology constitutions among IVDD, OA and RA. Finally, significant heterogeneity was noted in allele and recessive models of Fas (rs2234767), in allele model of FasL (rs5030772) and in allele, homozygote and dominant models of FasL (rs763110). Discrepancy among three types of MSDD might contribute to these heterogeneities. Other factors, such as ethnicity, sex distribution,

Table 4 Publication bias tests for association of the Fas (rs1800682) polymorphisms with musculoskeletal degenerative diseases

Comparisons	Egger's test			Begg's test
	t	95% CI	*P* value	*P* value
allele model	−0.58	(−2.91,1.72)	0.576	0.436
homozygote model	−0.53	(−3.70,2.29)	0.609	0.640
heterozygote model	0.41	(−1.56,2.24)	0.694	0.876
dominant model	0.05	(−2.03,2.11)	0.965	0.640
recessive model	−0.69	(−3.82,2.03)	0.508	1.000

Abbreviations: *CI* confidence interval

occupation and etc. might also be potential sources of heterogeneity.

What's more, the genotype distributions of controls in all of models were in accordance with HWE, except Sezgin et al. [22] in Fas (rs2234767) and Seyfi et al. [30] in FasL (rs5030772). However, the association was not significant change when ruled out these two studies by excluding one at a time. The quality assessment indicated that the enrolled studies were credible. No evidences of publication bias were observed by either Begg's or Egger's test in Fas (rs1800682). In order to analyze the stability of the overall results, sensitivity analysis by deleting each included studies was managed in this meta-analysis. Only one or two studies influenced the result of analysis in some models for Fas (rs1800682, rs2234767) and FasL (rs763110) and no study affects the results for FasL (rs5030772), suggesting the results were reliable in some extents. But more studies still need to be conducted in order to verify the outcome of the current meta-analysis. Overall, the results of this meta-analysis are credible and stable to a certain degree.

There are some limitations in the present study. Firstly, only three studies for FasL rs5030772 site were included in analysis and only one article was screened out for OA subgroup analysis due to shortage of original studies. Secondly, the heterogeneity was a little bit high ($I^2 > 50\%$) in some models for overall analyses, leading to a cautious acceptance of the results. So we performed subgroup analyses stratified by diagnosis to make the result more credible. What's more, some of the included articles did not match the confounding factors such as age, sex and ethnicity between case group and control group. And different factors for matching might also increase the probability of residual confounding. Such confounding factors might influence the final results. However, this meta-analysis has some strength. For example, to our best knowledge, this is the most comprehensive meta-analysis focused on the association of Fas/FasL gene polymorphism with the susceptibility of MSDD, including OA, IVDD and RA. Several strategies and rigid criteria were set to assess the methodological quality of each study; all of the included studies possessed high or moderate qualities.

Conclusions

In summary, the current meta-analysis suggested that Fas (rs1800682) and FasL (rs763110) polymorphism were associated with the susceptibility of IVDD. Fas (rs2234767) was correlated to the risk of OA and RA. Fas (rs1800682) and Fas (rs2234767) are more likely to be associated with MSDD for Chinese people. FasL (rs763110) is related to the progression of MSDD for both Caucasoid and Chinese race groups. However, FasL (rs5030772) might not be associated with MSDD. Because of the above-mentioned limitations, large-scale studies, including larger populations and considering more confounding factors, are required to verify the outcomes of this meta-analysis.

Additional files

Additional file1: Table S1. Summary of meta-analysis for the association of Fas rs1800682 and rs2234767 polymorphisms with musculoskeletal degenerative diseases leveled by diagnosis.

Additional file 2: Table S2. Summary of meta-analysis for the association of FAS rs1800682 and rs2234767 polymorphisms with musculoskeletal degenerative diseases leveled by race groups.

Additional file 3: Table S3. Summary of meta-analysis for the association of FasL rs5030772 and rs763110 polymorphisms with musculoskeletal degenerative diseases leveled by diagnosis.

Additional file 4: Table S4. Summary of meta-analysis for the association of FASL rs5030772 and rs763110 polymorphisms with musculoskeletal degenerative diseases leveled by race groups.

Abbreviations

CI: Confidence interval; CNKI: China National Knowledge Infrastructure; FasL: Fas ligand; HWE: Hardy-Weinberg equilibrium; IVD: Intervertebral disc; IVDD: Intervertebral disc degeneration; MSDD: Musculoskeletal degenerative diseases; OA: Osteoarthritis; OR: Odds ratio; RA: Rheumatoid arthritis; SNPs: Single nucleotide polymorphisms; WOS: Web of Science

Acknowledgments

We would like to thank all the people who helped us in the current study.

Funding

This study was supported by the National Key Research and Development Program of China (2016YFC1100100) and the Major Research Plan of National Natural Science Foundation of China (No.91649204).

Authors' contributions

Made substantial contributions to conception and design, or acquisition of data: HDH, XJR, SDY, WFS, LH; Analysis and interpretation of data: HDH, XJR, SDY, DXY; Been involved in drafting the manuscript; MKG, SZW, DXY, LH; Revising it critically for important intellectual content: MKG, SZW; Given final approval of the version to be published: SZW. Each author should have participated sufficiently in the work to take public responsibility for appropriate portions of the content and all authors have read and approved the manuscript, and ensure that this is the case.

Competing interests

The authors declare that they have no competing interests.

Author details

[1]Department of Orthopaedics, Union Hospital, Tongji Medical College, Huazhong University of Science and Technology, 1277 JieFang Avenue, Wuhan 430022, China. [2]Department of Epidemiology and Biostatistics, Ministry of Education Key Laboratory of Environment and Health, School of Public Health, Tongji Medical College, Huazhong University of Science and Technology, Wuhan 430030, Hubei, China.

References

1. Bailey AJ, Knott L. Molecular changes in bone collagen in osteoporosis and osteoarthritis in the elderly. Exp Gerontol. 1999;34(3):337–51.

2. Wegener T. Therapy of degenerative diseases of the musculoskeletal system with south African devil's claw (Harpagophytum procumbens DC). Wien Med Wochenschr (1946). 1999;149(8–10):254–7.
3. Denner SS. A review of the efficacy and safety of devil's claw for pain associated with degenerative musculoskeletal diseases, rheumatoid, and osteoarthritis. Holist Nurs Pract. 2007;21(4):203–7.
4. Glyn-Jones S, Palmer AJ, Agricola R, Price AJ, Vincent TL, Weinans H, Carr AJ. Osteoarthritis. Lancet. 2015;386(9991):376–87.
5. Raisz LG. Pathogenesis of osteoporosis: concepts, conflicts, and prospects. J Clin Invest. 2005;115(12):3318–25.
6. Smolen JS, Aletaha D, McInnes IB. Rheumatoid arthritis. Lancet. 2016; 388(10055):2023–38.
7. Spector TD, MacGregor AJ. Risk factors for osteoarthritis: genetics. Osteoarthr Cartil. 2004;12(Suppl A):S39–44.
8. Loughlin J. The genetic epidemiology of human primary osteoarthritis: current status. Expert Rev Mol Med. 2005;7(9):1–12.
9. Alenzi FQ. Apoptosis and diseases: regulation and clinical relevance. Saudi Med J. 2005;26(11):1679–90.
10. Itoh N, Yonehara S, Ishii A, Yonehara M, Mizushima S, Sameshima M, Hase A, Seto Y, Nagata S. The polypeptide encoded by the cDNA for human cell surface antigen Fas can mediate apoptosis. Cell. 1991;66(2):233–43.
11. Oehm A, Behrmann I, Falk W, Pawlita M, Maier G, Klas C, Li-Weber M, Richards S, Dhein J, Trauth BC, et al. Purification and molecular cloning of the APO-1 cell surface antigen, a member of the tumor necrosis factor/ nerve growth factor receptor superfamily. Sequence identity with the Fas antigen. J Biol Chem. 1992;267(15):10709–15.
12. Tan SC, Ismail MP, Duski DR, Othman NH, Ankathil R. FAS c.-671A>G polymorphism and cervical cancer risk: a case-control study and meta-analysis. Cancer Genet. 2017;211:18–25.
13. Ozdemirkiran FG, Nalbantoglu S, Gokgoz Z, Payzin BK, Vural F, Cagirgan S, Berdeli A. FAS/FASL gene polymorphisms in Turkish patients with chronic myeloproliferative disorders. Arch Med Sci. 2017;13(2):426–32.
14. Lee YH, Song GG. Associations between the FAS -670 a/G, −1377 G/a, and FASL −844 T/C polymorphisms and susceptibility to systemic lupus erythematosus: a meta-analysis. Clin Exp Rheumatol. 2016;34(4):634–40.
15. Goggs R, Carter SD, Schulze-Tanzil G, Shakibaei M, Mobasheri A. Apoptosis and the loss of chondrocyte survival signals contribute to articular cartilage degradation in osteoarthritis. Vet J. 2003;166(2):140–58.
16. Mobasheri A. Role of chondrocyte death and hypocellularity in ageing human articular cartilage and the pathogenesis of osteoarthritis. Med Hypotheses. 2002;58(3):193–7.
17. Salmon M, Scheel-Toellner D, Huissoon AP, Pilling D, Shamsadeen N, Hyde H, D'Angeac AD, Bacon PA, Emery P, Akbar AN. Inhibition of T cell apoptosis in the rheumatoid synovium. J Clin Invest. 1997;99(3):439–46.
18. Nagata S. Apoptosis by death factor. Cell. 1997;88(3):355–65.
19. Sun Z, Ling M, Chang Y, Huo Y, Yang G, Ji Y, Li Y. Single-nucleotide gene polymorphisms involving cell death pathways: a study of Chinese patients with lumbar disc herniation. Connect Tissue Res. 2013;54(1):55–61.
20. Park JB, Kim KW, Han CW, Chang H. Expression of Fas receptor on disc cells in herniated lumbar disc tissue. Spine (Phila Pa 1976). 2001;26(2):142–6.
21. Park JB, Chang H, Kim KW. Expression of Fas ligand and apoptosis of disc cells in herniated lumbar disc tissue. Spine (Phila Pa 1976). 2001;26(6):618–21.
22. Sezgin M, Barlas IO, Yildir S, Turkoz G, Ankarali HC, Sahin G, Erdal ME. Apoptosis-related Fas and FasL gene polymorphisms' associations with knee osteoarthritis. Rheumatol Int. 2013;33(8):2039–43.
23. Zhang YG, Zhang F, Sun Z, Guo W, Liu J, Liu M, Guo X. A controlled case study of the relationship between environmental risk factors and apoptotic gene polymorphism and lumbar disc herniation. Am J Pathol. 2013;182(1):56–63.
24. Zhu GB, Jiang XR, Xia CL, Sun YJ, Zeng QS, Wu XM, Li XC. Association of FAS and FAS ligand polymorphisms with the susceptibility and severity of lumbar disc degeneration in Chinese Han population. Biomarkers. 2011; 16(6):485–90.
25. Coakley G, Manolios N, Loughran TP Jr, Panayi GS, Lanchbury JS. A Fas promoter polymorphism at position −670 in the enhancer region does not confer susceptibility to Felty's and large granular lymphocyte syndromes. Rheumatol (Oxford). 1999;38(9):883–6.
26. Huang QR, Danis V, Lassere M, Edmonds J, Manolios N. Evaluation of a new Apo-1/Fas promoter polymorphism in rheumatoid arthritis and systemic lupus erythematosus patients. Rheumatol (Oxford). 1999;38(7):645–51.
27. Kobak S, Berdeli A. Fas/FasL promoter gene polymorphism in patients with rheumatoid arthritis. Reumatismo. 2012;64(6):374–9.
28. Lee YH, Kim YR, Ji JD, Sohn J, Song GG. Fas promoter −670 polymorphism is associated with development of anti-RNP antibodies in systemic lupus erythematosus. J Rheumatol. 2001;28(9):2008–11.
29. Mohammadzadeh A, Pourfathollah AA, Tahoori MT, Daneshmandi S, Langroudi L, Akhlaghi M. Evaluation of apoptosis-related gene Fas (CD95) and FasL (CD178) polymorphisms in Iranian rheumatoid arthritis patients. Rheumatol Int. 2012;32(9):2833–6.
30. Yildir S, Sezgin M, Barlas IO, Turkoz G, Ankarali HC, Sahin G, Erdal ME. Relation of the Fas and FasL gene polymorphisms with susceptibility to and severity of rheumatoid arthritis. Rheumatol Int. 2013;33(10):2637–45.
31. Zhu A, Wang M, Zhou G, Zhang H, Liu R, Wang Y. Fas/FasL, Bcl2 and Caspase-8 gene polymorphisms in Chinese patients with rheumatoid arthritis. Rheumatol Int. 2016;36(6):807–18.
32. Hao-ran L, Shang-li L, Dong-sheng H, Chun-hai L. The correlation between polymorphism in Fas gene and Degenerative disc disease. Acad J Guangzhou Med Coll. 2009;37(6):65–7.
33. Lee YH, Bae SC, Song GG. Association between the CTLA-4, CD226, FAS polymorphisms and rheumatoid arthritis susceptibility: a meta-analysis. Hum Immunol. 2015;76(2–3):83–9.
34. Srivastava K, Srivastava A, Sharma KL, Mittal B. Candidate gene studies in gallbladder cancer: a systematic review and meta-analysis. Mutat Res. 2011; 728(1–2):67–79.
35. Vrabel M. Preferred reporting items for systematic reviews and meta-analyses. Oncol Nurs Forum. 2015;42(5):552–4.
36. Higgins JP, Thompson SG. Quantifying heterogeneity in a meta-analysis. Stat Med. 2002;21(11):1539–58.
37. Begg CB, Mazumdar M. Operating characteristics of a rank correlation test for publication bias. Biometrics. 1994;50(4):1088–101.
38. Egger M, Davey Smith G, Schneider M, Minder C. Bias in meta-analysis detected by a simple, graphical test. BMJ. 1997;315(7109):629–34.
39. Martirosyan NL, Patel AA, Carotenuto A, Kalani MY, Belykh E, Walker CT, Preul MC, Theodore N. Genetic alterations in intervertebral disc disease. Frontiers Surg. 2016;3:59.
40. Mohan VK, Ganesan N, Gopalakrishnan R. Association of susceptible genetic markers and autoantibodies in rheumatoid arthritis. J Genet. 2014;93(2):597–605.
41. Zengini E, Finan C, Wilkinson JM. The genetic epidemiological landscape of hip and knee osteoarthritis: where are we now and where are we going? J Rheumatol. 2016;43(2):260–6.
42. Evangelou E, Kerkhof HJ, Styrkarsdottir U, Ntzani EE, Bos SD, Esko T, Evans DS, Metrustry S, Panoutsopoulou K, Ramos YF, et al. A meta-analysis of genome-wide association studies identifies novel variants associated with osteoarthritis of the hip. Ann Rheum Dis. 2014;73(12):2130–6.

19

Mild (not severe) disc degeneration is implicated in the progression of bilateral L5 spondylolysis to spondylolisthesis

Vivek A. S. Ramakrishna[1,2], Uphar Chamoli[1*], Luke L. Viglione[1], Naomi Tsafnat[3] and Ashish D. Diwan[1]

Abstract

Background: Spondylolytic (or lytic) spondylolisthesis is often associated with disc degeneration at the index-level; however, it is not clear if disc degeneration is the cause or the consequence of lytic spondylolisthesis. The main objective of this computed tomography based finite element modelling study was to examine the role of different grades of disc degeneration in the progression of a bilateral L5-lytic defect to spondylolisthesis.

Methods: High-resolution computed tomography data of the lumbosacral spine from an anonymised healthy male subject (26 years old) were segmented to build a 3D-computational model of an INTACT L1-S1 spine. The INTACT model was manipulated to generate four more models representing a bilateral L5-lytic defect and the following states of the L5-S1 disc: nil degeneration (NOR LYTIC), mild degeneration (M-DEG LYTIC), mild degeneration with 50% disc height collapse (M-DEG-COL LYTIC), and severe degeneration with 50% disc height collapse(S-COL LYTIC). The models were imported into a finite element modelling software for pre-processing, running nonlinear-static solves, and post-processing of the results.

Results: Compared with the baseline INTACT model, M-DEG LYTIC model experienced the greatest increase in kinematics (Fx range of motion: 73% ↑, Fx intervertebral translation: 53%↑), shear stresses in the annulus (Fx anteroposterior: 163%↑, Fx posteroanterior: 31%↑), and strain in the iliolumbar ligament (Fx: 90%↑). The S-COL LYTIC model experienced a decrease in mobility (Fx range of motion: 48%↓, Fx intervertebral translation: 69%↓) and an increase in normal stresses in the annulus (Fx Tensile: 170%↑; Fx Compressive: 397%↑). No significant difference in results was noted between M-DEG-COL LYTIC and S-COL LYTIC models.

Conclusions: In the presence of a bilateral L5 spondylolytic defect, a mildly degenerate index-level disc experienced greater intervertebral motions and shear stresses compared with a severely degenerate index-level disc in flexion and extension bending motions. Disc height collapse, with or without degenerative changes in the stiffness properties of the disc, is one of the plausible re-stabilisation mechanisms available to the L5-S1 motion segment to mitigate increased intervertebral motions and shear stresses due to a bilateral L5 lytic defect.

Keywords: Spondylolysis, Spondylolisthesis, Biomechanical instability, Disc degeneration, Intervertebral disc

* Correspondence: u.chamoli@unsw.edu.au
[1]Spine Service, Department of Orthopaedic Surgery, St. George & Sutherland Clinical School, University of New South Wales Australia, Kogarah, Sydney, NSW 2217, Australia
Full list of author information is available at the end of the article

Background

Isthmic spondylolysis (or lytic defect) is characterised by a bony defect of the pars interarticularis and occurs most commonly as a bilateral defect in the L5 vertebra [1, 2]. The mechanism for the progression of the lytic defect to spondylolisthesis remains unclear despite viable qualitative theories supported with clinical radiographic evidence [3–9].

Abnormal spinopelvic morphology and orientation measured through parameters such as pelvic incidence, sacral slope, pelvic tilt may create a biomechanical environment leading to the development of a pars defect and its progression to spondylolisthesis [3–6, 9]. In children and adolescents, the progression of the defect to spondylolisthesis is attributed to growth plate injury which may perpetuate to epiphyseal ring separation [8, 10]. Slippage in skeletally immature spines is not attributed to any disc degeneration, but rather growth plate lesions [7].

Lytic spondylolisthesis is often associated with disc degeneration at the olisthetic segment; however, it is not clear whether disc degeneration is the cause or consequence of lytic spondylolisthesis [11]. Clinical evidence suggests that disc degeneration occurs more rapidly and prematurely in the presence of lytic spondylolisthesis [11, 12]. Szypryt et al. (1988) compared disc degeneration at the olisthetic segment in 40 consecutive patients with an age-and-sex matched control group of 40 asymptomatic volunteers. The authors observed that over the age of 25 years, the prevalence of disc degeneration was significantly higher in the spondylolytic group compared with the control group [11]. Seitsalo et al. (1997) in their long-term follow-up study of operatively and conservatively treated isthmic spondylolisthesis patients reported a strong correlation between the severity of disc degeneration and the degree of slippage in the conservatively treated cohort. Progression to spondylolisthesis in adults is almost always attributed to disc degeneration [11, 13]. Case studies, however, have cited the rare progression of pars defect to vertebral slippage in adults without any associated disc degeneration, adding to the ambiguity around the role of disc degeneration in the pathomechanism for slippage progression [14, 15].

The intervertebral disc plays an important role in resisting shear and torsional forces acting on the spinal column during physiological bending motions. Biomechanical studies on cadaveric lumbar spines with healthy intervertebral discs have shown increased kinematics at the index-level following a bilateral lytic defect [16–18]. The loss of posterior tension band in the lumbar spine following the defect may redirect excessive shear and torsional forces on to the index-level disc, which may predispose the disc to accelerated or premature degeneration [19]. With progressive disc degeneration, the shear and torsional stiffness of the disc may get compromised, which in addition to the loss of posterior tension band, may perpetuate to spondylolisthesis. However, from a biomechanical standpoint, it remains unclear how different grades of disc degeneration may be implicated in the progression of a lytic defect to spondylolisthesis. Yong-Hing and Kirkaldy-Willis (1983) suggested that a degenerative progression occurs in the intervertebral disc from a state of hypermobility in the early stages of degeneration to hypomobility in the later stages [20]. Disc degeneration grades III and IV (Thomson's grading) characterised by nuclear clefts, radial and concentric tears in the annulus fibrosus have been reported to cause kinematic instability in lumbar motion segments, whereas grade V degeneration characterised by disc height collapse and osteophyte formation resulted in biomechanical stability in the segments [21].

Here we use computed tomography (CT) data from a healthy human subject and nonlinear finite element modelling (FE) to assemble three-dimensional models of the lumbosacral spine to investigate the role of different grades of disc degeneration in the progression of a bilateral L5 lytic defect to spondylolisthesis. We hypothesised that a mildly degenerated disc is not able to arrest hypermobility following a bilateral lytic defect in the L5 vertebra and therefore the defect is disposed to progress to spondylolisthesis; however, in a severely degenerated disc, hypomobility is sufficient to stabilise the motion segment and limit the progression of the defect to spondylolisthesis.

Methods

Image segmentation and 3D model generation from CT data

Prior approval from UNSW Human Research Ethics Advisory Panel was obtained for the use of retrospectively acquired CT data from a human subject (UNSW-NRR-HC16754). High-resolution lumbosacral spine CT data (437 axial cuts, 512 × 512 pixel resolution, voxel dimensions: 0.30 × 0.30 × 0.50 mm) from an anonymised healthy male subject (26 years old) were obtained in DICOM (Digital Imaging and Communications in Medicine) file format from Carl Bryan Radiology (St. George Private Hospital, Sydney, Australia). Using previously published protocols, the CT data were imported into image processing software Avizo Standard (vers. 8.1, FEI Visualization Sciences Group, Hillsboro, USA) for the segmentation of anatomical regions of interest, and subsequent generation and refinement of surface and volumetric meshes [22]. The segmented CT data were manipulated to generate a bilateral L5 spondylolytic defect model by deleting pixels from the L5 pars region (NOR LYTIC), creating an approximately 2-mm (mm) wide fracture gap between the bony fragments. Three more L5 spondylolysis models were built representing:

mild disc degeneration (M-DEG LYTIC), mild disc degeneration with a disc height collapse (M-DEG-COL LYTIC), and severe disc degeneration (S-COL LYTIC) as illustrated in Fig. 1.

The intervertebral disc is a composite structure comprising the annulus fibrosus and the nucleus pulposus, which degenerates accordingly with morphological and material property changes to both. In accordance with published material property data for normal and degenerated discs, the shear modulus for the annulus fibrosus (AF) was increased (mild: + 25%, severe: + 50%) and the Poisson's ratio for the nucleus pulposus (NP) was decreased (mild: – 13%, severe: – 34%) compared with the INTACT state in the FE models representing L5-S1 disc degeneration [23–25]. Disc height collapse was modelled as a 50% reduction in disc height measured in the mid-sagittal plane. The segmented CT data were manipulated to represent disc height collapse by moving the sacrum superiorly to reduce sagittal mid-disc height at the L5-S1 level from 14.35 mm to 6.64 mm while preserving the L5-S1 facet articulation.

Modelling annulus Fibres and ligaments

Volumetric meshes in Nastran file format (.nas) representing different variants of the lumbosacral spine model were imported into the FE modelling software Strand7 (vers. 2.4.6, Strand7 Pty. Ltd., Sydney, Australia). The annulus fibrosus was modelled per previously published protocols as a composite structure comprising concentric layers ($n = 4$) of criss-cross collagen fibres embedded within a homogenous ground substance, with the ends of the fibres rigidly anchored in the superior and inferior endplates [22]. Ligaments were modelled using cylindrical beam elements, with the attachment and insertion sites based on previously recorded anatomical observations and published protocols [22, 26]. The type and number of elements used in assembling the five FE models are presented in Table 1.

Facet joint articulations and pars Interarticularis fracture gap

The compressive load bearing characteristics of the bony articulating pillars at each facet joint was modelled using nonlinear *Point Contact-Tension* elements in Strand7 ($n = 5$ per joint), which were normally oriented and uniformly distributed over the bony articulating surfaces. The bilateral pars interarticularis fracture gap in the NOR LYTIC, M-DEG LYTIC, M-DEG-COL LYTIC, and S-COL LYTIC models was connected using nonlinear *Point Contact-Zero Gap* elements ($n = 25$ each side, compressive stiffness only) to allow for load transfer between the fractured fragments in the event of gap closure during simulated bending motions.

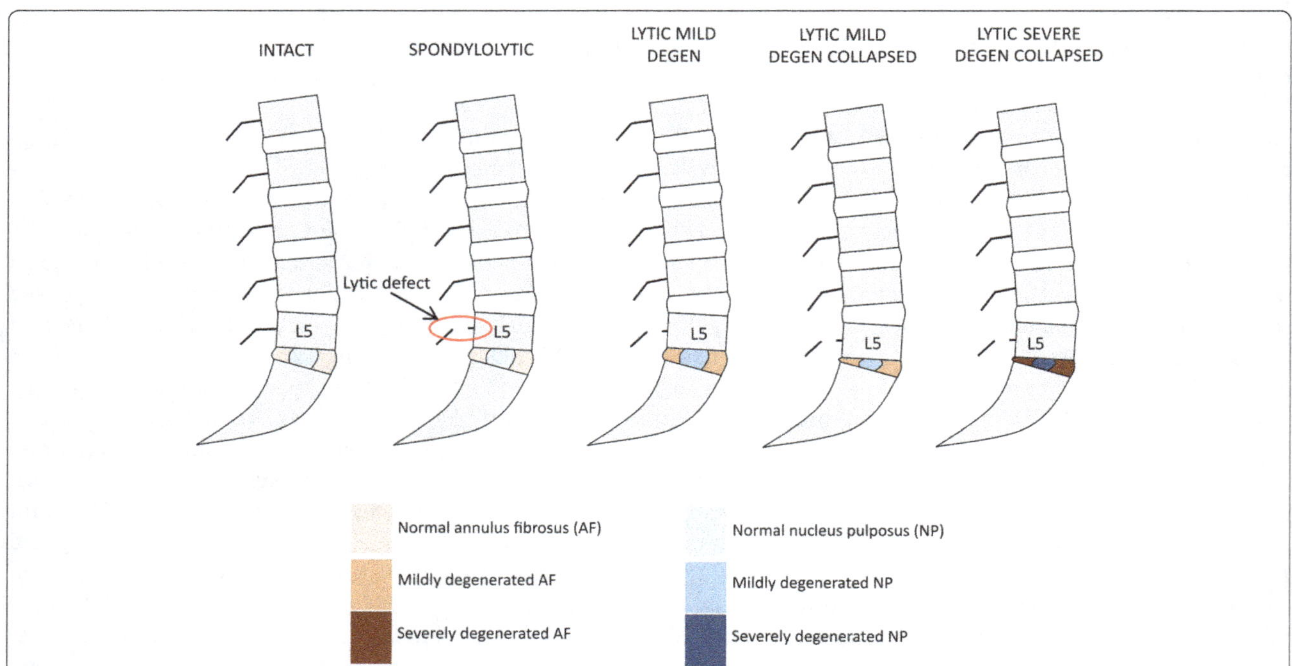

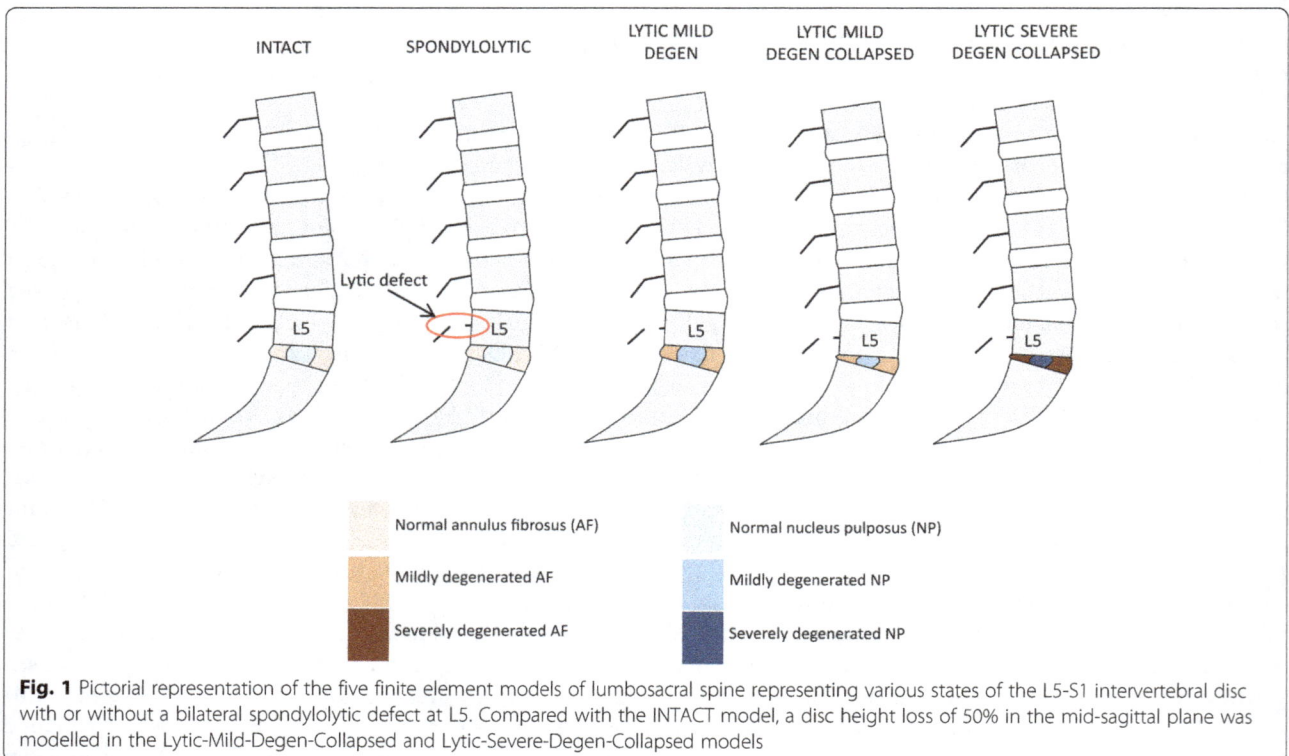

Fig. 1 Pictorial representation of the five finite element models of lumbosacral spine representing various states of the L5-S1 intervertebral disc with or without a bilateral spondylolytic defect at L5. Compared with the INTACT model, a disc height loss of 50% in the mid-sagittal plane was modelled in the Lytic-Mild-Degen-Collapsed and Lytic-Severe-Degen-Collapsed models

Table 1 Type and corresponding number of elements used in different finite element models of the lumbosacral spine

		INTACT	NOR LYTIC	M-DEG LYTIC	M-DEG-COL LYTIC	S-COL LYTIC
Nodes		308,539	320,256	320,256	382,025	382,025
Brick element (4-noded tetrahedrons)		1,454,554	1,522,196	1,522,196	1,811,798	1,811,798
Facet articulation (Nonlinear point contact elements)		5 per joint	5 per joint	5 per joint	5 per joint	5 per joint
Bilateral L5 lytic defect (Zero gap elements)		0	25 per side	25 per side	25 per side	25 per side
Annulus fibres (cylindrical beam elements)	L1-L2	(O) 312–321–293-266 (I)	(O) 289–272–229-224 (I)	(O) 289–272–229-224 (I)	(O) 350–311–279-262 (I)	(O) 350–311–279-262 (I)
	L2-L3	(O) 362–385–347-287 (I)	(O) 271–266–254-168 (I)	(O) 271–266–254-168 (I)	(O) 359–316–268-255 (I)	(O) 359–316–268-255 (I)
	L3-L4	(O) 330–298–232-240 (I)	(O) 265–244–212-189 (I)	(O) 265–244–212-189 (I)	(O) 395–318–269-258 (I)	(O) 395–318–269-258 (I)
	L4-L5	(O) 308–331–303-237 (I)	(O) 251–218–233-163 (I)	(O) 251–218–233-163 (I)	(O) 385–322–284-253 (I)	(O) 385–322–284-253 (I)
	L5-S1	(O) 243–258–236-219 (I)	(O) 202–192–169-167 (I)	(O) 202–192–169-167 (I)	(O) 436–352–341-291 (I)	(O) 436–352–341-291 (I)
Ligaments per level (cylindrical beam elements)	ALL	14	14	14	14	14
	PLL	6	6	6	6	6
	TL	16	16	16	16	16
	LF	18	18	18	18	18
	ISL	9	9	9	9	9
	SSL	4	4	4	4	4
	CL	24 per joint	24 per joint	24 per joint	24 per joint	24 per joint
	ILL	20	20	20	20	20
	LSL	22	22	22	22	22

The concentric rings of annulus fibres were modelled using nonlinear beam elements

(O) Layer1 (outermost)-Layer2-Layer3-Layer4 (innermost) (I); *ALL* Anterior Longitudinal Ligament, *PLL* Posterior Longitudinal Ligament, *TL* Transverse Ligament, *LF* Ligamentum Flavum, *ISL* Interspinous Ligament, *SSL* Supraspinous Ligament, *CL* Capsular Ligament, *ILL* Iliolumbar Ligament, *LSL* Lumbosacral Ligament

Loads and boundary constraints

In all the models, a centre node on the anterior surface of the sacral mass was fixed in all translational and rotational degrees of freedom (DOFs). Bending motions were simulated using a cross-beam construct accommodated on the L1 superior endplate by means of a surface cap, both of which were assigned material properties of stainless steel (E = 200 GPa, ν =0.25). A force couple was applied to the anterior and posterior ends of the cross-beam to simulate flexion (Fx) and extension (Ex) bending. The models were loaded in pure unconstrained moments (without any compressive preload) with step-wise increments in load from 1.0 N-metre (Nm) to 10 Nm. The pre-processed FE models were solved for geometry, material, and boundary nonlinearities using the nonlinear static solver in Strand7.

Material property values

Previously published material property values calibrated against in vitro biomechanical testing data were assigned to brick elements representing the intervertebral disc, beam elements representing the primary ligaments, and non-linear point contact elements representing facet articulation between the bony pillars (see Additional file 1). [22]

Results

All the results were analysed at peak Fx and Ex bending loads (10 Nm) in the five FE models.

L5-S1 range of motion (RoM)

The L5-S1 Fx and Ex RoM results are presented in Fig. 2. From the baseline INTACT state, the greatest increase in Fx and Ex RoMs was observed in the M-DEG LYTIC model (Fx: 7.2° (INTACT) to 12.4° (M-DEG LYTIC); Ex: 7.0° (INTACT) to 9.5° (M-DEG LYTIC)).

L5-S1 Interpedicular kinematics

The L5-S1 interpedicular kinematics in Fx and Ex were evaluated per published protocols [16, 27]. The in-plane component of the interpedicular travel (IPT) vector was projected onto the L5-S1 mid-discal plane to evaluate the relative posteroanterior translatory motions between the pedicles on the adjacent vertebrae.

The L5-S1 mid-discal plane projections of the IPT vector in Fx and Ex in the five models are presented in Fig. 3. From the baseline INTACT state, the greatest increase in IPT projections on to the mid-disc plane in Fx and Ex were observed in the M-DEG LYTIC model (Fx: 3.5 mm (INTACT) to 5.4 mm (M-DEG LYTIC); Ex: 1.9 mm (INTACT) to 2.7 mm (M-DEG LYTIC)).

Normal stresses in the L5-S1 AF

Colour coded compressive (−) and tensile (+) stress distribution in the L5-S1 AF in the mid-axial plane of the L5-S1 disc during Fx and Ex is presented in Fig. 4. The average values for the compressive and tensile stresses in the L5-S1 AF during Fx and Ex is presented in Fig. 5.

The greatest increase in the average normal stress from the baseline INTACT state was observed in M-DEG-COL LYTIC and S-COL LYTIC models. During Fx, average compressive stress increased from 0.11 (± 0. 20) MPa in the INTACT state to 0.54 (± 1.22) MPa in the M-DEG-COL LYTIC model and 0.56 (± 1.23) MPa in the S-COL LYTIC model. During Ex, average compressive stress increased from 0.15 (± 0.21) MPa in the INTACT state to 0.68 (± 1.60) MPa in the M-DEG-COL LYTIC model and 0.69 (± 1.57) MPa in the S-COL LYTIC model.

Shear stresses in the L5-S1 AF

Colour coded shear stress distribution in the L5-S1 AF in the mid-axial plane of the L5-S1 disc during Fx and Ex is presented in Fig. 6. The average values for the posteroanterior and anteroposterior shear stress in the L5-S1 AF during Fx and Ex is presented in Fig. 7.

The greatest increase in shear stresses from the baseline INTACT state was observed in M-DEG LYTIC models. During Fx, average anteroposterior shear stress increased from 0.015 (± 0.016) MPa in the INTACT state to 0.04 (± 0.046) MPa in the M-DEG LYTIC model. During Ex, average posteroanterior stress increased from 0.015 (± 0.014) MPa in the INTACT state to 0.029 (± 0.029) MPa in the M-DEG LYTIC model.

Axial strain in iliolumbar ligament (ILL) fibres

Table 2 Shows mean axial strain in the ILL fibres during peak Fx load. The ILL fibres did not experience any positive strain during peak ex load.

Discussions

The main objective of this biomechanical study was to examine the role of disc degeneration in the progression of a bilateral L5 spondylolytic defect to spondylolisthesis. The natural course of isthmic spondylolisthesis has been associated with disc degeneration and spontaneous stabilisation of the olisthetic segment, but the question whether disc degeneration is the cause or the consequence of vertebral slippage remains open [12].

The results from the present study confirm our hypothesis that in the presence of a bilateral L5 lytic defect, motion segments with a mildly degenerate index-level disc are at a greater risk for vertebral slippage compared to motion segments with a severely degenerate index-level disc. Compared with the baseline

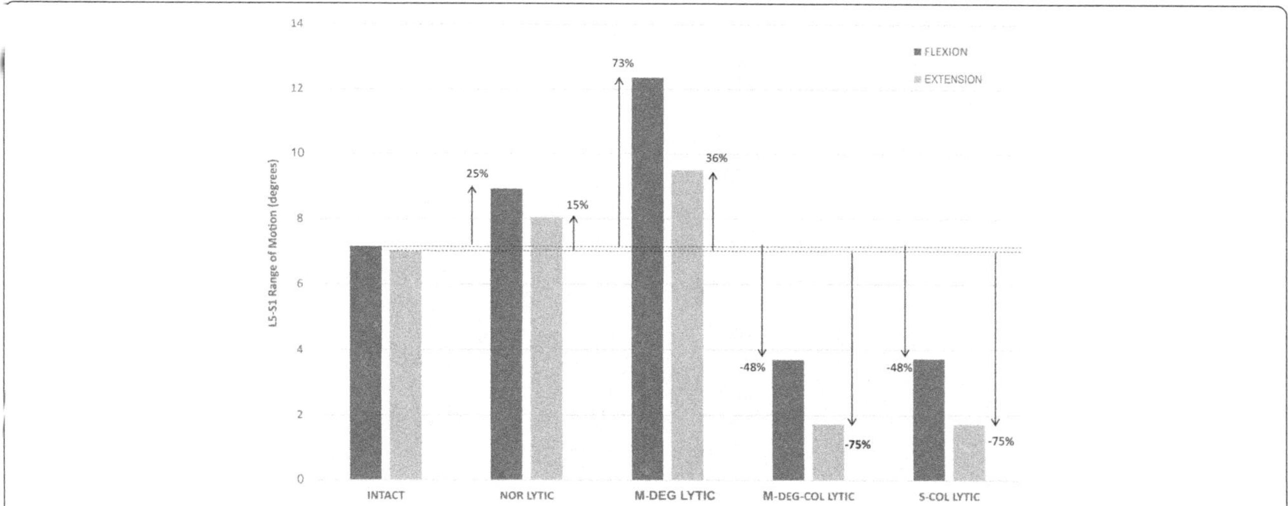

Fig. 2 L5-S1 range of motion (RoM) in flexion (Fx) and extension (Ex) bending at peak load of 10 Nm. Compared with the INTACT model, the greatest increase in Fx and Ex RoMs was observed in the mildly-degenerate lytic defect model (M-DEG-LYTIC)

INTACT model, M-DEG LYTIC model experienced the greatest increase in kinematics (Fx ROM: 73% ↑; Fx IPT mid-discal projection: 53%↑), shear stresses in the annulus (Fx anteroposterior: 163%↑; Fx posteroanterior: 31%↑), and average strain in the ILL fibres (Fx: 90%↑). The S-COL LYTIC model experienced a decrease in mobility (Fx ROM: 48% ↓; Fx IPT mid-discal projection: 69%↓) and an increase in normal stresses in the annulus (Fx Tensile: 170%↑; Fx Compressive: 397%↑) compared with the INTACT model. The results are corroborated by previous clinical findings for conservatively treated L5-S1 lytic defect patients which revealed immobility of the motion segment with severe degeneration of the index-level disc [12]. In the light of Kirkaldy-Willis model for degenerative changes in the lumbar spine and results from the present study, we posit that severe disc degeneration of the index-level disc is one of the restabilisation mechanisms available to the L5-S1 motion segment in order to mitigate increased intervertebral motions and shear stresses due to a bilateral L5 lytic defect [28]. The results also indicate that the disc height collapse and not the degenerative changes in the stiffness properties of the disc per se, play a predominant role in the restabilisation of the L5-S1 segment. With a 50% loss in disc height, the L5-S1 segment became less mobile, offloaded the ILL fibres, and experienced

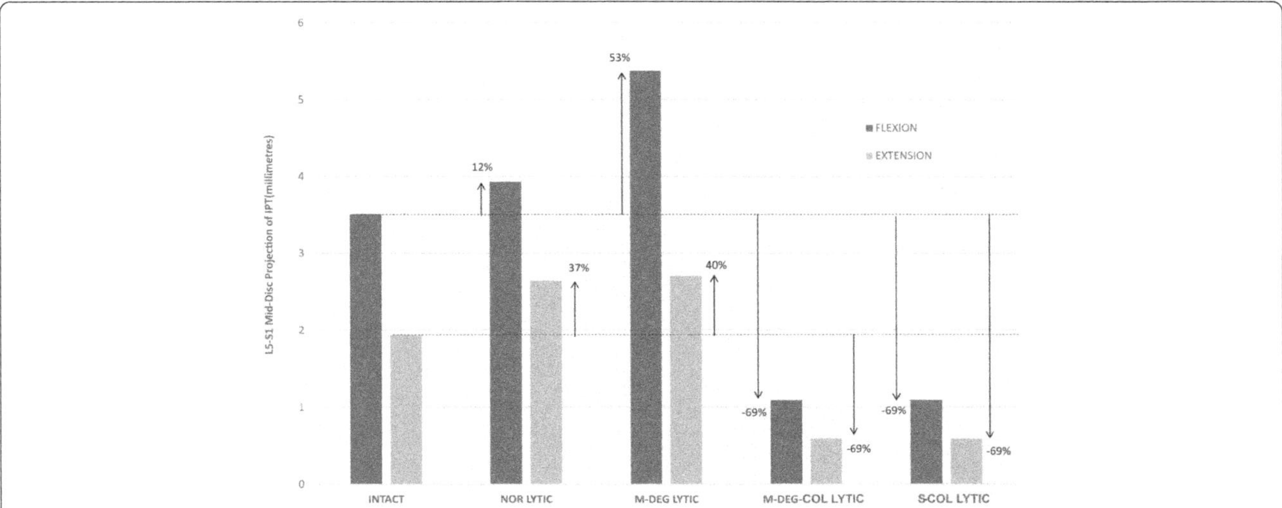

Fig. 3 Mid-discal plane projections of the L5-S1 interpedicular travel (IPT) vector in flexion (Fx) and extension (Ex) bending at peak load of 10 Nm. Compared with the INTACT state, the greatest increase in mid-discal plane IPT projections in Fx and Ex was observed in the mildly-degenerate lytic defect model (M-DEG-LYTIC)

FLEXION EXTENSION

Intact

L5 lytic

Mild degen L5 lytic

Mild degen L5 lytic collapsed

Severe degen L5 lytic collapsed

Brick Stress:ZZ (MPa)
5.000000×10^{-2}
2.772277×10^{-2}
-7.920792×10^{-3}
-4.356436×10^{-2}
-7.920792×10^{-2}
-1.148515×10^{-1}
-1.504950×10^{-1}
-1.861386×10^{-1}
-2.217822×10^{-1}
-2.574257×10^{-1}
-2.930693×10^{-1}
-3.287129×10^{-1}
-3.643564×10^{-1}
-4.000000×10^{-1}

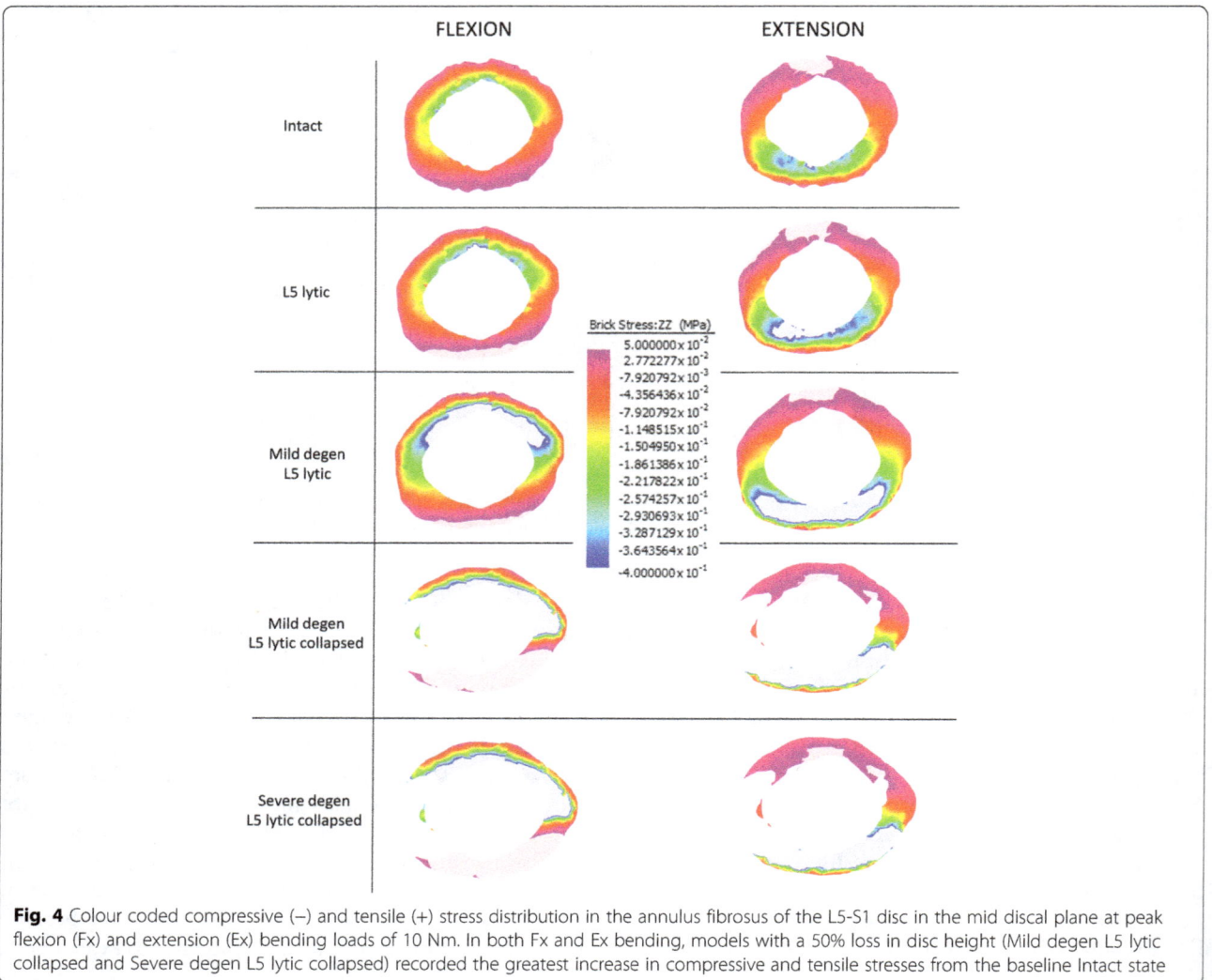

Fig. 4 Colour coded compressive (–) and tensile (+) stress distribution in the annulus fibrosus of the L5-S1 disc in the mid discal plane at peak flexion (Fx) and extension (Ex) bending loads of 10 Nm. In both Fx and Ex bending, models with a 50% loss in disc height (Mild degen L5 lytic collapsed and Severe degen L5 lytic collapsed) recorded the greatest increase in compressive and tensile stresses from the baseline Intact state

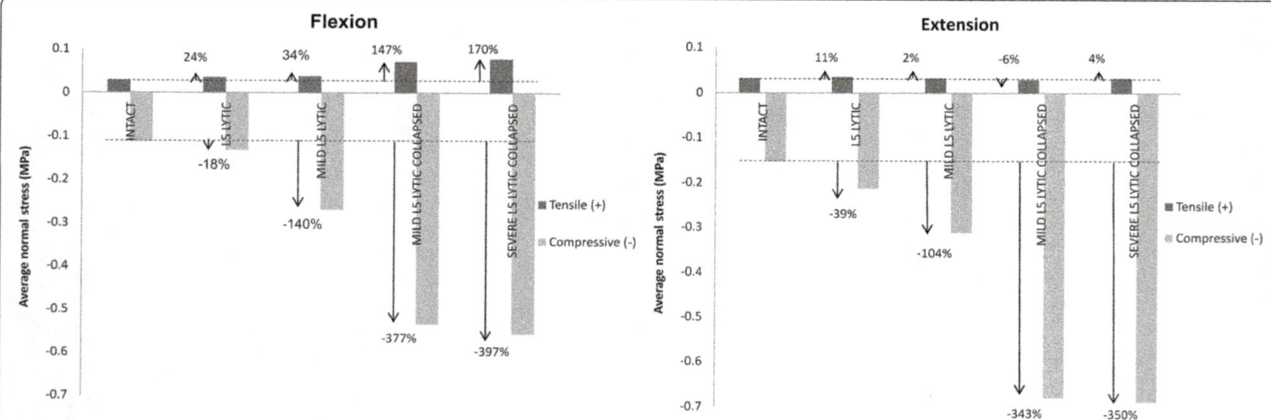

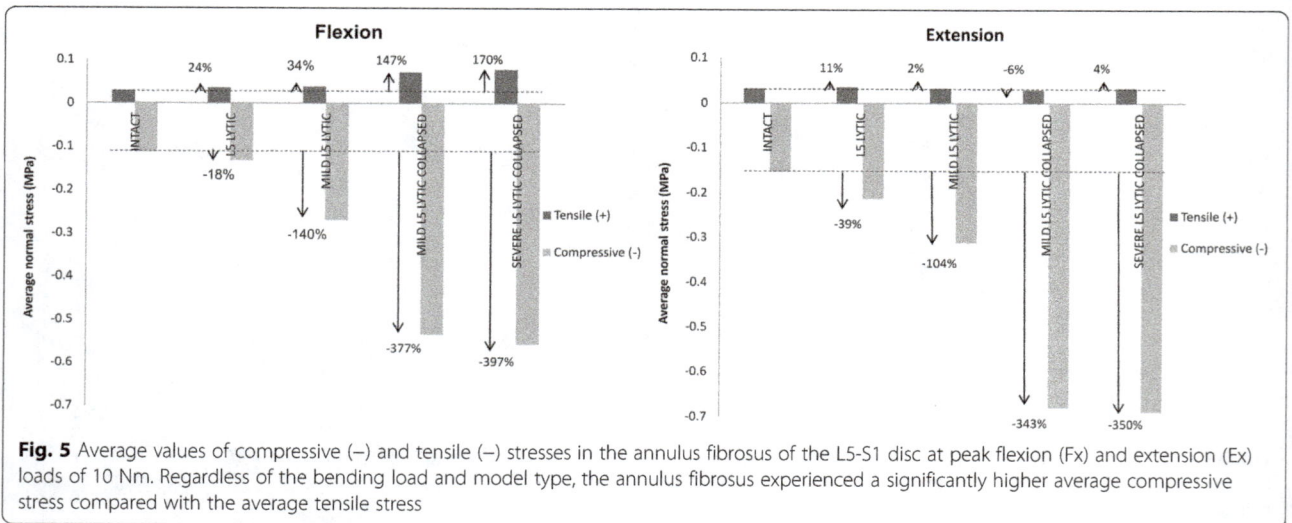

Fig. 5 Average values of compressive (–) and tensile (–) stresses in the annulus fibrosus of the L5-S1 disc at peak flexion (Fx) and extension (Ex) loads of 10 Nm. Regardless of the bending load and model type, the annulus fibrosus experienced a significantly higher average compressive stress compared with the average tensile stress

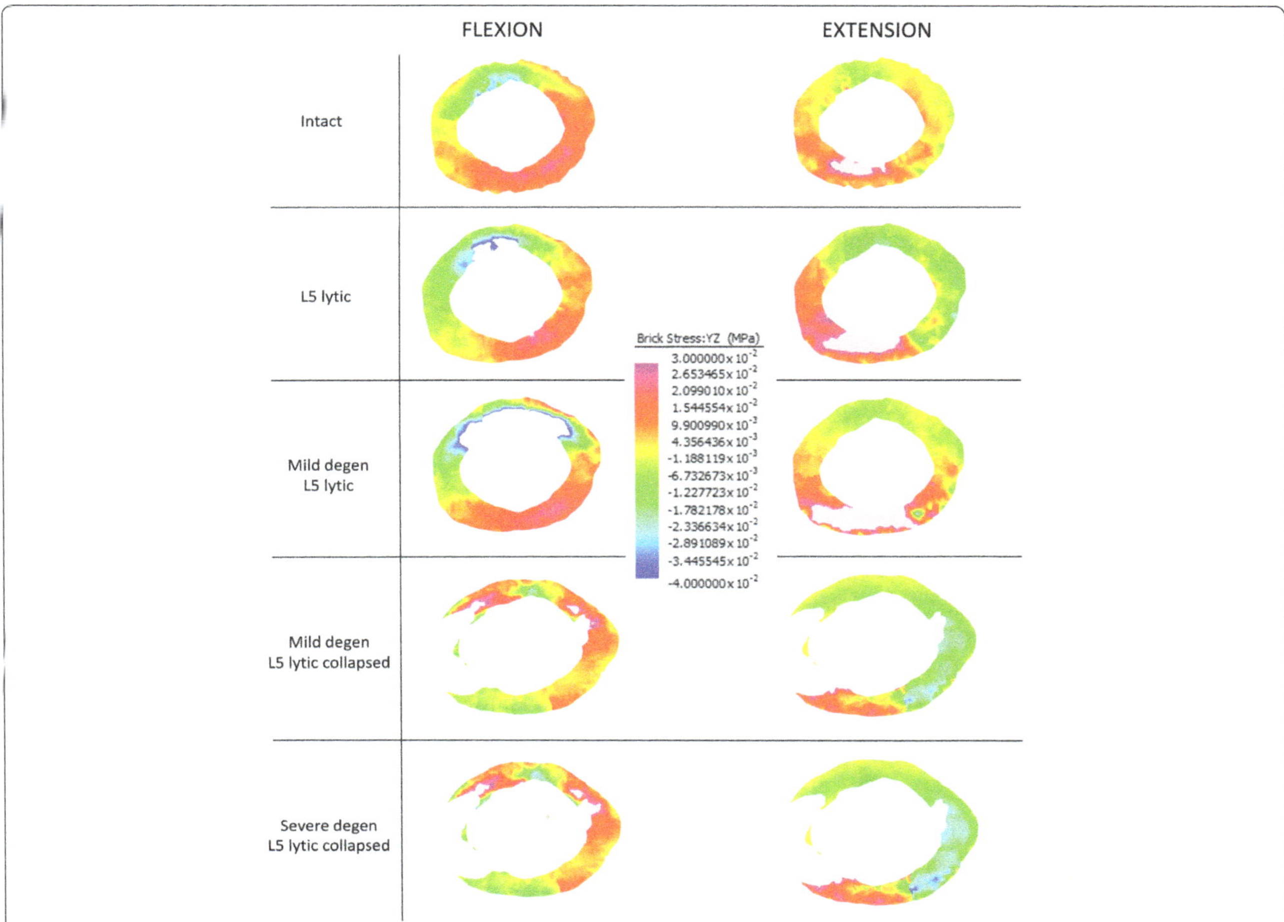

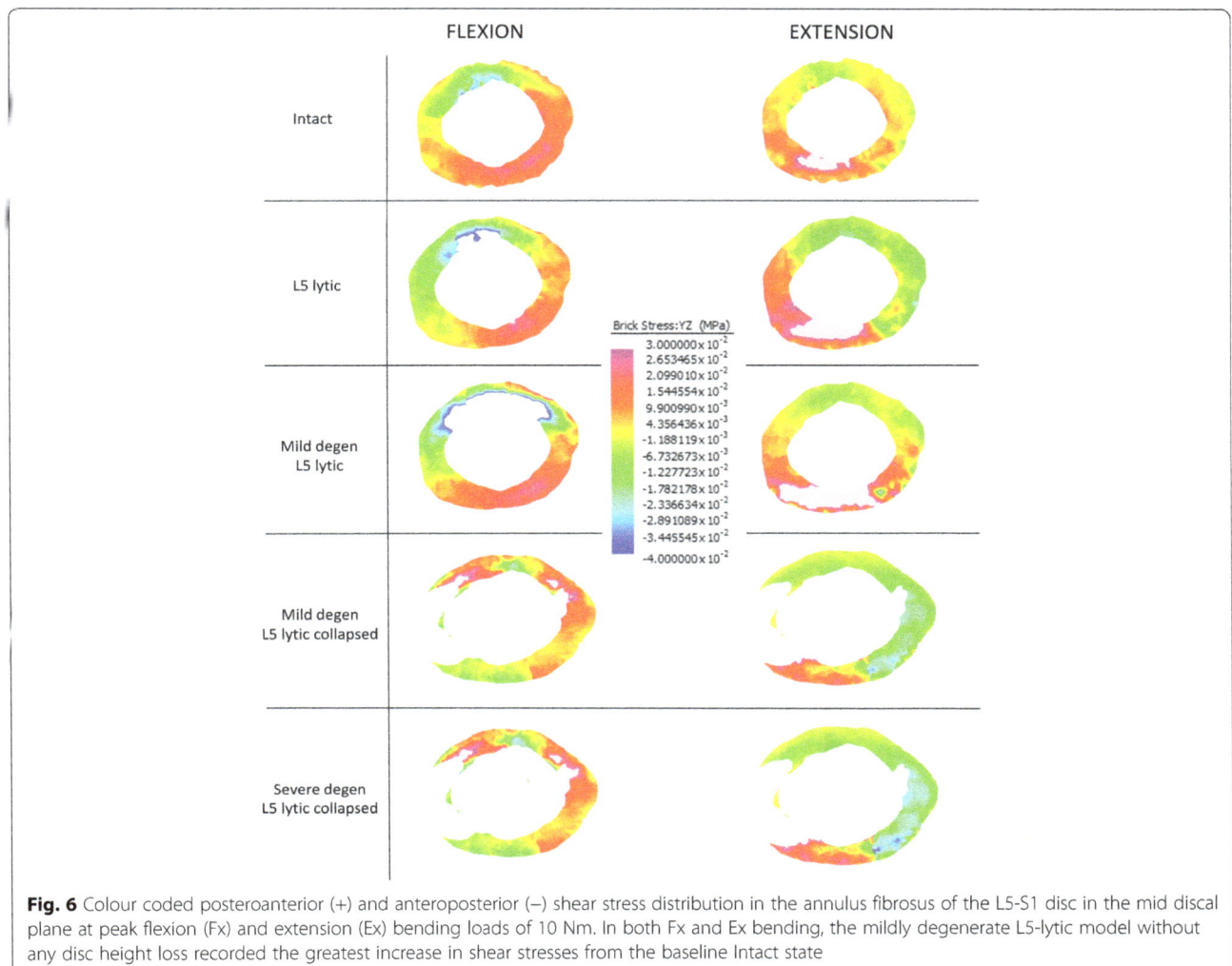

Fig. 6 Colour coded posteroanterior (+) and anteroposterior (–) shear stress distribution in the annulus fibrosus of the L5-S1 disc in the mid discal plane at peak flexion (Fx) and extension (Ex) bending loads of 10 Nm. In both Fx and Ex bending, the mildly degenerate L5-lytic model without any disc height loss recorded the greatest increase in shear stresses from the baseline Intact state

lower shear stresses compared with the intact disc height models. No significant difference in results was noted between M-DEG-COL LYTIC and S-DEG-COL LYTIC models. The collapsed disc height models, however, experienced high normal stresses compared with the intact disc height models suggesting that loss in disc height redistributed loads within the motion segment, decreasing the shear component of the intradiscal forces and increasing the normal component.

Over the age of 25 years, the prevalence of index-level disc degeneration in lytic defect patients was found to be significantly greater compared with an age-and-sex matched control group [11]. Although progression of a lytic defect to spondylolisthesis in adults depends on numerous factors such as spinopelvic balance, lower-lumbar muscle strength, repetitive flexion-extension activities, strength of the iliolumbar ligament; the most important structure resisting the vertebral slippage is the index-level disc [4, 6, 29, 30]. The health (or lack thereof) of the index-level disc is therefore critical to resisting the vertebral slippage. Two distinct pathways may be available to a L5-S1 segment with a bilateral lytic defect and a mildly degenerate index-level disc:

1) Within the limits of biomechanical stability provided by the active and passive spinal elements, the index-level disc may progressively lose height resulting in a decrease in intervertebral motions and redirection of the intradiscal shear stresses to normal stresses, until biomechanical stabilisation is achieved.
2) Beyond the limits of biomechanical stability provided by the active and passive spinal elements, the defect may progress to spondylolisthesis followed by a loss in disc height, in small and closed-loop increments, until biomechanical stabilisation is achieved.

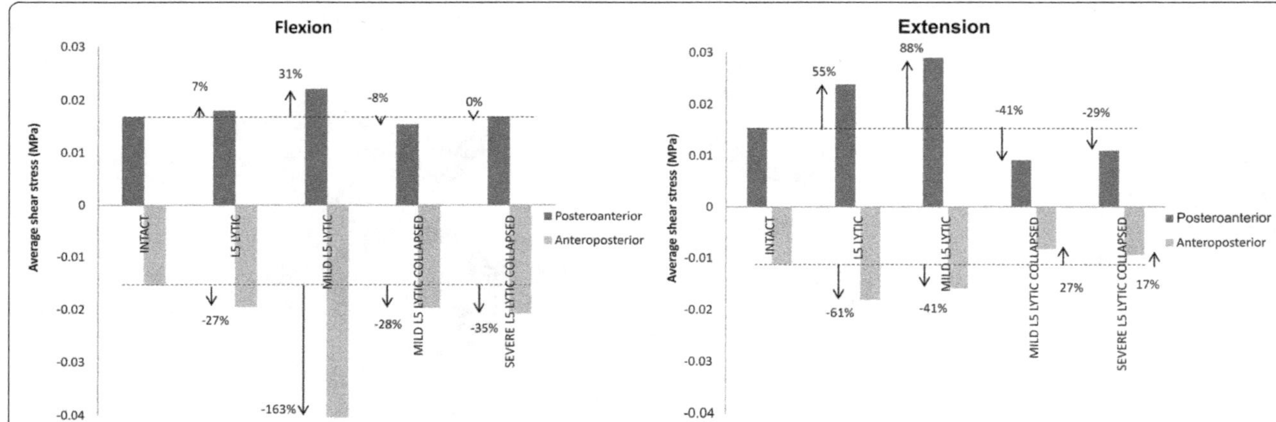

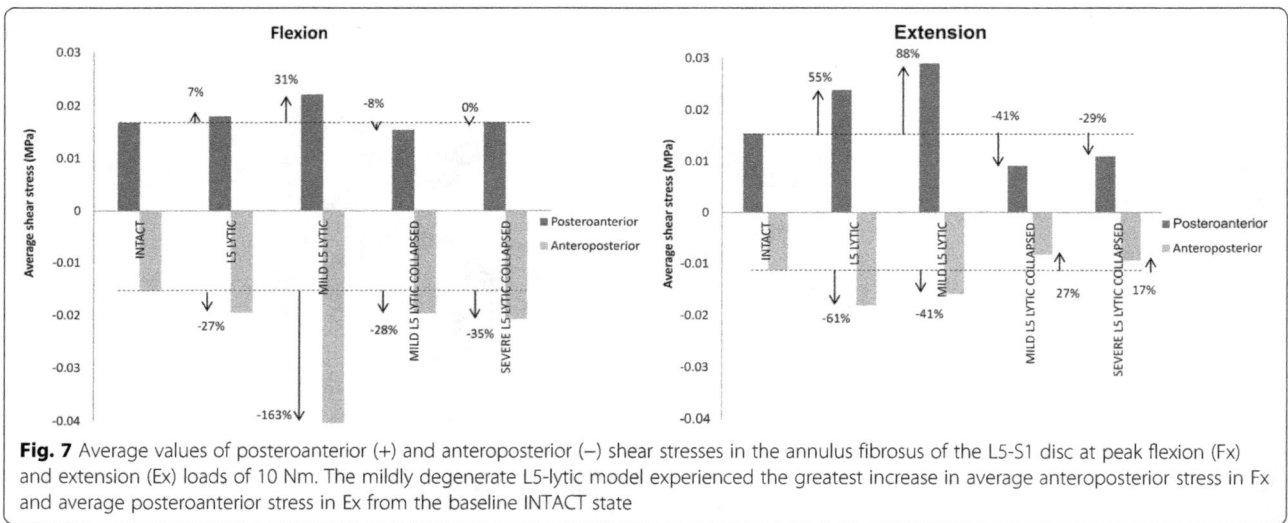

Fig. 7 Average values of posteroanterior (+) and anteroposterior (–) shear stresses in the annulus fibrosus of the L5-S1 disc at peak flexion (Fx) and extension (Ex) loads of 10 Nm. The mildly degenerate L5-lytic model experienced the greatest increase in average anteroposterior stress in Fx and average posteroanterior stress in Ex from the baseline INTACT state

From the onset of a bilateral L5 lytic defect, the exact duration of unstable and restabilisation phases may vary from patient to patient. Why some L5-S1 motion segments will adopt one pathway over the other may depend on genetic, anatomical, and lifestyle factors, and remains to be clinically explored. If the slippage progression is relatively rapid and intractable radicular pain associated with nerve root entrapment is evident, surgical intervention may be necessary to achieve biomechanical stability [12].

Progressive degeneration of the intervertebral disc is characterised by a cascade of cellular, biochemical, morphological, and functional changes. The sequence of these changes and the interplay between them are largely unknown. In the present study, a rather simplified approach was used to model progressive degeneration of the L5-S1 disc, altering only the structure (height) and material properties. The material properties of the AF and NP tissues were altered for different grades of disc degeneration in accordance with published data [25]. Whilst the shear modulus for the AF tissues was increased with progressive degeneration, Poisson's ratio for the NP tissues was decreased to simulate the loss in incompressibility with progressive degeneration. [25] A 50% loss in mid-sagittal plane disc height was modelled to simulate a collapsed disc.

Table 2 Mean axial strain in the iliolumbar ligament (ILL) fibres in different models during peak flexion load of 10 Nm

	Mean axial strain ILL fibres (± standard deviation)
Intact	5.91 (±1.87) %
Normal L5 Lytic	8.01 (±1.89)%
Mildly Degenerate L5 Lytic	11.25 (±1.91)%
Mildly Degenerate L5 Collapsed Lytic	1.91 (±0.91)%
Severely Degenerate L5 Collapsed Lytic	1.90 (±0.90)%

The greatest increase in mean axial strain from the baseline Intact state was observed in the mildly degenerate L5 lytic model

Some limitations to this study were noted. Poroelasticity and degeneration related structural defects (Schmorl's node, annular tears, nuclear clefts, and rim lesions) in the disc were not modelled, which may have a bearing on the results. Instead of assembling multiple FE models representing a gradual change in the disc height, only a 50% collapse in disc height was modelled. The AF was modelled as a composite structure with only four concentric layers of collagen fibres (without translamellar bridges) embedded within a homogenous ground substance.

Conclusions

In the presence of a bilateral L5 spondylolytic defect, a mildly degenerate index-level disc experienced greater intervertebral motions and shear stresses compared with a severely degenerate index-level disc during flexion and extension bending. Disc height collapse, with or without severe degenerative changes in the stiffness properties of the disc, is one of the plausible restabilisation mechanism available to the L5-S1 motion segment to mitigate increased intervertebral motions and shear stresses due to a bilateral L5 lytic defect.

Abbreviations

AF: Annulus Fibrosus; ALL: Anterior Longitudinal Ligament; CL: Capsular Ligament; CT: Computed Tomography; DICOM: Digital Imaging and Communications in Medicine; DOF: Degrees of Freedom; Ex: Extension; FE: Finite Element; Fx: Flexion; GPa: Giga Pascals; ILL: Iliolumbar Ligament; INTACT: An intact finite element model of L1-S1 spine without any defect or degeneration; IPT: Interpedicular Travel; ISL: Interspinous Ligament;

ITL: Intertransverse Ligament; L1: First Lumbar Vertebra; L5: Fifth Lumbar Vertebra; LF: Ligamentum Flavum; LSL: Lumbosacral Ligament; Lytic: A Spondylolytic Defect; M-DEG LYTIC: A finite element model of L1-S1 spine with a bilateral L5 lytic defect and mild degenerative changes in the stiffness properties of the L5-S1 disc; M-DEG-COL LYTIC: A finite element model of L1-S1 spine with a bilateral L5 lytic defect, mild degenerative changes in the stiffness properties of the L5-S1 disc and 50% disc height collapse; mm: Millimetre; Nm: Newton-Metre; NOR LYTIC: A finite element model of L1-S1 spine with a bilateral L5 lytic defect and a normal L5-S1 disc; NP: Nucleus Pulposus; PLL: Posterior Longitudinal Ligament; RoM: Range of Motion; S-COL LYTIC: A finite element model of L1-S1 spine with a bilateral L5 lytic defect, severe degenerative changes in the stiffness properties of the L5-S1 disc and 50% disc height collapse; SSL: Supraspinous Ligament; UNSW: University of New South Wales

Acknowledgements
The authors thank Emma Wheatley, Karen Ruut, and Carl Bryant from CJ Bryant Radiology, St. George Private Hospital, Sydney (Australia) for providing access to de-identified patient CT data.

Funding
This work was supported by a research grant from AO Spine Foundation Asia Pacific (AOSAUNZ(R) 2016-01) to ADD, a Taste of Summer Research Scholarship from UNSW Australia to VR, an International Postgraduate Research Scholarship from UNSW Australia and DIISRTE to UC, and internal research funds from Spine Service.

Authors' contributions
Conceived and designed the experiments: VASR, UC, ADD, NT. Performed the experiments: VASR, UC, LLV. Analysed the data: VASR, UC, ADD. Contributed materials and analysis tools: LLV, NT, ADD. Wrote the paper: VASR, UC, LLV, NT, ADD. All authors read and approved this version of the manuscript.

Consent for publication
A written consent was obtained from the patient for the use of their de-identified medical records for research purposes.

Competing interests
The authors declare that they have no competing interests.

Author details
[1]Spine Service, Department of Orthopaedic Surgery, St. George & Sutherland Clinical School, University of New South Wales Australia, Kogarah, Sydney, NSW 2217, Australia. [2]School of Biomedical Engineering, University of Technology Sydney, Ultimo, NSW 2007, Australia. [3]School of Mechanical and Manufacturing Engineering, University of New South Wales Australia, Kensington campus, Sydney, NSW 2052, Australia.

References

1. Fredrickson BE, Baker D, McHolick WJ, Yuan HA, Lubicky JP. The natural history of spondylolysis and spondylolisthesis. J Bone Joint Surg Am. 1984;36:699–707.
2. Leone A, Cianfoni A, Cerase A, Magarelli N, Bonomo L. Lumbar spondylolysis: a review. Skelet Radiol. 2011;40:683–700.
3. Hresko MT, Labelle H, Roussouly P, Berthonnaud E. Classification of high-grade spondylolistheses based on pelvic version and spine balance: possible rationale for reduction. Spine (Phila Pa 1976). 2007;32:2208–13.
4. Labelle H, Mac-Thiong JM, Roussouly P. Spino-pelvic sagittal balance of spondylolisthesis: a review and classification. Eur Spine J. 2011;20(Suppl 5):641–6.
5. Mac-Thiong JM, Labelle H. A proposal for a surgical classification of pediatric lumbosacral spondylolisthesis based on current literature. Eur Spine J. 2006;15:1425–35.
6. Roussouly P, Gollogly S, Berthonnaud E, Labelle H, Weidenbaum M. Sagittal alignment of the spine and pelvis in the presence of L5-s1 isthmic lysis and low-grade spondylolisthesis. Spine (Phila Pa 1976). 2006;31:2484–90.
7. Sairyo K, et al. Vertebral forward slippage in immature lumbar spine occurs following epiphyseal separation and its occurrence is unrelated to disc degeneration: is the pediatric spondylolisthesis a physis stress fracture of vertebral body? Spine (Phila Pa 1976). 2004;29:524–7.
8. Sairyo K, Katoh S, Sakamaki T, Inoue M, Komatsubara S, Ogawa T, et al. A review of the pathomechanism of forward slippage in pediatric spondylolysis: the Tokushima theory of growth plate slippage. J Med Investig. 2015;62:11–8.
9. Vialle R, Ilharreborde B, Dauzac C, Lenoir T, Rillardon L, Guigui P. Is there a sagittal imbalance of the spine in isthmic spondylolisthesis? A correlation study. Eur Spine J. 2007;16:1641–9.
10. Ikata T, Miyake R, Katoh S, Morita T, Murase M. Pathogenesis of sports-related spondylolisthesis in adolescents. Radiographic and magnetic resonance imaging study. Am J Sports Med. 1996;24:94–8.
11. Szypryt EP, Twining P, Mulholland C, Worthington BS. The prevalence of disc degeneration associated with neural arch defects of the lumbar spine assessed by magnetic resonance imaging. Spine (Phila Pa 1976). 1989;14:977–81.
12. Seitsalo S, Schlenzka Z, Poussa M, Österman K. Disc degeneration in young patients with isthmic spondylolisthesis treated operatively or conservatively: a long-term follow-up. Eur Spine J. 1996:393–7.
13. Floman Y. Progression of lumbosacral isthmic spondylolisthesis in adults. Spine (Phila Pa 1976). 2000;25:342–7.
14. Lyras DN, Tilkeridis K, Stavrakis T. Progression of spondylolysis to isthmic spondylolisthesis in an adult without accompanying disc degeneration: a case report. Acta Orthop Belg. 2008;74:141–4.
15. Stone AT, Tribus CB. Acute progression of spondylolysis to isthmic spondylolisthesis in an adult. Spine (Phila Pa 1976). 2002;27:E370–2.
16. Chamoli U, Chen AS, Diwan AD. Interpedicular kinematics in an in vitro biomechanical assessment of a bilateral lumbar spondylolytic defect. Clin Biomech (Bristol, Avon). 2014;29:1108–15.
17. Mihara H, Onari K, Cheng BC, David SM, Zbelick TA. The biomechanical effects of spondylolysis and its treatment. Spine (Phila Pa 1976). 2003;28:235–8.
18. Fan J, Yu GR, Liu F, Zhao J, Zhao WD. A biomechanical study on the direct repair of spondylolysis by different techniques of fixation. Orthop Surg. 2010;2:46–51.
19. Wiltse LL. The effect of the common anomalies of the lumbar spine upon disc degeneration and low back pain. Orthop Clin North Am. 1971;2:569–82.
20. Yong-Hing K, Kirkaldy-Willis WH. The pathophysiology of degenerative disease of the lumbar spine. Orthop Clin North Am. 1983;14:491–504.
21. Tanaka N, An HS, Lim T, Fujiwara A, Jeon C, Haughton VM. The relationship between disc degeneration and flexibility of the lumbar spine. Spine J. 2001;1:47–56.
22. Ramakrishna VAS, Chamoli U, Viglione LL, Tsafnat N, Diwan ADD. The role of sacral slope in the progression of a bilateral Spondylolytic defect at L5 to spondylolisthesis: a biomechanical investigation using finite element analysis. Global Spine Journal. 2017; https://doi.org/10.1177/2192568217735802.
23. Malandrino A, Planell JA, Lacroix D. Statistical factorial analysis on the poroelastic material properties sensitivity of the lumbar intervertebral disc under compression, flexion and axial rotation. J Biomech. 2009;42:2780–8.
24. Nguyen AM, Johannessen W, Yoder JH, Wheaton AJ, Vresilovic EJ, Borthakur A, Elliott DM. Noninvasive quantification of human nucleus pulposus pressure with use of T1rho-weighted magnetic resonance imaging. J Bone Joint Surg Am. 2008;90:796–802.
25. Wang Y, Chen H, Zhang L, Liu J, Wang Z. Influence of degenerative changes of intervertebral disc on its material properties and pathology. Chin J Traumatol. 2012;15:67–76.
26. Behrsin JF, Briggs CA. Ligaments of the lumbar spine: a review. Surg Radiol Anat. 1988;10:211–9.
27. Chamoli U, Chen AS, Diwan AD. Letter to the editor regarding the article " Interpedicular travel in the evaluation of spinal implants: an application in

posterior dynamic stabilization" by DJ Cook, MS Yeager, and BC Cheng: Spine 2012; 37(11): 923–931. Spine (Phila Pa 1976). 2014;39(11):921.

28. Kirkaldy-Willis WH, Farfan HF. Instability of the lumbar spine. Clin Orthop Relat Res. 1982:110–23.
29. Motley G, Nyland J, Jacobs J, Caborn DNM. The pars Interarticularis stress reaction, spondylolysis, and spondylolisthesis progression. J Athl Train. 1998;33:351–8.
30. Aihara T, Takahashi K, Yamagata M, Moriya H, Shimada Y. Does the iliolumbar ligament prevent anterior displacement of the fifth lumbar vertebra with defects of the pars? J Bone Joint Surg Br. 2000;82:846–50.

20

Effects of multilevel posterior ligament dissection after spinal instrumentation on adjacent segment biomechanics as a potential risk factor for proximal junctional kyphosis

Tobias Lange[1*†], Tobias L. Schulte[2†], Georg Gosheger[1], Albert Schulze Boevingloh[1], Raul Mayr[3] and Werner Schmoelz[3]

Abstract

Background: Spinous processes and posterior ligaments, such as inter- and supraspinous ligaments are often sacrificed either deliberately to harvest osseous material for final spondylodesis e.g. in deformity corrective surgery or accidentally after posterior spinal instrumentation. This biomechanical study evaluates the potential destabilizing effect of a progressive dissection of the posterior ligaments (PL) after instrumented spinal fusion as a potential risk factor for proximal junctional kyphosis (PJK).

Methods: Twelve calf lumbar spines were instrumented from L3 to L6 (L3 = upper instrumented vertebra, UIV) and randomly assigned to one of the two study groups (dissection vs. control group). The specimens in the dissection group underwent progressive PL dissection, followed by cyclic flexion motion (250 cycles, moment: + 2.5 to + 20.0 Nm) to simulate physical activity and range of motion (ROM) testing of each segment with pure moments of ±15.0 Nm after each dissection step. The segmental ROM in flexion and extension was measured. The control group underwent the same loading and ROM testing protocol, but without PL dissection.

Results: In the treatment group, the normalized mean ROM at L2-L3 (direct adjacent segment of interest, UIV/UIV + 1, PJK-level) increased to 104.7%, 107.3%, and 119.4% after dissection of the PL L4–L6, L3–L6, and L2–L6, respectively. In the control group the mean ROM increased only to 103.2%, 106.7%, and 108.7%. The ROM difference at L2-L3 with regard to the last dissection of the PL was statistically significant ($P = 0.017$) and a PL dissection in the instrumented segments showed a positive trend towards an increased ROM at UIV/UIV + 1.

Conclusions: A dissection of the PL at UIV/UIV + 1 leads to a significant increase in ROM at this level which can be considered to be a risk factor for PJK and should be definitely avoided during surgery. However, a dissection of the posterior ligaments within the instrumented segments while preserving the ligaments at UIV/UIV + 1 leads to a slight but not significant increase in ROM in the adjacent cranial segment UIV/UIV + 1 in the used experimental setup. Using this experimental setup we could not confirm our initial hypothesis that the posterior ligaments within a long posterior instrumentation should be preserved.

Keywords: Proximal junctional kyphosis, Posterior instrumentation, Posterior ligaments, Ligament dissection, Biomechanics

* Correspondence: tobias.lange@ukmuenster.de
†Equal contributors
[1]Department of Orthopedics and Tumor Orthopedics, Muenster University Hospital, Albert-Schweitzer-Campus 1, 48149 Muenster, Germany
Full list of author information is available at the end of the article

Background

Posterior instrumentation of the spine is one of the most frequently performed surgical procedures for various pathologies. According to a report by the Agency for Healthcare Research and Quality, approximately 488.000 spinal fusions were performed during U.S. hospital stays in 2011 (a rate of 15.7 stays per 10.000 population) [1]. In spinal deformity corrective surgery complication rates vary from 37 to 68% [2]. One of the major complications is proximal junctional kyphosis (PJK) with a varying incidence of 6 to 61.7% [3–7]. The rate of revision surgery due to PJK can be as high as 50% [5]. Numerous risk factors for PJK have been described in the literature, including:

- disruption of the posterior ligaments (supra- and interspinous ligaments, PL) and facet capsules [8]
- the type, stiffness, and combination of the implants selected [9–15]; wedging of the disc above or below an instrumentation [16]
- vertebral compression fractures in the upper instrumented vertebra (UIV) or the first proximal adjacent vertebra [17]
- the choice of the UIV in deformity correction [3, 18] and the influence of the sagittal parameters [19].

However, neither the precise pathophysiology of PJK nor clear strategies for preventing it have yet been established [3, 19].

One of the keys to PJK is the quality and integrity of the posterior tension banding [3, 8, 12]. This includes the supra- and interspinous ligaments. Many surgeons keep the spinous process of the UIV, the PL between the UIV and UIV + 1, as well as the facet joint capsules between UIV and UIV + 1 intact but sacrifice the spinous processes and PL caudal to the UIV, especially in deformity corrective surgery. The objective of this procedure is to facilitate a better deformity correction e.g. by Ponte osteotomies and to harvest osseous material which is used for the final spondylodesis.

The purpose of this biomechanical in vitro study was to evaluate the potential destabilizing effect of a progressive dissection of the PL, even within the fused segments caudal to UIV following posterior instrumentation on the segmental biomechanics at UIV/UIV + 1. It was hypothesized, that the PL even within the fused segments caudal to UIV are relevant for sagittal stability, that a dissection could therefore lead to an increase of range of motion (ROM) at UIV/UIV + 1 and could possibly represent a risk factor for the development of PJK and that the PL should therefore be preserved during surgery.

Methods

Specimen preparation

Twelve L1–L6 calf lumbar spines (aged 12–18 months) obtained from a local slaughterhouse were used according to established biomechanical testing protocols [15, 20, 21]. The specimens were stored at – 20 °C and thawed overnight at 4 °C before testing. All soft tissue was removed, leaving the PL, capsules, and other supporting ligamentous structures intact. The specimens were embedded in polymethylmethacrylate (PMMA; Technovit 3040, Heraeus Kulzer, Wehrheim, Germany) at the upper half of the L1 and the lower half of the L6 vertebrae. They were mounted in a well-established spine tester [22, 23] with the middle disc (L3–L4) aligned horizontally. Screws for fixation of the three-dimensional motion analysis system (Winbiomechanics, Zebris Medical Ltd., Isny, Germany) were fixed to the ventral side of the PMMA blocks and vertebrae L2, L3, and L4.

Posterior instrumentation at L3–L6 was performed by an experienced spine surgeon using a bilateral polyaxial pedicle screw rod system (screws: 6.0 × 45 mm for the L3, L4, and L5 vertebrae, 7.0 × 45 mm for L6; rod: titanium, diameter 5.5 mm; Expedium® System, DePuy Synthes, Raynham, MA, USA).

The specimens were randomly assigned to one of the two study groups (treatment vs. control group). The tests were performed at room temperature, and the specimens were kept moist with physiological saline solution during testing.

Biomechanical test setup

In the treatment group, six specimens underwent stepwise dissection of PL (supra- and interspinous ligaments, from caudal to cranial) within the fused segments and at last also at UIV/UIV + 1. After each level of ligament dissection (four states: intact, PL L4–L6, PL L3–L6, and PL L2–L6), the specimens underwent cyclic flexion motion of 250 cycles in which a flexural moment of + 2.5 to + 20.0 Nm was applied (triangular loading function, 2.5°/sec) to simulate physical activity. The number of load cycles was limited to 250 cycles due to time constraints of in vitro testing with cadaveric specimens (maximal one day of testing before degradation sets in). The load magnitudes were chosen rather high to provoke an effect of stretching ligamentous structures beyond the elastic region to cause an increased motion in the segment to simulate the genesis of PJK. This was followed by a flexibility test with pure moments of ±15.0 Nm in flexion/extension for three load cycles measuring the ROM of each segment.

In the control group, six specimens underwent the same test protocol with cyclic motion and flexibility tests, but without PL dissection (Figs. 1 and 2).

Flexibility tests and cyclic flexion motion were done in the same setup of a six degree of freedom spine tester. The specimens were loaded with pure moments, applied by a stepper motor. A six-component load cell with feedback control was connected to the stepper motor to

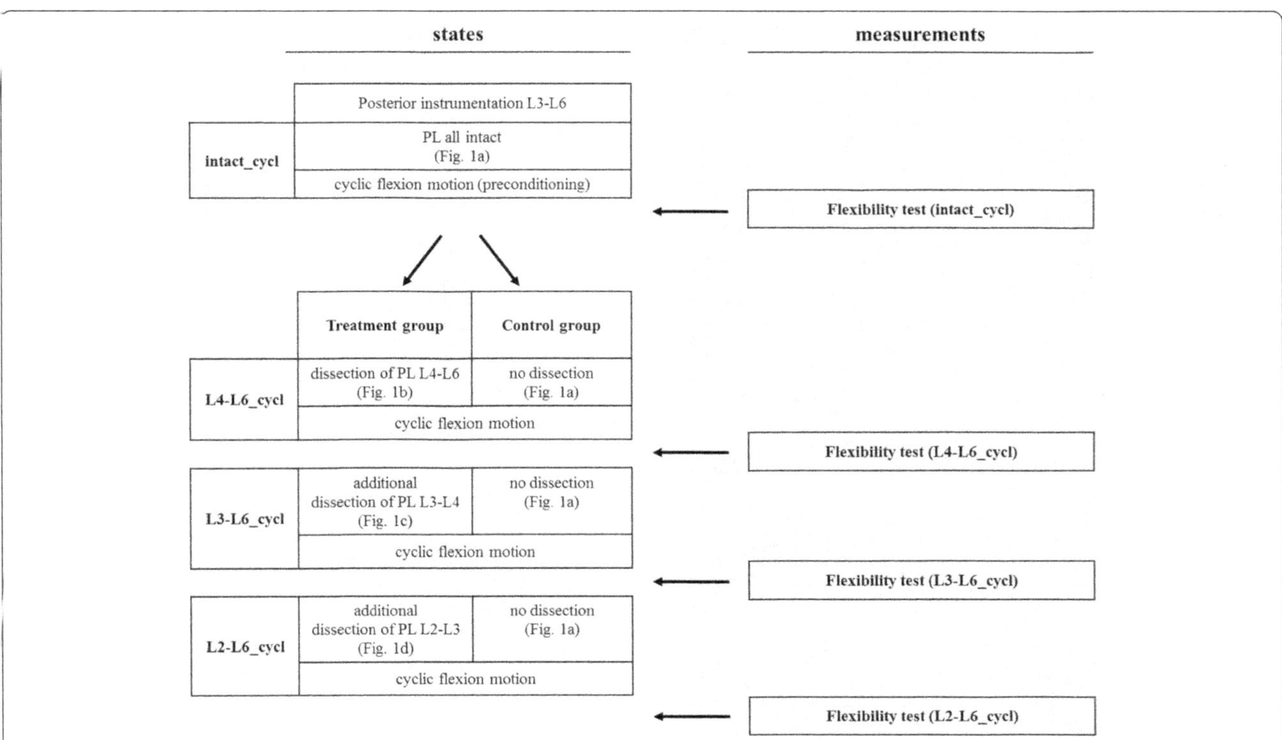

Fig. 1 The sequence of the experiment. For each state, flexibility tests were carried out after cyclic flexion motion, and the data obtained were used for statistical analysis

control the loading of the specimens (Fig. 3). No preload or specific preconditioning was applied to the specimens. The test speed was 0.7°/sec. Intersegmental motions were measured using an ultrasound-based motion analysis system. From the recorded data, the ROM was measured during the third load cycle for segments L1–L2, L2–L3, L3–L4, and L4–L6.

Data evaluation

After instrumentation, a baseline flexibility test was performed. To facilitate data comparison, subsequent ROM measurements were normalized to the initial ROM. Statistical analysis was performed using IBM SPSS Statistics® for Windows, version 22.0 (IBM Corporation, Armonk, New York). For data comparison analysis, two-way analysis of variance (ANOVA) with repeated measures was performed (four states: intact_cycl, PL L4–L6_cycl, PL L3–L6_cycl, and PL L2–L6_cycl) with post hoc analysis using Bonferroni correction. To account for possible sphericity violation among the states, P values were corrected using the Greenhouse–Geisser method [24]. The significance level was set at $p < 0.05$.

Results

The ROM for each segment (L1-L2, L2-L3, L3-L4, L4–L6) was measured for each state (intact_cycl, PL L4–L6_cycl, PL L3–L6_cycl, PL L2–L6_cycl) (Table 1).

The most important approval of this study is that a dissection of the PL including L2-L3 (UIV/UIV + 1) leads to a significant increase of ROM at the adjacent segment L2-L3 (UIV/UIV + 1) itself, whereas dissection of PL within the instrumented segments (keeping PL of UIV/UIV + 1 intact) results in a slight but not significant increment of ROM at the segment L2-L3 (UIV/UIV + 1) (Fig. 4).

In the treatment group, the normalized mean ROM in segment L2-L3 (direct adjacent segment of interest, UIV/UIV + 1, PJK-level) increased to 104.7%, 107.3% and 119.4% after dissection of the L4–L6, L3–L6 and L2–L6 PL, respectively (Fig. 4). In the control group, the mean ROM increased only to 103.2%, 106.7% and 108.7%, respectively, without dissections for each state. The difference in the L2-L3 segment with regard to changes in ROM across testing states between the two groups was statistically significant ($p = 0.017$). The interaction between treatment (dissection or control) and state (intact, PL L4–L6, PL L3–L6 and PL L2–L6) was also statistically significant ($p = 0.002$).

The normalized mean ROM of segment L1-L2 (second adjacent segment, UIV + 1/UIV + 2) increased to 105.5%, 108.6%, and 113.9% after dissection of the L4–L6, L3–L6, and L2–L6 PL, respectively (Fig. 4) in the treatment group. Whereas in the control group, an increase to 103.3%, 108.3%, and 111.0% was seen after cyclic flexion

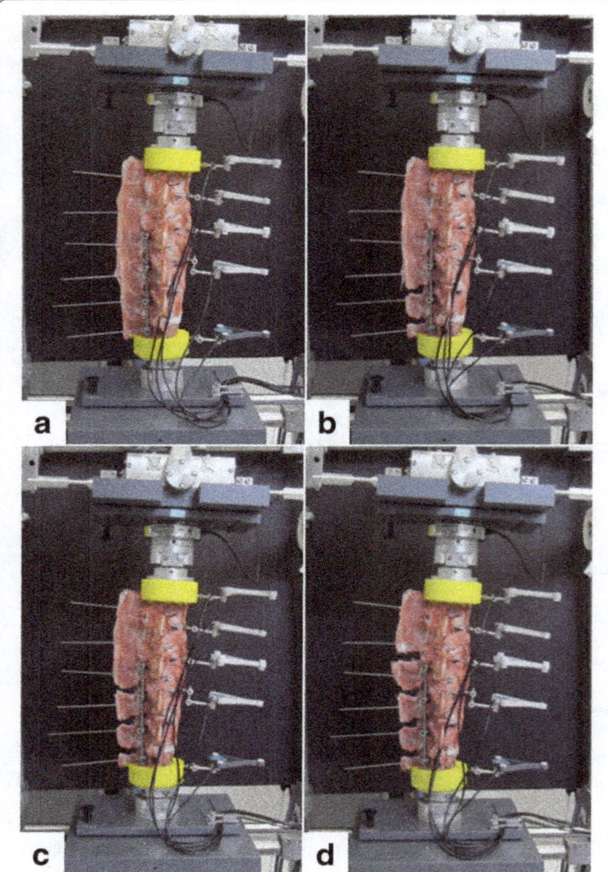

Fig. 2 States of the specimens during testing in the treatment group. **a** Instrumented (intact). **b** Dissection of supraspinous and interspinous ligaments L4–L6. **c** Additional dissection of supraspinous and interspinous ligaments L3–L4. **d** Additional dissection of supraspinous and interspinous ligaments L2–L3

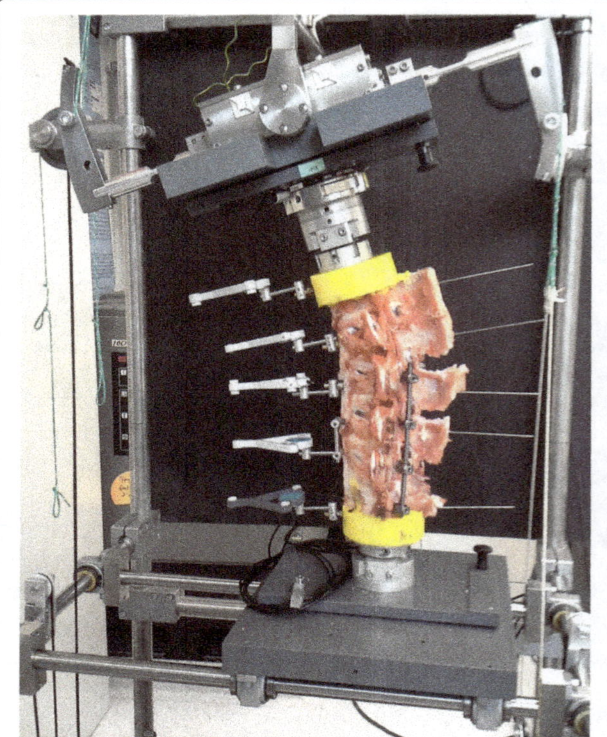

Fig. 3 Six degrees of freedom spine simulator for in vitro biomechanical testing

motion without dissections for each state. The differences between the two groups with regard to changes in ROM across the testing states were not significant (p = 0.154). The interaction between treatment (dissection or control) and state (intact, PL L4–L6, PL L3–L6, and PL L2–L6) was also not significant (p = 0.171).

The segments L4-L6 and L3-L4 (segments within the rigid posterior instrumentation) show only small absolute values of ROM (Table 1) and they do not show any significant changes within the treatment group after PL dissection (L4-L6: p = 0.496, L3-L6: p = 0.245) compared to the native state. The reason is the rigid posterior instrumentation spanning from L3-L6.

Table 1 Absolute values of range of motion (ROM)

Segment	State	Treatment group		Control group	
		Mean (°)	SD (°)	Mean (°)	SD (°)
L1–L2	intact_cycl	9.88	3.68	9.51	1.18
	L4-L6_cycl	10.44	3.97	9.83	1.25
	L3-L6_cycl	10.73	4.07	10.29	1.23
	L2-L6_cycl	11.25	4.22	10.56	1.34
L2–L3	intact_cycl	10.47	2.56	11.27	1.65
	L4-L6_cycl	10.97	2.74	11.64	1.69
	L3-L6_cycl	11.24	2.83	12.02	1.74
	L2-L6_cycl	12.50	3.47	12.25	1.70
L3–L4	intact_cycl	1.53	0.73	1.71	0.26
	L4-L6_cycl	1.60	0.72	1.75	0.25
	L3-L6_cycl	1.66	0.75	1.82	0.24
	L2-L6_cycl	1.71	0.76	1.85	0.24
L4–L6	intact_cycl	2.58	0.81	3.16	0.84
	L4-L6_cycl	2.81	0.87	3.30	0.85
	L3-L6_cycl	2.87	0.89	3.43	0.83
	L2-L6_cycl	2.84	0.80	3.47	0.80

Absolute values of range of motion (ROM) in degrees during testing of segments L1–L2, L2–L3, L3–L4, and L4–L6 in the treatment and control groups

Discussion

This study shows that a dissection of the posterior ligaments (the supraspinous and interspinous ligaments) at UIV/UIV + 1 does have a significant influence on the

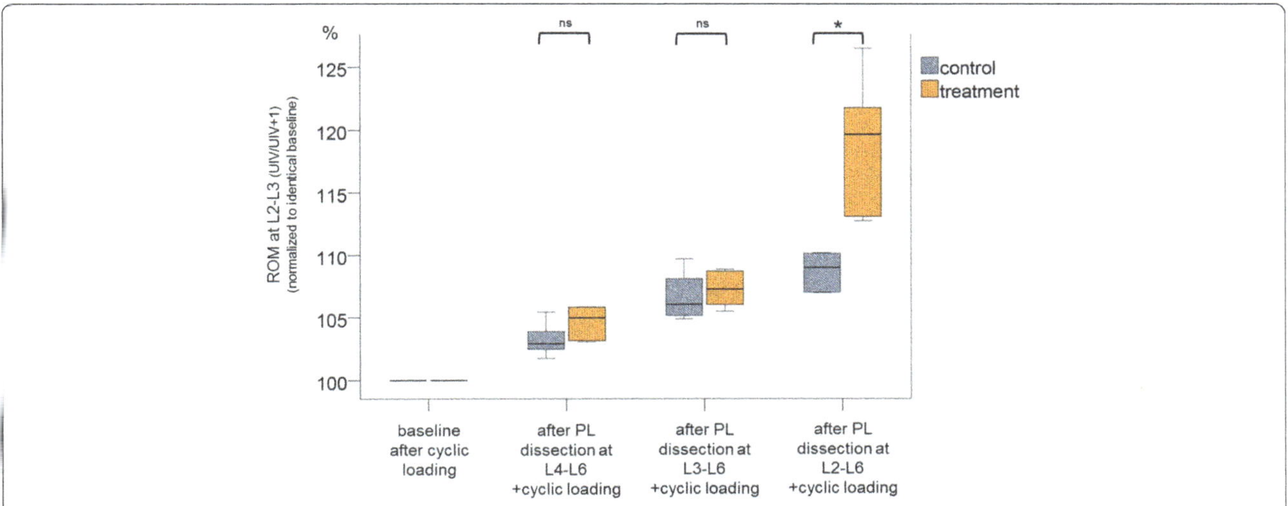

Fig. 4 Changes in range of motion (ROM) at segment L2–L3 (UIV/UIV + 1) after stepwise dissection of the posterior ligaments (L4–L6, L3–L6, L2–L6), normalized to the initial flexibility test as basis (intact_cycl) in percentages, after preconditioning by cyclic loading. * Significant at $P < 0.05$, ns: not significant

ROM in the adjacent segment and is therefore definitely a risk factor for PJK.

PJK is defined as pathologic kyphosis in the first mobile proximal adjacent segment after instrumentation. Whereas some authors define PJK radiographically as kyphosis greater than 10° between the upper instrumented vertebra and the vertebral body two levels above it (UIV/UIV + 2) [4], others require this angle to be additionally at least 10° greater than the corresponding preoperative measurement [25]. According to Arlet and Aebi, PJK is a junctional kyphosis of 15° or more above a previous instrumentation [3]. Various failure modes have been proposed [3]: progressive deformity above a previous instrumentation, representing the natural course of the deformity; wedging of the disc above or below an instrumentation [16]; vertebral compression fractures in the upper instrumented vertebra or the first proximal adjacent vertebra [17]; failure of proximal fixation (screw pull-out, screw ploughing, screw cutting into end plates); dislocation of the spine above the instrumentation; disc degeneration in the adjacent segment; and in particular, elongation with or without disruption of the PL [8].

The incidence of PJK is reported to be in the range of 6–61.7% [3–6]. In most cases, PJK develops during the first 3 months after surgery [25], and this may represent evidence for failure of the posterior ligament complex intraoperatively or immediately postoperatively.

Various risk factors have been suggested in the literature as being responsible for PJK. Some of these cannot be controlled or influenced by the surgeon, but others can [3, 8, 26–28]. One of the key factors that can be influenced by the surgeon is the amount of tissue disruption [3, 8]. In addition to the facet joint capsules at the UIV + 1/UIV level and the PL are relevant posterior tension banding structures. The practical question during surgery is whether to sacrifice spinous processes in the upper part of the instrumentation or whether to keep them — and thus the ligamentous tension banding — intact. The ligaments distal to the spinous process of the UIV and also the spinous processes of UIV-1 and below are often resected in order to harvest material for posterior spondylodesis. During surgery, a sudden loss of tension in the adjacent inter- and supraspinous ligaments was occasionally observed during dissection of supraspinous and interspinous ligaments, even far away within the instrumentation. It is a fact that the fibers of the supraspinous ligament are attached multisegmental to the spinous processes [29] and it was therefore hypothesized that these ligaments and spinous processes distal to the UIV are relevant for sagittal stability and should be preserved in order to prevent PJK.

Cahill et al. have shown in a finite element modeling an increased angular displacement and nucleus pressure immediately after dissection of the posterior ligamentous complex at the level above the construct [8]. Different dissection procedures of the facet joints and ligaments at the level UIV + 1/UIV have been analyzed already by Cammarata et al., they carried out a virtual biomechanical analysis of PJK using computer simulation and also showed that dissection of the PL, bilateral facetectomy, and a combination of the two between UIV and UIV + 1 lead to increases in the proximal junctional angle of 10%, 28%, and 53%, respectively [12]. Liu et al. have also shown protective effects of a preservation of the posterior complex (complete laminectomy vs. hemi-laminectomy vs. facet joint resection only) on the development of adjacent segment degeneration after lumbar fusion [28]. Additionally, Pham et al. proposed an application of a tendon graft as an interspinous ligament reinforcement between UIV + 1 and UIV-2 as a preventive strategy for proximal junctional kyphosis [30].

However, there is no previous biomechanical study with an experimental setup evaluating the effect of a dissection of the posterior ligaments even within the instrumented levels, far away from the junction level, and not only at the adjacent level itself. Therefore, we conducted this biomechanical study which at least supports the theory that there is an important tension band effect of the PL preventing PJK in the adjacent segment. In our study a small, nonsignificant increase in ROM at UIV/UIV + 1 was detected after PL dissection even within the fused segments of the spine. Most notably, a PL dissection at UIV/UIV + 1 itself has a significant impact on the ROM in this segment (+ 18.9%) and therefore on the potential development of PJK.

As an increase in ROM is only an indicator and not equal to an increased kyphosis, i.e. PJK, the hysteresis curves (applied moment vs resulting angular displacement) of the flexibility tests were further evaluated to emphasize the effect of posterior ligament dissection on segmental alignment. The ROM mainly increased in flexion, while the ROM in extension did not substantially change. With this the mean neutral zone as an indicator of the segmental alignment also shifted in the kyphotic direction. This became even more pronounced with an increasing dissection of the posterior ligaments (Fig. 5) and the difference between the control and dissection group became significant ($p < 0.02$) at the final dissection. To simulate a physical activity a cyclic flexion motion was performed in both groups. Therefore, all ligamentous structures and other tissues are strained and might lose their tension over time. This can explain the increase of the ROM in the treatment group as well as the small increase in the control group over time.

A limitation of the present study is the use of calf instead of human spines. These specimens do not represent the same sagittal profile as humans and therefore the absolute ROM values cannot be directly transferred to the situation in humans. However, the relative effects of the various states that were tested should be similar in humans. Previous studies have shown that the use of calf lumbar spines does allow accurate biomechanical studies comparable to human spines [20, 31]. The obvious difference between quadrupeds and humans is the everyday loading of the spine, while the human spine is loaded more in axial compressions whereas the spine of quadrupeds is subjected to more bending. It can therefore be assumed that there is an even more pronounced effect in human spines, which have greater thoracic kyphosis due to the upright body position. It might also be speculated that the spine in elderly humans is more susceptible to the development of PJK in comparison with younger spines, due to age-related tissue degenerative effects [32]. In this study, nonkyphotic lumbar spines were used. As PJK is mainly present in the thoracic spine, with its natural precondition of kyphosis, it may be speculated that the effect of an increase in ROM in the adjacent segment that is demonstrated here is even more distinctive in the kyphotic thoracic spine. We are well aware that we are not able to control the influence of sagittal parameters on the risk of development of PJK in this test setup. Even in case of sagittal parameter

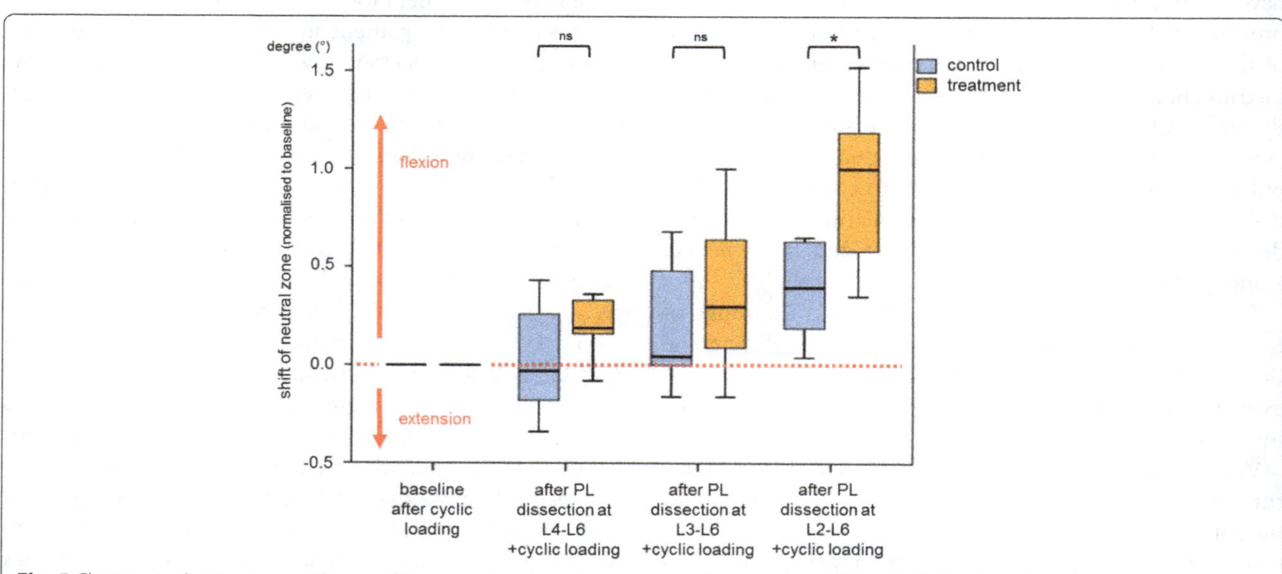

Fig. 5 Changes in the mean neutral zone of the control and treatment group of the segment L2-L3 (UIV/UIV + 1). A change in the positive direction represents a shift towards kyphosis. * Significant at $P < 0.05$, ns: not significant

evaluation it could be speculated that these data would be of limited value as our setup is a bovine in vitro model.

Obviously, the biomechanical experiments were carried out with a limited number of specimens. However, due to the controlled laboratory environment the common confounding variables occurring in a clinical trial can be excluded. Therefore it can be assumed that if the biomechanical effect of an intervention cannot be shown in a controlled laboratory environment with a limited sample size, it is deemed to be unlikely to have a clinical impact.

Furthermore a more extensive cyclic flexion motion after each PL dissection simulating a higher and longer physical activity could have been resulted in an even more increased ROM at UIV/UIV + 1 coming to statistical significance, especially for the ligament dissection within the instrumented segments and should be evaluated in the future.

Conclusions

Dissection of posterior ligaments (supraspinous and interspinous ligaments) of the adjacent segment (UIV/UIV + 1) cranial to a posterior instrumentation leads to a significant increase in ROM in the adjacent segment itself. Therefore, an accidental injury to or an intentional dissection of the posterior ligaments at UIV/UIV + 1 could be a risk factor for PJK and should definitively be avoided.

Dissection of the posterior ligaments within the instrumented segments while preserving the ligaments at UIV/UIV + 1 leads to a slight but not significant increase in ROM in the adjacent cranial segment UIV/UIV + 1 in the used experimental setup. Using this experimental setup we could not confirm our initial hypothesis that the posterior ligaments within a long posterior instrumentation should be preserved.

Further clinical evaluation is needed to finally answer the question of the role of the posterior ligaments regarding sagittal stability after posterior instrumentation.

Abbreviations

e.g.: for example; PJK: Proximal junctional kyphosis; PL: Posterior ligaments; PMMA: Polymethylmethacrylate; ROM: Range of motion; UIV + 1: one vertebra above the upper instrumented vertebra; UIV: Upper instrumented vertebra

Acknowledgements

Not applicable.

Funding

We acknowledge support by Open Access Publication Fund of University of Muenster.

Authors' contributions

TL review of literature, conception and design, acquisition of data, analysis and interpretation of date, drafting of the manuscript, statistical analysis, obtaining funding; TS review of literature, conception and design, acquisition of data, analysis and interpretation of date, drafting of the manuscript, critical revision of the manuscript; GG conception and design, critical revision of the manuscript, supervision; AS critical revision of the manuscript, supervision; RM conception and design, acquisition of data, analysis and interpretation of date, statistical analysis, critical revision of the manuscript; WS conception and design, acquisition of data, analysis and interpretation of date, drafting of the manuscript, statistical analysis, administrative, technical and material support, critical revision of the manuscript, supervision. All authors read and approved the final manuscript.

Consent for publication

Not applicable.

Competing interests

Each author certifies that he has no commercial associations (e.g., consultancies, stock ownership, equity interest, patent/licensing arrangements, etc.) that might pose a conflict of interest in connection with the submitted article. Each author certifies that he has no non-commercial interests.

Author details

[1]Department of Orthopedics and Tumor Orthopedics, Muenster University Hospital, Albert-Schweitzer-Campus 1, 48149 Muenster, Germany. [2]Department of Orthopedics and Trauma Surgery, St. Josef-Hospital, University Hospital, Ruhr-University Bochum, Gudrunstrasse 56, 44791 Bochum, Germany. [3]Department of Trauma Surgery, Medical University of Innsbruck, Anichstrasse 35, 6020 Innsbruck, Austria.

References

1. Weiss AJ, Elixhauser A, Andrews RM. Characteristics of Operating Room Procedures in U.S. Hospitals, 2011: Statistical Brief #170. In: Anonymous Healthcare Cost and Utilization Project (HCUP) Statistical Briefs. Rockville (MD):; 2006.
2. De la Garza-Ramos R, Jain A, Kebaish KM, Bydon A, Passias PG, Sciubba DM. Inpatient morbidity and mortality after adult spinal deformity surgery in teaching versus nonteaching hospitals. J Neurosurg Spine. 2016; doi:https://doi.org/10.3171/2015.11.SPINE151021 [doi].
3. Arlet V, Junctional AM. Spinal disorders in operated adult spinal deformities: present understanding and future perspectives. Eur. Spine J. 2013; https://doi.org/10.1007/s00586-013-2676-x [doi].
4. Kim HJ, Lenke LG, Shaffrey CI, Van Alstyne EM, Proximal SAC. Junctional kyphosis as a distinct form of adjacent segment pathology after spinal deformity surgery: a systematic review. Spine (Phila Pa 1976). 2012; https://doi.org/10.1097/BRS.0b013e31826d611b [doi].
5. Lau D, Clark AJ, Scheer JK, Daubs MD, Coe JD, Paonessa KJ, LaGrone MO, Kasten MD, Amaral RA, Trobisch PD, Lee JH, Fabris-Monterumici D, Anand N, Cree AK, Hart RA, Hey LA, Ames CP, SRS Adult Spinal deformity committee. Proximal junctional kyphosis and failure after spinal deformity surgery: a systematic review of the literature as a background to classification development. Spine (Phila Pa 1976) 2014; doi:https://doi.org/10.1097/BRS.0000000000000627 [doi].
6. Kim HJ, Lee HM, Kim HS, Moon ES, Park JO, Lee KJ, Life MSH. Expectancy after lumbar spine surgery: one- to eleven-year follow-up of 1015 patients. Spine (Phila Pa 1976). 2008; https://doi.org/10.1097/BRS.0b013e31817e1022 [doi].
7. Cho SK, Shin JI, Proximal KYJ. Junctional kyphosis following adult spinal deformity surgery. Eur. Spine J. 2014; https://doi.org/10.1007/s00586-014-3531-4 [doi].
8. Cahill PJ, Wang W, Asghar J, Booker R, Betz RR, Ramsey C, Baran G. The use of a transition rod may prevent proximal junctional kyphosis in the thoracic spine after scoliosis surgery: a finite element analysis. Spine (Phila Pa 1976). 2012; https://doi.org/10.1097/BRS.0b013e318246d4f2 [doi].
9. Thawrani DP, Glos DL, Coombs MT, Bylski-Austrow DI, Transverse SPF. Process hooks at upper instrumented vertebra provide more gradual motion transition than pedicle screws. Spine (Phila Pa 1976). 2014; https://doi.org/10.1097/BRS.0000000000000367 [doi].
10. Kim YJ, Lenke LG, Bridwell KH, Kim J, Cho SK, Cheh G, Proximal YJ. Junctional kyphosis in adolescent idiopathic scoliosis after 3 different types

of posterior segmental spinal instrumentation and fusions: incidence and risk factor analysis of 410 cases. Spine (Phila Pa 1976). 2007; https://doi.org/10.1097/BRS.0b013e31815a7ead [doi].

11. Helgeson MD, Shah SA, Newton PO, Clements DH. 3rd, Betz RR, marks MC, Bastrom T, harms study group. Evaluation of proximal junctional kyphosis in adolescent idiopathic scoliosis following pedicle screw, hook, or hybrid instrumentation. Spine (Phila Pa 1976). 2010; https://doi.org/10.1097/BRS.0b013e3181c77f8c [doi].
12. Cammarata M, Aubin CE, Wang X, Biomechanical M-TJM. Risk factors for proximal junctional kyphosis: a detailed numerical analysis of surgical instrumentation variables. Spine (Phila Pa 1976). 2014; https://doi.org/10.1097/BRS.0000000000000222 [doi].
13. Hassanzadeh H, Jain A, El Dafrawy MH, Mesfin A, Neubauer PR, Skolasky RL, Clinical KKM. Results and functional outcomes of primary and revision spinal deformity surgery in adults. J Bone Joint Surg Am. 2013; https://doi.org/10.2106/JBJS.L.00358 [doi].
14. Kim HJ, Bridwell KH, Lenke LG, Park MS, Song KS, Piyaskulkaew C, Patients CT. With proximal junctional kyphosis requiring revision surgery have higher postoperative lumbar lordosis and larger sagittal balance corrections. Spine (Phila Pa 1976). 2014; https://doi.org/10.1097/BRS.0000000000000246 [doi].
15. Lange T, Schmoelz W, Gosheger G, Eichinger M, Heinrichs CH, Boevingloh AS, Schulte TL. Is a gradual reduction of stiffness on top of posterior instrumentation possible with a suitable proximal implant? A biomechanical study. Spine J. 2017; doi:S1529-9430(17)30129-8 [pii]
16. Sun Z, Qiu G, Zhao Y, Guo S, Wang Y, Zhang J, Risk SJ. Factors of proximal junctional angle increase after selective posterior thoracolumbar/lumbar fusion in patients with adolescent idiopathic scoliosis. Eur. Spine J. 2015; https://doi.org/10.1007/s00586-014-3639-6 [doi].
17. Kebaish KM, Martin CT, O'Brien JR, LaMotta IE, Voros GD, Use BSM. Of vertebroplasty to prevent proximal junctional fractures in adult deformity surgery: a biomechanical cadaveric study. Spine J. 2013; https://doi.org/10.1016/j.spinee.2013.06.039 [doi].
18. Denis F, Sun EC, Incidence WRB. Risk factors for proximal and distal junctional kyphosis following surgical treatment for Scheuermann kyphosis: minimum five-year follow-up. Spine (Phila Pa 1976). 2009; https://doi.org/10.1097/BRS.0b013e3181ae2ab2 [doi].
19. Diebo BG, Henry J, Lafage V, Sagittal BP. Deformities of the spine: factors influencing the outcomes and complications. Eur. Spine J. 2015; https://doi.org/10.1007/s00586-014-3653-8 [doi].
20. Wilke HJ, Krischak S, Biomechanical CL. Comparison of calf and human spines. J Orthop Res. 1996; https://doi.org/10.1002/jor.1100140321 [doi].
21. Wilke HJ, Wenger K, Claes L. Testing criteria for spinal implants: recommendations for the standardization of in vitro stability testing of spinal implants. Eur Spine J. 1998;
22. Schmoelz W, Erhart S, Unger S, Biomechanical DAC. Evaluation of a posterior non-fusion instrumentation of the lumbar spine. Eur. Spine J. 2012; https://doi.org/10.1007/s00586-011-2121-y [doi].
23. Schmoelz W, Onder U, Martin A, Non-fusion v SA. Instrumentation of the lumbar spine with a hinged pedicle screw rod system: an in vitro experiment. Eur. Spine J. 2009; https://doi.org/10.1007/s00586-009-1052-3 [doi].
24. Greenhouse S, Geisser S. On methods in the analysis of profile data. Psychometrika. 1959;24:95–112.
25. Yagi M, King AB, Boachie-Adjei O. Incidence, risk factors, and natural course of proximal junctional kyphosis: surgical outcomes review of adult idiopathic scoliosis. Minimum 5 years of follow-up. Spine (Phila Pa 1976). 2012; https://doi.org/10.1097/BRS.0b013e31824e4888 [doi].
26. Metzger MF, Robinson ST, Svet MT, Liu JC, Biomechanical Analysis AFL. Of the proximal adjacent segment after multilevel instrumentation of the thoracic spine: do hooks ease the transition? Global. Spine J. 2016; https://doi.org/10.1055/s-0035-1563611 [doi].
27. Senteler M, Weisse B, Rothenfluh DA, Farshad MT, Fusion SJG. Angle affects intervertebral adjacent spinal segment joint forces-model-based analysis of patient specific alignment. J Orthop Res. 2017; https://doi.org/10.1002/jor.23357 [doi].
28. Liu H. Wu W, li Y, Liu J, Yang K, Chen Y. Protective effects of preserving the posterior complex on the development of adjacent-segment degeneration after lumbar fusion: clinical article. J Neurosurg Spine. 2013; https://doi.org/10.3171/2013.5.SPINE12650 [doi].
29. Behrsin JF, Briggs CA. Ligaments of the lumbar spine: a review. Surg Radiol Anat. 1988;
30. Pham MH, Tuchman A, Smith L, Jakoi AM, Patel NN, Mehta VA, Semitendinosus Graft AFL. For Interspinous ligament reinforcement in adult spinal deformity. Orthopedics. 2017; https://doi.org/10.3928/01477447-20161006-05 [doi].
31. Wilke HJ, Krischak ST, Wenger KH, Claes LE. Load-displacement properties of the thoracolumbar calf spine: experimental results and comparison to known human data. Eur Spine J. 1997;
32. Liu FY, Wang T, Yang SD, Wang H, Yang DL, Incidence DWY. Risk factors for proximal junctional kyphosis: a meta-analysis. Eur. Spine J. 2016; https://doi.org/10.1007/s00586-016-4534-0 [doi].

Towards defining muscular regions of interest from axial magnetic resonance imaging with anatomical cross-reference: cervical spine musculature

James M. Elliott[1,2,3*], Jon Cornwall[4], Ewan Kennedy[5], Rebecca Abbott[2] and Rebecca J. Crawford[6]

Abstract

Background: It has been suggested that the quantification of paravertebral muscle composition and morphology (e.g. size/shape/structure) with magnetic resonance imaging (MRI) has diagnostic, prognostic, and therapeutic potential in contributing to overall musculoskeletal health. If this is to be realised, then consensus towards standardised MRI methods for measuring muscular size/shape/structure are crucial to allow the translation of such measurements towards management of, and hopefully improved health for, those with some musculoskeletal conditions. Following on from an original paper detailing methods for measuring muscles traversing the lumbar spine, we propose new methods based on anatomical cross-reference that strive towards standardising MRI-based quantification of anterior and posterior cervical spine muscle composition.

Methods: In this descriptive technical advance paper we expand our methods from the lumbar spine by providing a detailed examination of regional cervical spine muscle morphology, followed by a comprehensive description of the proposed technique defining muscle ROI from axial MRI. Cross-referencing cervical musculature and vertebral anatomy includes an innovative comparison between axial E12 sheet-plastinates derived from cadaveric material to a series of axial MRIs detailing commonly used sequences. These images are shown at different cervical levels to illustrate differences in regional morphology. The method for defining ROI for both anterior (scalenes group, sternocleidomastoid, longus colli, longus capitis) and posterior (multifidus, semispinalis cervicis, semispinalis capitis, splenius capitis) cervical muscles is then described and discussed in relation to existing literature.

Results: A series of steps towards standardising the quantification of cervical spine muscle quality are described, with concentration on the measurement of muscle volume and fatty infiltration (MFI). We offer recommendations for imaging parameters that should additionally inform a priori decisions when planning investigations of cervical muscle tissues with MRI.

Conclusions: The proposed method provides an option rather than a final position for quantifying cervical spine muscle composition and morphology using MRI. We intend to stimulate discussion towards establishing measurement consensus whereby data-pooling and meaningful comparisons between imaging studies (primarily MRI) investigating cervical muscle quality becomes available and the norm.

Keywords: Cervical spine, Paravertebral muscles, Muscle fat infiltration, Magnetic resonance imaging, Region of interest, Manual segmentation

* Correspondence: jim.elliott@sydney.edu.au
[1]Faculty of Health Sciences, The University of Sydney, Northern Sydney Local Health District, St Leonards, Australia 75 East Street Lidcombe NSW, Sydney 2141, Australia
[2]Department of Physical Therapy and Human Movement Sciences, Feinberg School of Medicine, Northwestern University, Chicago, USA
Full list of author information is available at the end of the article

Background

Magnetic resonance imaging (MRI) has been widely and variably utilised to qualify and quantify musculoskeletal pathology involving a number of soft-tissues in both traumatic [1–6] and non-traumatic [7, 8] neck disorders. Such methods have provided convergent [9, 10] and divergent [11–15] evidence around insight into tissue composition, disease characterisation, response to injury, and changes in somatic and nervous structures potentially due to biological, psychological, and socioenvironmental stresses. Advances in MRI technology have raised the number of investigations quantifying skeletal muscle composition (MFI) and structure (volume, cross-sectional area (CSA)), but not without equivocal results [9]. This variability in findings is likely the result of methodological differences across research groups, including variables such as study design, participant demographics (trauma vs. non-trauma; sex, sociocultural, age range), measurement techniques, and MR parameters used by investigators.

In order to better understand the influence of muscle composition and structure on cervical spine health, it is imperative that clinical research communities explore and establish common methodologies in order to facilitate standardisation and accurate comparison of data between studies. Doing so should ultimately result in an improved understanding of the aetiological features of muscle composition and facilitate an improved prognostic, diagnostic, and theranostic landscape.

While data for age-related, degenerative changes of tissues (e.g. vertebrae, joints, discs, muscles) of the lumbar and cervical spine have been published [16–27], studies assessing age-related alterations in paravertebral muscle morphology [19, 28, 29] remain unique to the healthy lumbar spine. Such normative data, to our knowledge, does not exist for the cervical spine. While cross-sectional and longitudinal studies indicate a positive relationship between MFI and traumatic neck pain (e.g. whiplash associated disorders) [1–3, 5, 6, 30], inconsistent associations are also reported [11–14]. Such inconsistencies have not improved our mechanistic understanding of changes in muscle composition in both traumatic and non-traumatic neck pain. Future works must collectively control for what might be considered normative age-related changes [19, 29, 31], degenerative features of the vertebrae or discs [13, 26, 31–34], and spinal curvature [35–37].

A way forward through standardisation of methodology

In order to facilitate widespread adoption of agreed and time-efficient techniques for measuring cervical spine muscle quality, a standardised, reliable, and replicable method is urgently required. While there is a general trend toward optimising automated methodologies that quantify muscle composition based on differential tissue signal intensities of paravertebral muscle, even the latest, time-efficient tools require a degree of manual input for defining regions of interest (ROI) [3, 5, 6, 38–41]. A standardised ROI method is arguably most important for these studies where it has been speculated that difficulties identifying morphology of both the cervical and lumbar musculature results in poorer repeatability [6, 38]. With continued improvements in both the uptake of, and imaging quality from, MRI technology, an agreed analysis plan utilising a common research measurement method for the identification of ROIs could result in meaningful comparisons with a target towards knowledge transfer and clinical translation of muscle imaging. Following on from the recent manuscript detailing a method for determining ROI in the lumbar spine [42], the purpose of this proposed method is to provide a standardised MRI procedure for measuring cervical spine muscle composition. The method also serves to initiate and continue discussion on the analysis of skeletal muscle composition amongst and between the global clinical and scientific communities.

Method

Challenges for producing a region of interest of cervical muscles using MRI

A number of conventional MRI applications (T1, T2, proton-density, Gradient Echo) are available and have been used to qualitatively and quantitatively measure the water and fat species of healthy and diseased soft-aqueous skeletal muscle tissue [1, 3, 41, 43–49]. Technological advancements have also produced alternatives that can be used to image muscle, such as dual acquisition methods, where frequency is selectively excited to produce a water image [50] and a standard image of fat and water. This, however, produces a challenge when measuring a redundant and anatomically complex set of multi-layered (and small) muscles in the cervical spine. The challenge is further compounded by the advent of higher field scanners (e.g. 3–7 Tesla), where a uniform frequency difference between fat and water content may be difficult, but certainly not impossible, to achieve.

Despite recent technological advances that have permitted further insight into muscle composition, the mechanisms underlying muscle degeneration and their influence on outcomes in neck disorders remain elusive. In addition, the vast majority of symptomatic and asymptomatic population-based studies examining pathoanatomical features (e.g. the intervertebral disc, ligaments, and the skeletal vertebral column) of the cervical spine have used a variety of conventional MRI sequences [1, 2, 12, 13, 26, 30, 34, 51–55]. Despite the large repository of available works, the data derived from these imaging investigations have not revealed a consistent structural lesion(s), or response to said lesion(s), that have clarified the clinical presentation of traumatic or non-traumatic neck disorders. This has, in our opinion, created a clinical (and research) impasse that we believe is due partly to the heterogeneous methods across a number of high quality studies investigating the usefulness of imaging for understanding spinal pathology. Ultimately, the clinical value of imaging findings of spinal pathology and/or muscle degeneration will be realised if such findings predict important outcomes or help to identify patients likely to respond to specific interventions (e.g. spinal phenotypes).

Research efforts that focus on the consistent assessment of spinal muscle quality with MRI may improve our collective biological understanding of traumatic and non-traumatic neck disorders and why some, but not others, recover spontaneously. Accordingly, a robust and easily-replicated platform for acquiring, assessing, measuring, analysing, and interpreting imaging data on muscle composition and morphology is needed. Currently a wide variety of methods are used to describe the composition and morphology of cervical spine muscles (see Table 1 for a non-exhaustive summary). This represents a key challenge for both producing consistent regions of interest of cervical spine muscles and allowing comparison between research studies.

Anatomically defining the muscles of interest

The muscles spanning the mid-to-lower cervical spine that are typically examined include: multifidus, semispinalis cervicis, semispinalis capitis, splenius capitis, scalenes, levator scapulae, sternocleidomastoid, and longus capitis and longus colli. We do not describe muscles of the suboccipital region (rectus capitis posterior major and minor, and the superior and inferior obliquus muscles [56]) as it is not possible to accurately measure a clinically useful ROI of the suboccipital muscles from the typically employed transverse images used for assessing cervical musculature. This is because no suboccipital muscle has a long axis close to perpendicular to the transverse plane, thus making measurement of useful cross-sectional ROI impractical. Further, fan shaped muscles such as both rectus capitii muscles require special consideration in order to validate useful measures, given a single cross-sectional measurement along the length of either muscle would pose difficulty for determining whole muscle volume. Future work should include developing imaging protocols for the suboccipital muscles as they require more nuanced imaging methods and measures with careful consideration around the highest resolution possible within a reasonable scan time.

The anatomical study we use and recommend for reference are those detailed in Au et al. [57]. They have provided a comprehensive series of labelled axial MR images from one individual to serve as a reference atlas of the cervical spine musculature to guide clinicians and researchers in the accurate identification of these muscles on MR imaging. We have further reinforced by cross-referencing with the E-12 plastinates that have previously been used to assist morphological studies [42, 58].

Anterior muscles

Sternocleidomastoid (SCM)

The SCM arises from the manubrium and medial clavicle inferiorly, and angles laterally and posteriorly towards its superior attachments at the mastoid process and superior nuchal line. This superficial muscle is readily identifiable in cross-section. While the SCM has four portions, [59] as they cross and blend, they are not separable in cross-section along their length on MRI. The muscle has an oval appearance inferiorly, and superiorly forms a distinctive 'comma' shape (Fig. 1).

Scalenus muscles

Scalenus anterior arises from the scalene tubercle on the first rib as a thin tendon antero-lateral to the lung and pleural cavities, and extends superiorly to attach to the anterior tubercles of the C4–6 (and frequently C3) transverse processes. At the level of the first rib the subclavian vein passes anterior to scalenus anterior, while the subclavian artery passes between scalenus anterior and medius, visibly separating these two muscles. At this level scalenus anterior appears rounded in cross-section. Scalenus medius arises from the first rib posterior to the groove for the subclavian artery and extends superiorly to attach to the transverse processes of C1–7.

Longus capitis

This muscle is largest at C1, and has a flattened appearance immediately anterior to the lateral masses on each side of the midline. Inferiorly, it remains anterior to the anterior tubercles of the transverse processes, which allows it to be differentiated from longus colli and the scalenus muscles, particularly scalenus anterior (Fig. 2) [60].

Longus colli

Longus colli is recognised by its location in the groove formed between the vertebral bodies and transverse processes of the vertebrae, extending between C1 and T2/3. While longus colli is described as having superior, vertical, and inferior oblique portions, these are based on attachment sites and are not discernible in cross-section [61]. The muscle first becomes visible at C2, emerging

Table 1 A non-systematic summary of methods across investigations describing cervical spine muscle analysis using magnetic resonance imaging (MRI)

Citation	Reliability	MRI Sequence	Slice Selection	Muscles of Interest	ROI Selection	Fat Detection	Measure
Elliott et al., 2006 [1] Elliott et al., 2008 [7] Elliott et al., 2009 [78] Elliott et al., 2011 [2]	Inter-rater (0.94) Intra-rater (0.94)	T1	Axial images aligned parallel to C2–3 disc; Measured at single slice per level C3-C7; most cephalad slice of each vertebral body selected	MF SSCerv SSCap SpCap UT	Manual	Quantitative Pixel Intensity	Fat Infiltration %MFI = (muscle signal)/(fat signal)*100
Fernandez De Las Penas et al., 2007 [79]	Inter-rater (0.80–0.98)	T1	Axial images aligned parallel to C2–3 disc; measured at single slice per level; most cephalad slice of each vertebral body selected	SSCap SpCap	Manual	N/A	CSA
Elliott et al., 2007 [47]	Intra-rater (0.84–0.99) Inter-rater (0.89–0.96)	T1	Axial images aligned parallel to C2–3 disc; measured at single slice per level C3-C7; most cephalad slice of each vertebral body selected	MF SSCerv SSCap SpCap UT	Manual	N/A	CSA
Okada et al., 2011 [80] Matsumoto et al., 2012 [12]	Intra- rater (0.90) Inter-rater (0.844)	T2	Measurements from a single axial slice aligned parallel to each IVD C3–4, C4–5, and C5–6	MF SSCerv SSCap SpCap	Manual	N/A	CSA
Ulbrich et al., 2012 [14]	Inter-rater (0.79–0.98)	STIR	Axial images aligned perpendicular to the vertebral body in the middle of a 20-slice slab. 2 or 3 overlapping slabs used; measurements from single slice per vertebral level C2, C4, and C5	Deep Extensors All Extensors SCM	Manual	N/A	CSA
Elliott et al., 2013 [41]	Inter-rater for fat-water sequence (0.83–0.99)	T1 vs. Dixon	Axial images aligned perpendicular to the spinal cord at the C2-C3 IVD; measurement from single slice per vertebral level C3-C7	MF	Manual	Quantitative Pixel Intensity vs. Fat (F)-Water (W)	Fat Infiltration % MFI = (fat signal)/(fat signal + water signal) *100
Elliott et al., 2014 [8]	From Elliott et al., 2007 [47] for CSA Intra- rater (0.84–0.99) Inter-rater (0.89–0.96)	T1	Axial images aligned parallel to C2–3 IVD; measurements from single slice crossing IVDs C2-C3 and C5-C6	MF SSCerv SSCap SpCap LCap/LCol SCM	Manual	Quantitative Pixel Intensity	Fat Infiltration %MFI = (fat signal)/(fat signal + water signal)*100 CSA
Elliott et al., 2015 [3]	Not reported	Dixon	Measurements from single slice per vertebral level C3-C7; alignment and slice selection not reported	MF	Manual	Fat-Water	Fat Infiltration %MFI = (fat signal)/(fat signal + water signal)*100
Abbott et al., 2015 [6]	Intra-rater (0.98) Inter-rater (0.93)	Dixon	Measurements averaged over 5 slices for each vertebral level C3-C7; Slab alignment not reported.	MF + SSCerv (combined)	Manual with automatic quartile measure	Fat-Water	Fat Infiltration %MFI = (fat signal)/(fat signal + water signal)*100

Table 1 A non-systematic summary of methods across investigations describing cervical spine muscle analysis using magnetic resonance imaging (MRI) (*Continued*)

Citation	Reliability	MRI Sequence	Slice Selection	Muscles of Interest	ROI Selection	Fat Detection	Measure
Karlsson et al., 2016 [5]	For muscle fat Intra-rater (0.81–0.93) Inter-rater (0.82–0.97)	Dixon	Axial images aligned parallel to vertebral segments; measurements averaged over 5 slices for each vertebral level C4-C7	MF	Manual	Fat-Water	Fat Infiltration %MFI = (fat signal)/(fat signal + water signal)*100 CSA
Au et al., 2016 [57]	Not reported	T1	Axial images aligned parallel to C2–3 intervertebral disc; 3D reconstruction	IC, IS, LS, LoCap, LoC, LCap, LCol, MF, LoCap, LoCerv, SSCap, SSCerv, SCM, UT	Manual	N/A	N/A
Fortin et al., 2017 [27] Fortin et al., 2018 [81]	From [81]: Intra-rater (0.83–0.99) Inter-rater (0.38–0.98)	T2	3D multiplanar reconstruction to align images perpendicular to muscle mass; measurements from a single slice per IVD C2–3 through C6–7	MF SSCerv SSCap SpCap	Manual ROI with semi-automatic muscle/fat thresholding technique	Gray-scale threshold technique to calculate CSA of fat within total muscle CSA; gray-scale range determined for each slice individually	Total CSA Functional CSA (FCSA) (= fat free area) Fatty Infiltration = FCSA/ Total CSA
Inoue et al., 2012 [82]	Intra-rater (0.85)	T1 T2-fat suppression	Measured from single slice per level; most caudal slice of C3 and most cephalad slice of each vertebral body C4-C7 selected; slab alignment not reported	MF	Manual	Lean muscle CSA: ROI drawn on T1-W images not including fat Total muscle CSA: ROI drawn on fat suppression T2-W image including fat Fat CSA = Total CSA – Lean Muscle CSA	Fatty Infiltration = (Fat CSA)/(Total muscle CSA)
Mitsutake et al., 2016 [83]	Intra-rater 0.85–0.94 Inter-rater (0.84–0.89)	T1	Measured from single, most cephalad slice at level of injury (C4, C5, or C6)	MF	Manual	Quantitative Pixel Intensity	MFI index = Muscle signal/Fat signal
Abbott et al., 2017 [67]	Intra-rater (0.77–0.88) Inter-rater (0.67–0.82)	Dixon	Axial images aligned parallel to each IVD; measured from 5 slices across each vertebral level C4-C7	MF	Manual	Qualitative grading (0, 1, 2) for each 8 regions within visualized ROI on fat image	Fat Infiltration MFI Score: 0 = no or marginal fat 1 = light fat 2 = distinct fat Sum of scores Total # of 2's
Choi et al., 2016 [84]	Inter-rater (0.82)	T1	Axial images aligned parallel to the inferior end plate of each vertebral body from C4–5 to C7-T1; measured from single slice per vertebral level	Flexor Group: LCap + LCol Extensor Group: MF + SSCerv	Manual	N/A	CSA Normalized Extensor CSA = (Extensor Muscle CSA)/(Vertebral body CSA) *100

Table 1 A non-systematic summary of methods across investigations describing cervical spine muscle analysis using magnetic resonance imaging (MRI) *(Continued)*

Citation	Reliability	MRI Sequence	Slice Selection	Muscles of Interest	ROI Selection	Fat Detection	Measure
Cagnie et al., 2009 [85]	Inter-rater (0.91)	T1	Measured from a single slice aligned parallel IVD at C4-C5	LCap LCol UT LS SpCap SSCerv MF	Manual	Quantitative Pixel Intensity	Muscle/Fat Index = Muscle signal/Fat signal
Uthaikup et al., 2017 [86]	Intra-rater (0.75–0.96) Inter-rater (0.84–0.99)	T1	Axial images aligned parallel to the C2–3 IVD; measured from a single slice at each vertebral level C2-C3	MF SSCap SpCap LCap LCol SCM	Manual	Quantitative Pixel Intensity	Fat Infiltration MFI = Muscle signal/ Fat signal

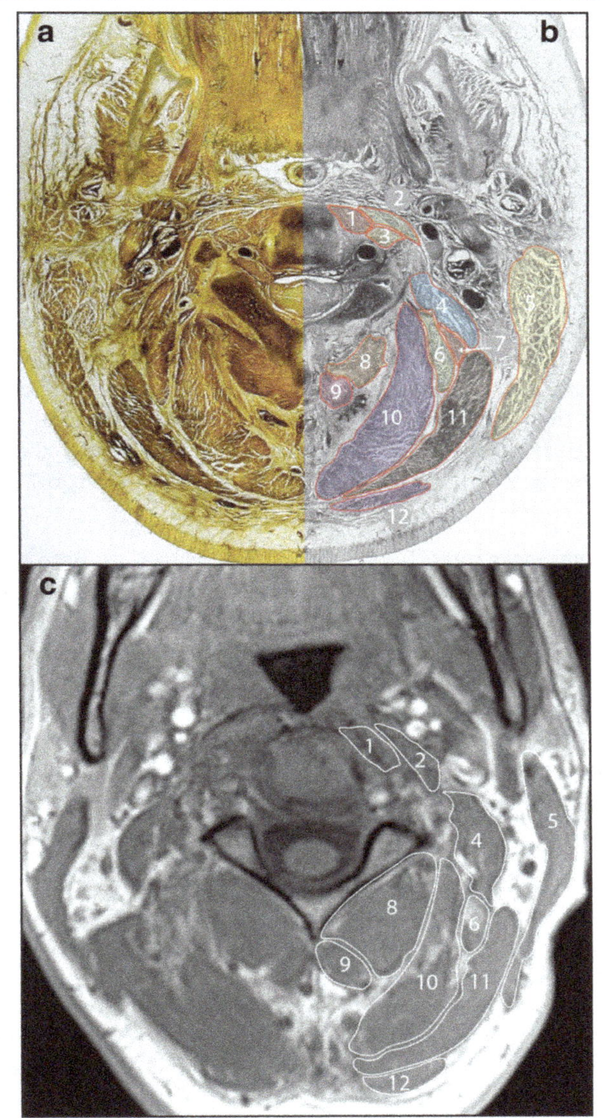

Fig. 1 Axial E12 plastinated section (**a**) with schematic illustration (**b**) and in-phase magnetic resonance image (**c**) at approximately C2/3 identifying musculature at this vertebral level. 1. Longus colli; 2. Longus capitis; 3. Intertransversarii; 4. Levator scapulae; 5. Sternocleidomastoid; 6. Longissimus capitis; 7. Splenius cervicis; 8. Inferior obliquus; 9. Rectus capitis posterior major; 10. Semispinalis capitis; 11. Splenius capitis; 12. Trapezius

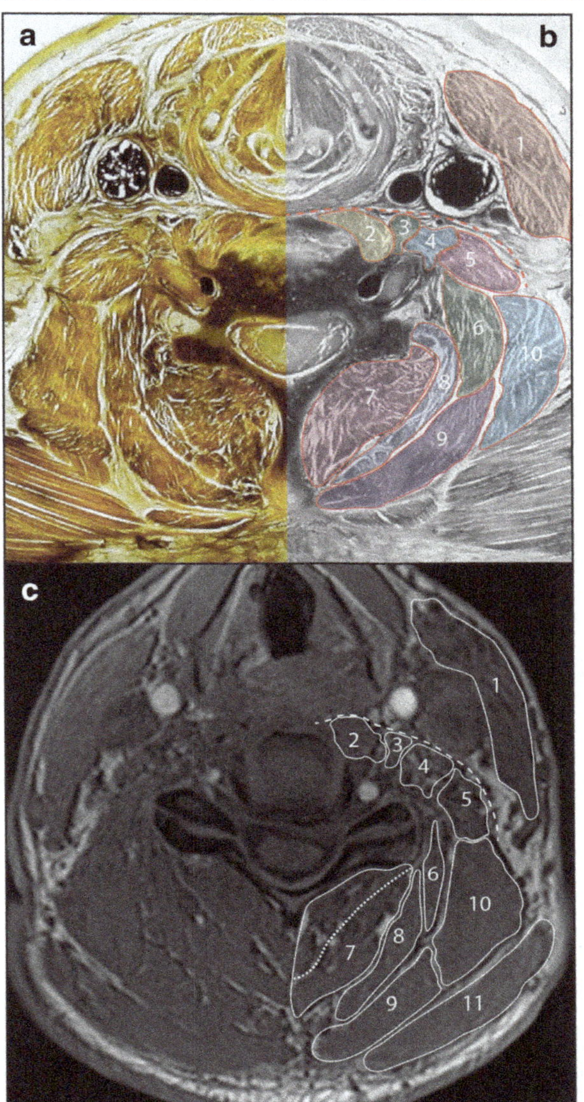

Fig. 2 Axial E12 plastinated section (**a**) with schematic illustration (**b**) and in-phase magnetic resonance image (c) at approximately C5/6 identifying musculature at this vertebral level. Dashed red (**b**) and white (**c**) line indicates an anatomical plane which can be used as a reference point for identifying some anterior muscles. Dashed white line in (**c**) indicates likely border between multifidus and semispinalis cervicis. 1. Sternocleidomastoid; 2. Longus colli; 3. Longus capitis; 4. Scalenus anterior; 5. Scalenus medius; 6. Splenius cervicis; 7. Multifidus / semispinalis cervicis; 8. Semispinalis capitis; 9. Splenius capitis; 10. Levator scapulae; 11. Trapezius

medial to longus capitis and initially with a more rounded appearance. Inferior to C7 the muscle thins and moves towards the midline, before attaching to the anterolateral vertebral bodies. Fascial borders between longus colli and the intertransversarii muscles may not be readily apparent between any of the cervical levels on MRI. This should not, however, present difficulties as long as the bony transverse processes are well visualised. Longus colli remains immediately anterior and medial to the bony transverse processes. The intertransversarii muscles are only seen in slices between transverse processes (Fig. 1).

Posterior muscles

Multifidus and rotatores

Deep against the vertebra, these architecturally complex muscles fill the space between the spinous and transverse processes. Multifidus is present along the length of the spine below C2, forming the deepest layer (Figs. 2, 3). Rotatores can be considered together with multifidus in this deep muscle layer, as these muscles are small and do not form a distinct layer able to be identified in cross-section. Together with semispinalis cervicis, multifidus sits in the paravertebral gutter between the spinous and transverse processes. Because of the intimate relationship between these two muscles [62], it can be difficult to identify them as separate entities on both E12s and MRI.

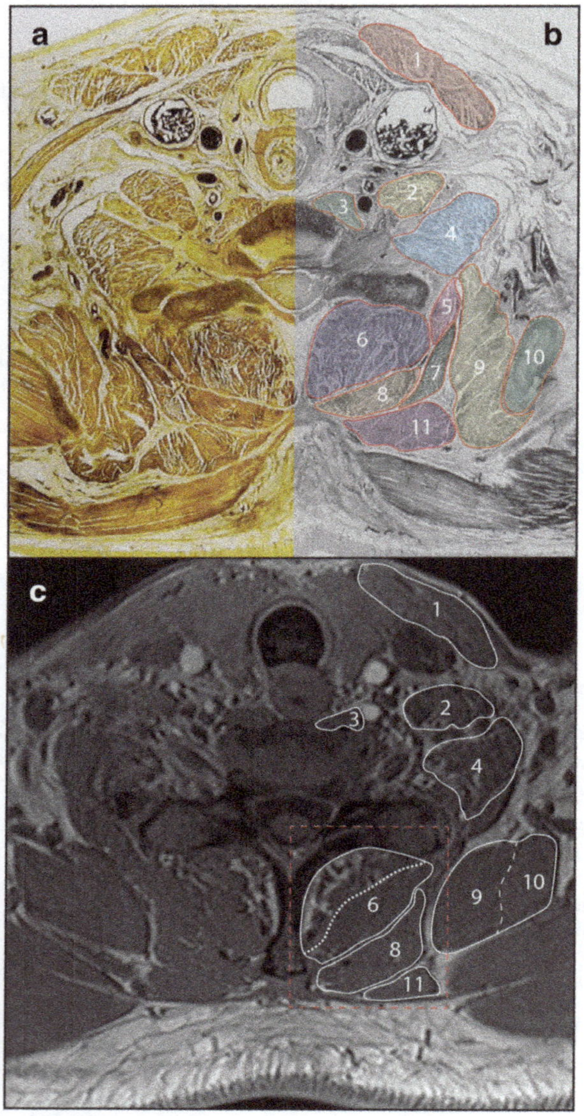

Fig. 3 Axial E12 plastinated section (**a**) with schematic illustration (**b**) and in-phase magnetic resonance image (**c**) at approximately C7/T1 identifying musculature at this vertebral level. Red box indicates boundary for Fig. 4. 1. Sternocleidomastoid; 2. Scalenus anterior; 3. Longus colli; 4. Scalenus medius; 5. Iliocostalis cervicis; 6. Multifidus / semispinalis cervicis; 7. Serratus posterior superior; 8. Splenius capitis / cervicis; 9. Levator scapulae; 10. Serratus anterior; 11. Rhomboid minor

Semispinalis cervicis

Semispinalis cervicis extends between the spinous processes of C2–5 and the transverse processes of T1-T5 [63] (Figs. 1, 2, 3). It overlies multifidus along with other cervical-attaching erector spinae (longissimus cervicis, iliocostalis cervicis). The semispinalis cervicis and erector spinae muscles are difficult, if not impossible, to adequately distinguish in cross-section. The close approximation, similar alignment and attachments of multifidus, semispinalis and erector spinae fascicles are such that a distinct layer will not always be clear on MRI. In this situation it is reasonable to consider these muscles together as a single group (seen [64] and [6]).

Semispinalis capitis

Semispinalis capitis is a major muscle of the cervical spine, overlying semispinalis cervicis and forming a large and distinct muscle layer. While semispinalis capitis spans between the occiput and T6–7 [63], in cross-section this layer is most apparent between the occiput and C6/7. Below this level this muscle layer becomes less distinct as semispinalis thins and becomes tendinous towards the thoracic transverse processes (Figs. 1, 2).

Erector spinae

Longissimus cervicis extends between the thoracic transverse processes of T1–4 and the C2–6 transverse processes, while iliocostalis cervicis passes between the angles of ribs 3–4 and the transverse processes of C4–6 [63]. As noted, erector spinae muscles attaching to the cervical spine are unlikely to be differentiated from semispinalis cervicis. Longissimus capitis is more distinct, extending between the mastoid process and the transverse processes of approximately C4-T4 (Fig. 1) [63].

Splenius capitis and cervicis

Splenius capitis and cervicis form a single layer and overlie semispinalis capitis. Splenius capitis spans between the C7-T4 spinous processes and the mastoid process / occiput, while splenius cervicis spans between the T3–6 spinous processes and the transverse processes of C1–3 [63]. In cross-section, splenius capitis forms a distinct layer between trapezius and semispinalis capitis. Splenius cervicis can be identified between C2–6 on the antero-lateral edge of this layer (Figs. 1, 2, 3), as it diverges from splenius capitis towards its cervical attachments. Below the level of approximately C5 splenius cervicis is unlikely to be visibly separate from splenius capitis in cross-section.

Levator scapulae

Levator scapulae have a presence throughout the cervical spine, and its presence is worth noting as one of the larger and more distinctive muscles in the region. It passes from the upper aspect of the medial scapula to the transverse processes of C1–4 [63]. In cross-section levator scapulae is well-defined at lower levels, sitting anterior to trapezius and lateral to splenius (Figs. 2, 3). Superiorly, levator scapulae extends towards the transverse processes of C1–4 in close relation to the scalenus and longus capitis muscles (Fig. 1).

Results

Our method provides anatomical reference between MRI imaging and E12 plastinates (derived from cadavers) to advance ROI identification and definition to improve standardised measurement of musculature traversing the cervical spine. The E12 plastinates provide a unique opportunity to detail specific tissues that may be MR invisible, [65] leading to natural disagreement across studies where fat-water separation is a target. To follow, we also include suggestions on operational characteristics for acquiring MR images.

Defining the regions of interest from MRI

Similar to that reported for the lumbar spine, [42] a standard scout image from the sagittal localiser or conventional T2-weighted scan can be used to cross-reference and discern cervical level from axial MR. Users will also find it useful to scroll between the adjacent axial slices to accurately landmark anatomical structures when producing ROIs. The method is applicable to studies examining paravertebral ROIs for single (cross-sectional) or multiple (volumetric) slices. Previous work from the lumbar spine suggests a randomised approach for starting with either the left or right side, and/or separate muscles can influence repeatability when creating ROIs [38, 66]. The same randomised approach is suggested for the cervical spine.

Definitions for ROI measures from MRI for the multifidus, semispinalis cervicis, semispinalis capitis, longissimus capitis, splenius capitis and cervicis, levator scapulae, longus colli, longus capitis, scalenus and sternocleidomastoid are included, describing the anatomical borders (cross referenced to Figs. 1, 2, 3). ROI definitions are detailed with particular reference to cervical levels C2/3, C5/6, and C7/T1. Technical notes are also provided where identifying the guided ROI on MRI may be difficult.

Anterior muscles

It is worth noting that an anatomical plane that passes laterally and posteriorly in an arc from the anterior aspect of the vertebral body presents a reliable reference point for identifying the anterior aspect of all anterior muscles apart from the sternocleidomastoid (Fig. 2).

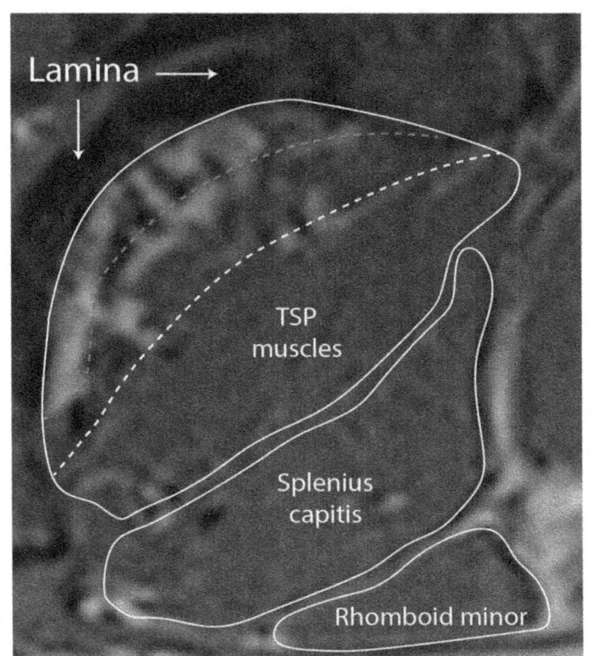

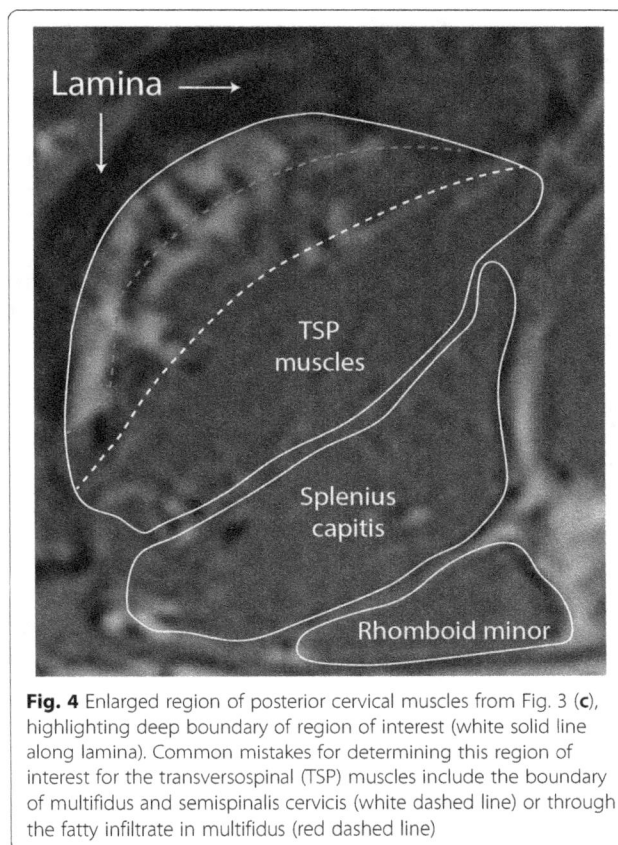

Fig. 4 Enlarged region of posterior cervical muscles from Fig. 3 (**c**), highlighting deep boundary of region of interest (white solid line along lamina). Common mistakes for determining this region of interest for the transversospinal (TSP) muscles include the boundary of multifidus and semispinalis cervicis (white dashed line) or through the fatty infiltrate in multifidus (red dashed line)

Sternocleidomastoid

This definition can be applied along the full extent of sternocleidomastoid, from the occiput to approximately T2/3. The anatomical boundaries of sternocleidomastoid are straight forward, and tracing should present few challenges. Some care is needed to trace along the full occipital extent at higher levels (Fig. 1).

Scalenus muscles

This definition is best applied at the C6-T2 levels. The scalenus muscles are best identified at their inferior extent arising from the first rib. Superiorly scalenus anterior and scalenus medius converge, and may be difficult to differentiate above the level of C6 on MRI. Differentiation is aided by the angle each muscle approaches the cervical transverse processes, as each muscle follows a straight course. Sequentially from anterior to posterior: longus capitis is seen anterior to the anterior tubercles, scalenus anterior angles to attach to the anterior tubercles slightly more laterally, scalenus medius angles between the anterior and posterior tubercles, scalenus posterior (if present) angles towards the posterior tubercles, and (above C4) levator scapulae also angles to attach to the posterior tubercles (Fig. 2).

Longus capitis

This definition is best applied at the C1–5 levels. Longus capitis is largest and most distinct superiorly, just below where it attaches to the basi-occiput. As such, the muscle is best tracked inferiorly from this point. At its superior extent longus capitis has a rounded appearance, which flattens and thins out over the lateral masses of C1. By the level of C2/3 longus capitis is a relatively thin slip immediately anterior to the anterior tubercles of transverse processes C3–6. As for the scalenus muscles, identification is aided by identifying the transverse processes (in particular the anterior tubercles) and remaining posterior to the prevertebral fascia (Fig. 2).

Longus colli

This definition is best applied at C2-T1 levels. As noted anatomically, longus colli sits in the groove between the vertebral bodies and transverse processes of the vertebrae. Thus, these bony landmarks must be well visualised to accurately identify the muscle. As described for multifidus, the ROI should closely follow the bony vertebrae to include fat adjacent to the bone. If the anterior aspect of the transverse processes are not visible, or slices above and below are not reviewed to clarify the position of bony landmarks, a ROI for longus colli may be inaccurate.

Posterior muscles

Multifidus and semispinalis Cervicis

This definition is best applied at the caudal portion of the C4 vertebral body through the entire T1 vertebral body. With current technology it is generally not possible to consistently delineate between the cervical portions of the semispinalis cervicis and multifidus on the axial slices. While measuring the two muscles independently is recommended, they can be combined to form one measure (Figs. 2, 3). As evidenced from the lumbar spine [42], the same approach of approximating the spinous process or lamina is recommended and should be included within the ROI defining cervical multifidus (Fig. 4). A challenge for both novice and expert clinicians remains what to do when creating ROIs between the spinous processes. Whether referencing the lumbar [42] or cervical spine, fat commonly overlies the interspinous space, remains defined, and should be included when generating ROIs on these slices. Finally, when the interspinous ligaments are clearly distinct with a slightly irregular and darkened edge, their lateral contour can be followed rather than the spinous process in defining the medial border [42].

Semispinalis capitis

This definition is best applied at the occiput-C6 levels. The muscle forms a distinct anatomical layer and can be traced consistent with the anatomy described. As semispinalis capitis is clearest at higher levels, difficulties identifying this muscle at lower cervical levels would benefit from reviewing and toggling between multiple slices from superior to inferior. As the E12 slices highlight, it may not be realistic to identify this muscle below approximately C7.

Longissimus capitis

This definition is best applied at the C1–4 levels. Longissimus capitis is most easily identified as a rounded muscle at its superior extent, just below the mastoid process. Towards C4 the muscle flattens, and below approximately C4 it becomes difficult to distinguish from other muscles.

Splenius capitis and cervicis

This definition is best applied at the C1-T3 levels. Splenius capitis is identifiable as a distinct layer located between trapezius / sternocleidomastoid and the semispinalis capitis. Care is needed around the level of the mastoid process not to confuse the superior extent of splenius capitis with sternocleidomastoid or longissimus capitis, which share attachment to the mastoid process. Just below the mastoid process at the level of C1/2 the muscles appear closely layered from superficial to deep: sternocleidomastoid, splenius capitis (both an elongated comma shape), and longissimus capitis (rounded in appearance). Below this level the muscles diverge. Ideally, splenius cervicis will be able to be distinguished from splenius capitis at the levels of C2–6 (Figs. 1, 2). However, this may not be realistic with current MRI technology. In this situation, it is reasonable to include splenius capitis and cervicis together as a single ROI.

Levator scapulae

This definition is best applied at the C2- T1 levels. While not part of the intrinsic cervical spine musculature, cross-sectional views highlight the presence and size of levator scapulae throughout the cervical spine. This muscle is largest inferiorly above where it arises from the upper part of the medial scapula border, and as such is best tracked superiorly from this point. Care is needed to distinguish levator scapulae from serratus anterior as they converge on the scapula (Fig. 3). Attention to slices above and below the level of interest will help resolve their borders.

MR imaging - operational parameters

The type, quality, and output of images acquired from MR scans are highly influenced by many factors including, but not limited to, user-prescribed parameters. Similar to our previous paper covering the lumbar spine, [42] we endorse consistency in the adoption of MR imaging parameters to facilitate standardised operational procedures that allow intra-study/–institutional comparison and future pooling of results for meta-analyses.

The parameters listed here are based on those widely utilised in literature (refer to Table 1), and are adapted from those published in a previous paper on ROI for lumbar spine muscles [42]. The parenthetical values given with each parameter are not definitive or unique to a cervical spine study; rather they are displayed as an example of the consistent reporting style we propose. At a minimum, we believe the following information should be reported in all submitted manuscripts: Field strength (e.g. 3 Tesla); sequence type (e.g. 2-point DIXON (3D fast-field echo T1) whole body); repetition time (e.g. TR 4.2 ms); echo time (e.g. TE 1.2 and 3.1 ms); flip angle (e. g. 5°); field of view (e.g. FOV 560 × 352 mm); acquired voxel dimensions (e.g. 2.0 × 2.0 × 4.0 mm); reconstructed voxel dimensions (e.g. 1.0 × 1.0 × 2.0 mm); bandwidth (e.g. 240 Hz/Px), acquisition time (e.g. TA 5 min 22 s) and slice thickness (e.g. 4.0 mm). Additionally, the description should include axial slice alignment (e.g. *aligned parallel to C2–3 intervertebral disc*), slice selection (e.g. *measurements taken at most cephalad slice per vertebral level*), and subject body position including any support materials that may influence cervical spine posture/curvature (e.g. *subjects positioned supine with arms at sides and 2 in. foam cushion under head*).

Discussion

A foundational edict for defining lumbar paravertebral ROI's from MRI studies has previously been published [42]. Here, we expand the previous methods [57] for the cervical pre- and para-vertebral muscles using a number of MRI and E12 sheet plastinate illustrations of vertebral morphology with the aim of standardising muscle ROI definitions. The E12 plastinates provide a unique opportunity to detail specific tissues that may be MR invisible, [65] leading to natural disagreement across studies where fat-water separation is a target. Also unique to this work is the included suggestions on operational characteristics for acquiring MR images.

Similar to the proposed approach in the lumbar spine, [42] we consider that if fat is occupying space deep to the epimysial sheath and close to the spinous processes, laminae, zygapophyseal joints, it has a potential biomechanical consequence on muscle function, [6, 67] and should be included in the ROI (Fig. 4). We base this decision in part on previous work in the cervical spine [3, 5, 6, 27, 41]. Such an approach has revealed not only improved inter- and intra-rater reliability when following the spinous process and/or lamina in the cervical spine, but also the ability to discriminate between clinical groups [6]. This improved repeatability for defining MF over ES in the lumbar spine has also been demonstrated [38].

Measures of muscle size and fat

Measures of muscle size are frequently reported in MRI and other imaging-based studies (e.g. ultrasound). In both the lumbar and cervical regions, methods employing a single cross-sectional MR slice are time efficient for determining muscle size and fat proportion within an ROI. However, a CSA measure from a single-slice should not be taken to constitute a whole muscle size or fat measure [15, 68]. Accordingly, volumetric measures, may be more appropriate [15, 69, 70]. We therefore recommend a multi-slice approach that derives muscle size and fat content based on a three-dimensional volume across the levels of interest. In going forward, such measures should be accurately categorised as a 3-dimensional volume of the entire muscle as 3D acquisition methods with MRI have evolved and are not as sensitive to the radio frequency slice profile as is 2D imaging [15].

It is of course acknowledged that acquiring such data with both semi-automated or automated programmes for both the lumbar [42] and cervical spines is time-consuming. However, with the evolution of higher-resolution imaging techniques a more time-efficient capture of cervical muscle volumes from a single vertebral level may correspond to a representative marker of MFI across the entire cervical column. While this has been demonstrated in the healthy lumbar spine [29] where the fat content at L4 best represents that of the entire lumbar region, future research should continue to systematically include the entire cervical spine in healthy and symptomatic cohorts to build a stronger body of evidence regarding age-aggregated cervical paravertebral muscle composition.

Another issue with longitudinal designs, where muscle measures are produced over time, remains a general lack of reporting on how the MRI slices are aligned in plane. A failure to do so could potentially result in registration discrepancies depending how the angle through each muscle was performed. Using some standard anatomical reference (e.g. vertebral bone) that is not expected to appreciably change over time could control for this. Errors of this type can be further minimised by reporting muscle volume over the full length of the muscle (from origin to insertion), as suggested above, rather than a single-slice CSA.

Measures of muscle fat with MRI

The demonstration of neck muscle fatty infiltrates on T1- weighted imaging in acute [2, 3] and chronic traumatic neck pain [1, 5, 8, 30] has been reported in cross-sectional and longitudinal fashion and across three countries (Australia, [2] Sweden, [5] and the United States [3, 6]). Such findings are not present to the same magnitude for those with chronic idiopathic neck pain [7] and it has been postulated that these muscle changes represent one neurophysiologic basis for the transition to chronic pain in this population [71]. A variety of newer and more rapid high resolution MRI techniques (3D Fat/Water Separation and Proton-Density Fat Fraction, Fat suppression) [65, 72–77] and analyses (FCSA/CSA, Fat Signal Fraction, MFI %) could help better visualise and quantify physiologic changes at the level of the muscle cell or other disease processes when compared to other conventional clinical imaging sequences (e.g. T1- and T2-weighted). However, such variety across methods and techniques also complicates comparison among studies. Accordingly, we call for all authors to clearly detail their fat infiltration measurements to ensure that future pooling of data efforts is possible. Further, with the number of proprietary semi-automated or automated methods appearing in the literature, and of which descriptions are limited due to commercial sensitivity, we contend it will be helpful for authors to include enough technical detail for comparisons to the fundamental literature to be made.

Participant positioning

It is our recommendation that participants should lie supine inside the magnet with a foam pad under their knees and foam padding placed on the right and left of the head to minimise head movement. A neutral position, visually determined by ensuring that a horizontal position of the forehead to the chin is parallel to the MRI table, is also recommended.

Conclusion

We follow on from, and have expanded, an original paper of manually defining ROIs of lumbar spine musculature [42] to now include the cervical muscles. While the method aims to permit accurate and reliable comparison of cervical muscle quality between studies in (and beyond) this field, we further suggest journals adopt a more robust reporting of imaging parameters used to assist consistency and allow accurate comparison between studies.

It is imperative to note that we are cognisant the application methods are not definitive end-points on 'how to' and that there is potential for much repetition across body regions. Rather, we hope that with time, and new research findings, these methods will be modified, expanded, and refined and ultimately result in an established common methodology towards facilitating consistent and accurate definitions of lumbar, cervical, and upper/lower limb muscle ROIs on axial imaging, particularly MRI.

Abbreviations

CSA: Cross-sectional area; FCSA: Functional cross-sectional area; FSPGR: Fast-spoiled gradient echo; IC: Iliocostalis cervicis; IP: In-phase (water); IS: Interspinalis cervicis; IVD: Intervertebral disc; LCap: Longus capitis; LCol: Longus colli; LoCap: Longissimus capitis; LoCerv: Longissimus cervicis; LS: Levator scapulae; MF: Multifidus; MFI: Muscle fat infiltration; OP: Opposed-phase (Fat); SCap: Spinalis capitis; SCerv: Spinalis cervicis; SCM: Sternocleidomastoid; SI: Signal intensity; SpCap: Splenius capitis; SSCap: Semispinalis capitis; SSCerv: Semispinalis cervicis; UT: Upper trapezius

Authors' contributions

JME and RJC conceived the study, while RJC, JC, EK, RA, and JME each made substantial contributions to its design. RJC, JC, EK, RA, and JME have been involved in drafting the manuscript or revising it critically for important intellectual content and each given final approval of the version to be published. RJC, JC, EK, RA, and JME agree to be accountable for all aspects of the work in ensuring that questions related to the accuracy or integrity of any part of the work are appropriately investigated and resolved.All authors read and approved the final manuscript.

Consent for publication

Approval to use images of the E-plastinated sections was granted by Department of Anatomy, University of Otago. All MRIs were derived from the same informed and consenting adult subject.

Competing interests

Authors RJC, JC, EK, and RA have no disclosures to declare. In unrelated activities, JME is principal investigator on NIH grant [HD079076-01A1; 09/2014–05/2019].

Author details

[1]Faculty of Health Sciences, The University of Sydney, Northern Sydney Local Health District, St Leonards, Australia 75 East Street Lidcombe NSW, Sydney 2141, Australia. [2]Department of Physical Therapy and Human Movement Sciences, Feinberg School of Medicine, Northwestern University, Chicago, USA. [3]Honorary Fellow School of Health and Rehabilitation Sciences, The University of Queensland, St. Lucia, Australia. [4]Centre for Early Learning in Medicine, Otago Medical School, University of Otago, Dunedin, New Zealand. [5]School of Physiotherapy, University of Otago, Dunedin, New Zealand. [6]Faculty of Health Sciences, Curtin University, Perth, Australia.

References

1. Elliott J, Jull G, Noteboom JT, Darnell R, Galloway G, Gibbon WW. Fatty infiltration in the cervical extensor muscles in persistent whiplash-associated disorders: a magnetic resonance imaging analysis. Spine (Phila Pa 1976). 2006;31(22):E847–55.
2. Elliott J, Pedler A, Kenardy J, Galloway G, Jull G, Sterling M. The temporal development of fatty infiltrates in the neck muscles following whiplash injury: an association with pain and posttraumatic stress. PLoS One. 2011; 6(6):e21194.
3. Elliott JM, Courtney DM, Rademaker A, Pinto D, Sterling MM, Parrish T. The rapid and progressive degeneration of the cervical multifidus in whiplash: a MRI study of fatty infiltration. Spine (Phila Pa 1976). 2015;40(12):E694–700.
4. Elliott JM, Pedler AR, Theodoros D, Jull GA. Magnetic resonance imaging changes in the size and shape of the oropharynx following acute whiplash injury. J Orthop Sports Phys Ther. 2012;42(11):912–8.
5. Karlsson A, Dahlqvist Leinhard O, West J, Romu T, Aslund U, Smedby O,

Zsigmond P, Peolsson A. An investigation of fat infiltration of the multifidus muscle in patients with severe neck symptoms associated with chronic whiplash associated disorder. J Orthop Sports Phys Ther. 2016;46(10):886–93.

6. Abbott R, Pedler A, Sterling M, Hides J, Murphey T, Hoggarth M, Elliott J. The geography of fatty infiltrates within the cervical multifidus and semispinalis Cervicis in individuals with chronic whiplash-associated disorders. J Orthop Sports Phys Ther. 2015;45(4):281–8.
7. Elliott J, Sterling M, Noteboom JT, Darnell R, Galloway G, Jull G. Fatty infiltrate in the cervical extensor muscles is not a feature of chronic, insidious-onset neck pain. Clin Radiol. 2008;63(6):681–7.
8. Elliott JM, Pedler AR, Jull GA, Van Wyk L, Galloway GG, O'Leary S. Differential changes in muscle composition exist in traumatic and non-traumatic neck pain. Spine (Phila Pa 1976). 2014;39(1):39–47.
9. De Pauw R, Coppieters I, Kregel J, De Meulemeester K, Danneels L, Cagnie B. Does muscle morphology change in chronic neck pain patients? - a systematic review. Man Ther. 2016;22:42–9.
10. Thakar S, Mohan D, Furtado SV, Sai Kiran NA, Dadlani R, Aryan S, Rao AS, Hegde AS. Paraspinal muscle morphometry in cervical spondylotic myelopathy and its implications in clinicoradiological outcomes following central corpectomy: clinical article. J Neurosurg Spine. 2014;21(2):223–30.
11. Anderson SE, Boesch C, Zimmermann H, Busato A, Hodler J, Bingisser R, Ulbrich EJ, Nidecker A, Buitrago-Tellez CH, Bonel HM, et al. Are there cervical spine findings at MR imaging that are specific to acute symptomatic whiplash injury? A prospective controlled study with four experienced blinded readers. Radiology. 2012;262(2):567–75.
12. Matsumoto M, Ichihara D, Okada E, Chiba K, Toyama Y, Fujiwara H, Momoshima S, Nishiwaki Y, Takahata T. Cross-sectional area of the posterior extensor muscles of the cervical spine in whiplash injury patients versus healthy volunteers - 10year follow-up MR study. Injury. 2012;43(6):912–6.
13. Matsumoto M, Okada E, Ichihara D, Chiba K, Toyama Y, Fujiwara H, Momoshima S, Nishiwaki Y, Hashimoto T, Inoue T, et al. Prospective ten-year follow-up study comparing patients with whiplash-associated disorders and asymptomatic subjects using magnetic resonance imaging. Spine (Phila Pa 1976). 2010;35(18):1684–90.
14. Ulbrich EJ, Aeberhard R, Wetli S, Busato A, Boesch C, Zimmermann H, Hodler J, Anderson SE, Sturzenegger M. Cervical muscle area measurements in whiplash patients: acute, 3, and 6 months of follow-up. J Magn Reson Imaging. 2012;36(6):1413–20.
15. Elliott JM, Kerry R, Flynn T, Parrish T. Content not quantity is a better measure of muscle degeneration in whiplash. Man Ther. 2013;18(6):578–82.
16. Brinjikji W, Luetmer PH, Comstock B, Bresnahan BW, Chen LE, Deyo RA, Halabi S, Turner JA, Avins AL, James K, et al. Systematic literature review of imaging features of spinal degeneration in asymptomatic populations. Am J Neuroradiol. 2015;36(4):811–6.
17. Crawford RJ, Volken T, Valentin S, Melloh M, Elliott J. Rate of lumbar paravertebral muscle fat infiltration versus spinal degeneration in asymptomatic populations: an age- aggregated cross-sectional simulation study. BMC Scoliosis Spinal Disord. 2016;11(1):21.
18. Fortin M, Yuan Y, Battie MC. Factors associated with paraspinal muscle asymmetry in size and composition in a general population sample of men. Phys Ther. 2013;93(11):1540–50.
19. Valentin S, Licka T, Elliott J. Age and side-related morphometric MRI evaluation of trunk muscles in people without back pain. Man Ther. 2015; 20(1):90–5.
20. Valentin S, Licka TF, Elliott J. MRI-determined lumbar muscle morphometry in man and sheep: potential biomechanical implications for ovine model to human spine translation. J Anat. 2015;227(4):506–13.
21. Hancock M, Maher C, Macaskill P, Latimer J, Kos W, Pik J. MRI findings are more common in selected patients with acute low back pain than controls? Eur Spine J. 2012;21(2):240–6.
22. Hancock MJ, Kjaer P, Kent P, Jensen RK, Jensen T. Is the number of different MRI findings more strongly associated with low back painthan single MRI findings? Spine. 2017;42(17):1283–8.
23. Panagopoulos J, Hush J, Steffens D, Hancock M. Do MRI findings change over a period of up to one year in patients with low back pain and/or sciatica? A Systematic Review. *Spine*. 2017;42(7):504–12.
24. Steffens D, Hancock MJ, Maher CG, Williams C, Jensen TS, Latimer J. Does magnetic resonance imaging predict future low back pain? A systematic review. Eur J Pain. 2014;18(6):755–65.
25. Wan Q, Lin C, Li X, Zeng W, Ma C. MRI assessment of paraspinal muscles in patients with acute and chronic unilateral low back pain. Br J Radiol. 2015; 88(1053):20140546.
26. Nakashima H, Yukawa Y, Suda K, Yamagata M, Ueta T, Kato F. Abnormal findings on magnetic resonance images of the cervical spines in 1211 asymptomatic subjects. Spine (Phila Pa 1976). 2015;40(6):392–8.
27. Fortin M, Dobrescu O, Courtemanche M, Sparrey CJ, Santaguida C, Fehlings MG, Weber M. Association between paraspinal muscle morphology, clinical symptoms and functional status in patients with degenerative cervical myelopathy. Spine. 2017;42(4):232–9.
28. Amabile C, Moal B, Chtara OA, Pillet H, Raya JG, Iannessi A, Skalli W, Lafage V, Bronsard N: Estimation of spinopelvic muscles' volumes in young asymptomatic subjects: a quantitative analysis. Surgical and radiologic anatomy: SRA. 2016;39(4): 393–403.
29. Crawford R, Filli L, Elliott J, Nanz D, Fischer M, Marcon M, Ulbrich E. Age- and level-dependence of fatty infiltration in lumbar paravertebral muscles of healthy volunteers. Am J Neuroradiol. 2016;37(4):742–8.
30. Elliott JM, O'Leary S, Sterling M, Hendrikz J, Pedler A, Jull G. Magnetic resonance imaging findings of fatty infiltrate in the cervical flexors in chronic whiplash. Spine (Phila Pa 1976). 2010;35(9):948–54.
31. Bhadresha A, Lawrence OJ, McCarthy MJ. A comparison of magnetic resonance imaging muscle fat content in the lumbar Paraspinal muscles with patient-reported outcome measures in patients with lumbar degenerative disk disease and focal disk prolapse. Glob Spine J. 2016;6(4):401–10.
32. Teichtahl AJ, Urquhart DM, Wang Y, Wluka AE, Wijethilake P, O'Sullivan R, Cicuttini FM. Fat infiltration of paraspinal muscles is associated with low back pain, disability, and structural abnormalities in community-based adults. Spine J. 2015;15(7):1593–601.
33. Kalichman L, Hodges P, Li L, Guermazi A, Hunter DJ. Changes in paraspinal muscles and their association with low back pain and spinal degeneration: CT study. Eur Spine J. 2010;19(7):1136–44.
34. Matsumoto M, Ichihara D, Okada E, Toyama Y, Fujiwara H, Momoshima S, Nishiwaki Y, Takahata T. Modic changes of the cervical spine in patients with whiplash injury: a prospective 11-year follow-up study. Injury. 2013;44(6):819–24.
35. Meakin JR, Fulford J, Seymour R, Welsman JR, Knapp KM. The relationship between sagittal curvature and extensor muscle volume in the lumbar spine. J Anat. 2013;222(6):608–14.
36. Pezolato A, de Vasconcelos EE, Defino HL, Nogueira-Barbosa MH. Fat infiltration in the lumbar multifidus and erector spinae muscles in subjects with sway-back posture. Eur Spine J. 2012;21(11):2158–64.
37. Johansson MP, Baann Liane MS, Bendix T, Kasch H, Kongsted A. Does cervical kyphosis relate to symptoms following whiplash injury. Man Ther. 2011;16(4):378–83.
38. Mhuiris AN, Volken T, Elliott JM, Hoggarth M, Samartzis D, Crawford RJ. Reliability of quantifying the spatial distribution of fatty infiltration in lumbar paravertebral muscles using a new segmentation method for T1-weighted MRI. BMC Musculoskelet Disord. 2016;17(1):234.
39. Putzier M, Hartwig T, Hoff EK, Streitparth F, Strube P. Minimally invasive TLIF leads to increased muscle sparing of the multifidus muscle but not the longissimus muscle compared with conventional PLIF-a prospective randomized clinical trial. Spine Journal. 2016;16(7):811–9.
40. Valenzuela W, Ferguson SJ, Ignasiak D, Diserens G, Vermathen P, Boesch C, Reyes M. Correction tool for active shape model based lumbar muscle segmentation. PLoS One. 2015;2015:3033–6.
41. Elliott JM, Walton DM, Rademaker A, Parrish T. Quantification of cervical spine muscle fat: a comparison between T1-weighted and multi-echo gradient echo imaging using a variable projection algorithm (VARPRO). BMC Med Imaging. 2013;11:13–30. https://doi.org/10.1186/1471-2342-13-30.
42. Crawford RJ, Cornwall J, Abbott R, Elliott J. Manually defining regions of interest when quantifying paravertebral muscles fatty infiltration from axial magnetic resonance imaging: a proposed method for the lumbar spine with anatomical cross-reference. BMC Musculoskelet Disord. 2017:18(25).
43. Fleckenstein JL, Watamull D, Conner KE, Ezaki M, Greenlee RG Jr, Bryan WW, Chason DP, Parkey RW, Peshock RM, Purdy PD. Denervated human skeletal muscle: MR imaging evaluation. Radiology. 1993;187(1):213–8.
44. Fritz RC, Domroese ME, Carter GT. Physiological and anatomical basis of muscle magnetic resonance imaging. Phys Med Rehabil Clin N Am. 2005; 16(4):1033–51. x

45. Wokke BH, Bos C, Reijnierse M, van Rijswijk CS, Eggers H, Webb A, Verschuuren JJ, Kan HE. Comparison of Dixon and T1-weighted MR methods to assess the degree of fat infiltration in duchenne muscular dystrophy patients. J Magn Reson Imaging. 2013;38(3):619–24.
46. Elliott JM, Galloway GJ, Jull GA, Noteboom JT, Centeno CJ, Gibbon WW. Magnetic resonance imaging analysis of the upper cervical spine extensor musculature in an asymptomatic cohort: an index of fat within muscle. Clin Radiol. 2005;60(3):355–63.
47. Elliott JM, Jull GA, Noteboom JT, Durbridge GL, Gibbon WW. Magnetic resonance imaging study of cross-sectional area of the cervical extensor musculature in an asymptomatic cohort. Clin Anat. 2007;20(1):35–40.
48. Sinclair CD, Morrow JM, Miranda MA, Davagnanam I, Cowley PC, Mehta H, Hanna MG, Koltzenburg M, Yousry TA, Reilly MM, et al. Skeletal muscle MRI magnetisation transfer ratio reflects clinical severity in peripheral neuropathies. J Neurol Neurosurg Psychiatry. 2012;83(1):29–32.
49. Sinclair CD, Morrow JM, Janiczek RL, Evans MR, Rawah E, Shah S, Hanna MG, Reilly MM, Yousry TA, Thornton J. Stability and sensitivity of water T2 obtained with IDEAL-CPMG in healthy and fat-infiltrated skeletal muscle. NMR Biomed. 2016;29(12):1800–12.
50. Haase A, Frahm J, Hänicke W, Matthaei D. 1H NMR chemical shift selective (CHESS) imaging. Phys Med Biol. 1985;30:341–4.
51. Kaale BR, Krakenes J, Albrektsen G, Wester K. Whiplash-associated disorders impairment rating: neck disability index score according to severity of MRI findings of ligaments and membranes in the upper cervical spine. J Neurotrauma. 2005;22(4):466–75.
52. Krakenes J, Kaale BR. Magnetic resonance imaging assessment of craniovertebral ligaments and membranes after whiplash trauma. Spine. 2006;31(24):2820–6.
53. Krakenes J, Kaale BR, Moen G, Nordli H, Gilhus NE, Rorvik J. MRI assessment of the alar ligaments in the late stage of whiplash injury–a study of structural abnormalities and observer agreement. Neuroradiology. 2002; 44(7):617–24.
54. Myran R, Kvistad KA, Nygaard OP, Andresen H, Folvik M, Zwart JA. Magnetic resonance imaging assessment of the alar ligaments in whiplash injuries: a case-control study. Spine. 2008;33(18):2012–6.
55. Ronnen HR, de Korte PJ, Brink PR, van der Bijl HJ, Tonino AJ, Franke C. Acute whiplash injury: is there a role for MR imaging?–a prospective study of 100 patients. Radiology. 1996;201(1):93–6.
56. Cornwall J, Farrell SF, Sheard P. Fibre types of human suboccipital muscles. Eur J Anat. 2016;20(1):31–6.
57. Au J, Perriman DM, Pickering MR, Buirski G, Smith PN, Webb AL. Magnetic resonance imaging atlas of the cervical spine musculature. Clin Anat. 2016; 29(5):643–59.
58. Farrell SF, Osmotherly PG, Cornwall J, Sterling M, Rivett D. Cervical spine meniscoids: an update on their morphological characteristics and potential clinical significance. Eur Spine J. 2017;26(4):939–47.
59. Kennedy E, Albert M, Nicholson H. The fascicular anatomy and peak force capabilities of the sternocleidomastoid muscle. Surg Radiol Anat. 2017;39(6): 629–45.
60. Cornwall J, Kennedy E. Fiber types of the anterior and lateral cervical muscles in elderly males. Eur Spine J. 2015;24(9):1986–91.
61. Miller A, Woodley SJ, Cornwall J. Fibre type composition of female longus capitis and longus colli muscles. Anat Sci Int. 2016;91(2):163–8.
62. Cornwall J, Stringer MD, Duxson M. Functional morphology of the thoracolumbar transversospinal muscles. Spine (Phila Pa 1976). 2011;36(16):E1053–61.
63. Standring S, Anand N, Birch R, Collins P, Crossman AR, Gleeson M, et al: Gray's anatomy : the anatomical basis of clinical practice., 41st edn. New York: Elsevier; 2016.
64. Smith AC, Parrish TB, Hoggarth MA, McPherson JG, Tysseling VM, Wasielewski M, Kim H, Hornby TG, Elliott J. Potential associations between chronic whiplash and incomplete spinal cord injury. Spinal Cord Ser Cases. 2015;2015:15024. https://doi.org/10.1038/scsandc.2015.24.
65. Reeder SB, Hu HH, Sirlin CB. Proton density fat-fraction: a standardized mr-based biomarker of tissue fat concentration. J Magn Reson Imaging. 2012;36(5):1011–4.
66. Valentin S, Yeates TD, Licka T, Elliott J. Inter-rater reliability of trunk muscle morphometric analysis. J Back Musculoskeletal Rehabil. 2015;28(1):181–90.
67. Abbott R, Peolsson A, West J, Elliott JM, Aslund U, Karlsson A, Dahlqvist Leinhard O: The qualitative grading of muscle fat infiltration in whiplash using fat/water magnetic resonance imaging. Spine J 2017, Sep 5. pii: S1529–9430(17)30907–5. https://doi.org/10.1016/j.spinee.2017.08.233. [Epub ahead of print].
68. Elliott JM, Pedler AR, Jull GA, Van Wyk L, Galloway GG, O'Leary SP. Differential changes in muscle composition exist in traumatic and nontraumatic neck pain. Spine. 2014;39(1):39–47.
69. Boom HP, van Spronsen PH, van Ginkel FC, van Schijndel RA, Castelijns JA, Tuinzing DB. A comparison of human jaw muscle cross-sectional area and volume in long- and short-face subjects, using MRI. Arch Oral Biol. 2008;53(3):273–81.
70. Abbott R, Pedler A, Sterling M, Hides J, Murphey T, Hoggarth M, Elliott J. The geography of fatty infiltrates within the cervical multifidus and semispinalis cervicis in individuals with chronic whiplash-associated disorders. J Orthop Sports Phys Ther. 2015;45(4):8.
71. Elliott J. Are there implications for morphological changes in neck muscles after whiplash injury? Spine (Phila Pa 1976). 2011;1(36(25 Suppl)):S205–10. Review
72. Bley TA, Wieben O, Francois CJ, Brittain JH, Reeder SB. Fat and water magnetic resonance imaging. J Magn Reson Imaging. 2010;31(1):4–18.
73. Reeder SB, McKenzie CA, Pineda AR, Yu H, Shimakawa A, Brau AC, Hargreaves BA, Gold GE, Brittain JH. Water-fat separation with IDEAL gradient-echo imaging. J Magn Reson Imaging. 2007;25(3):644–52.
74. Costa DN, Pedrosa I, McKenzie C, Reeder SB, Rofsky NM. Body MRI using IDEAL. Am J Roentgenol. 2008;190(4):1076–84.
75. Gerdes CM, Kijowski R, Reeder SB. IDEAL imaging of the musculoskeletal system: robust water fat separation for uniform fat suppression, marrow evaluation, and cartilage imaging. AJR Am J Roentgenol. 2007;189(5):W284–91.
76. Romu T, Dahlqvist Leinhard O, Dahlström N, Borga M. Robust water fat separated dual-Echo MRI by phase-sensitive reconstruction. Magn Reson Med. 2017;78(3):1208–16.
77. Gerdle B, Forsgren MF, Bengtsson A, Leinhard OD, Soren B, Karlsson A, Brandejsky V, Lund E, Lundberg P. Decreased muscle concentrations of ATP and PCR in the quadriceps muscle of fibromyalgia patients - a (31) P-MRS study. Eur J Pain. 2013;17(8):1205–15.
78. Elliott J, Sterling M, Noteboom JT, Treleaven J, Galloway G, Jull G. The clinical presentation of chronic whiplash and the relationship to findings of MRI fatty infiltrates in the cervical extensor musculature: a preliminary investigation. Eur Spine J. 2009;18(9):1371–8.
79. Fernandez-de-Las-Penas C, Bueno A, Ferrando J, Elliott JM, Cuadrado ML, Pareja JA. Magnetic resonance imaging study of the morphometry of cervical extensor muscles in chronic tension-type headache. Cephalalgia. 2007;27(4):355–62.
80. Okada E, Matsumoto M, Ichihara D, Chiba K, Toyama Y, Fujiwara H, Momoshima S, Nishiwaki Y, Takahata T. Cross-sectional area of posterior extensor muscles of the cervical spine in asymptomatic subjects: a 10-year longitudinal magnetic resonance imaging study. Eur Spine J. 2011;20(9):1567–73.
81. Fortin M, Dobrescu O, Jarzem P, Ouellet J, Weber MH. Quantitative magnetic resonance imaging analysis of the cervical spine extensor muscles: Intrarater and interrater reliability of a novice and an experienced rater. Asian Spine J. 2018;12(1):94–102.
82. Inoue H, Montgomery S, Aghdasi B, Tan Y, Tian H, Jian X, Terrell R, Singh V, Wang J. Analysis of relationship between Paraspinal muscle fatty degeneration and cervical spine motion using kinetic magnetic resonance imaging. Glob Spine J. 2012;2(1):33–8.
83. Mitsutake T, Sakamoto M, Chyuda Y, Oka S, Hirata H, Matsuo T, Oishi T, Horikawa E. Greater cervical muscle fat infiltration evaluated by magnetic resonance imaging is associated with poor postural stability in patients with cervical Spondylotic radiculopathy. Spine. 2016;41:1.
84. Choi MK, Kim SB, Park CK, Lee SH, Jo DJ. Relation of deep Paraspinal Muscles' cross-sectional area of the cervical spine and bone Union in Anterior Cervical Decompression and Fusion: a retrospective study. World Neurosurg. 2016;96:91–100.
85. Cagnie B, Barbe T, Vandemaele P, Achten E, Cambier D, Danneels L. MRI analysis of muscle/fat index of the superficial and deep neck muscles in an asymptomatic cohort. Eur Spine J. 2009;18(5):704–9.
86. Uthaikhup S, Assapun J, Kothan S, Watcharasaksilp K, Elliott JM. Structural changes of the cervical muscles in elder women with cervicogenic headache. Musculoskelet Sci Pract. 2017;29:1–6.

22

Epidemiology of arthritis, chronic back pain, gout, osteoporosis, spondyloarthropathies and rheumatoid arthritis among 1.5 million patients in Australian general practice: NPS MedicineWise MedicineInsight dataset

David Alejandro González-Chica[1*], Simon Vanlint[1], Elizabeth Hoon[2] and Nigel Stocks[1]

Abstract

Background: Previous estimates for the prevalence of musculoskeletal conditions (MSK) and chronic pain in Australia have been based on self-report. We aimed to determine the prevalence and distribution of arthritis, chronic back pain, gout, osteoporosis, spondyloarthropathies and rheumatoid arthritis and current consultations for chronic pain among adults attending Australian general practice, and describe their distribution according to sociodemographic characteristics and presence of co-morbidities.

Methods: We investigated 1,501,267 active adult patients (57.6% females; 22.5% ≥65y) evaluated between 2013 and 2016 and included in the MedicineInsight database (a National Prescribing Service MedicineWise program), a large general practice data program that extracts longitudinal de-identified electronic medical record data from 'active' patients in over 550 practices. Three main groups of outcomes were investigated: 1) "prevalence" of arthritis, chronic back pain, gout, osteoporosis, spondyloarthropathies, and/or rheumatoid arthritis between 2000 and 2016; 2) "current" diagnosis/encounter for the same conditions occurring between 2013 and 2016, and; 3) "current" consultations for chronic pain of any type occurring between 2013 and 2016.

Results: The combined "prevalence" of the investigated MSK (diagnosis between 2000 and 2016) among adults attending Australian general practice was 16.8% (95%CI 15.9;17.7) with 21.3% (95%CI 20.2;22.4) of the sample consulting for chronic pain between 2013 and 2016. The investigated MSK with the highest "prevalence" were arthritis (9.5%) and chronic back pain (6.7%). Patients with some of these MSK attended general practices more frequently than those without these conditions (median 2.0 and 1.0 contacts/year, respectively). The "prevalence" of the investigated MSK and "current" consultations for chronic pain increased with age, especially in women, but chronic pain remained stable at 22% for males aged > 40 years. The investigated MSK and chronic pain were more frequent among those in lower socioeconomic groups, veterans, Aboriginal and Torrent Strait Islanders, current and ex-smokers, and patients with chronic obstructive pulmonary disease or heart failure.
(Continued on next page)

* Correspondence: david.gonzalez@adelaide.edu.au
[1]Discipline of General Practice, Adelaide Medical School, NHMRC Centre of Research Excellence to Reduce Inequality in Heart Disease, The University of Adelaide, Adelaide, SA, Australia
Full list of author information is available at the end of the article

(Continued from previous page)

Conclusions: The investigated MSK are more frequent among lower socioeconomic groups and the elderly. Based on information collected from adults attending Australian general practices, MedicineInsight provided similar estimates to those obtained from population-based studies, with the advantage of being based on medical diagnosis and including a national sample.

Keywords: Pain, chronic, Back pain, Musculoskeletal, Arthritis, Epidemiology, Population health

Background

Musculoskeletal conditions (MSK) and chronic pain represent an increasing public health problem worldwide [1–5]. According to the Australian Institute of Health and Welfare (AIHW) and the National Health Survey (NHS), in 2011 they affected 28% of Australian adults (6.1 million) [6]. Due to their chronicity and impact on health status and quality of life, they represent the fourth most expensive group of diseases in Australia, accounting for 9% of total health-care expenditure related to hospitalisations, out-of-hospital health care, and prescribed medications (approximately AUD$5.7 billion of the AUD$65 billion spent for all diseases) [7]. In terms of health service use, in 2010 they were among the ten most frequent problems managed by general practitioners (GPs) (2.7 per 100 encounters for osteoarthritis and 2.6 for back pain), only after metabolic conditions and depression [8].

A few surveys have used self-reported data to investigate the prevalence of these conditions among Australian adults [6, 9, 10], while the Bettering the Evaluation and Care of Health (BEACH) program reported encounter rates and medication use for MSK and chronic pain in adults attending a random sample of Australian general practices [11, 12]. Estimates for MSK and chronic pain vary across studies and information bias has been highlighted as one of the reasons for these differences [13–15]. Self-report for chronic pain and some MSK is less accurate than for sociodemographic characteristics, lifestyle, or other chronic conditions, thus affecting the ability of population-based surveys to provide accurate estimates for the total burden of MSK [14, 15]. On the other hand, studies on this topic using nationally representative samples and based on medical diagnosis are scarce in the scientific literature [3–5, 13].

The Australian Government have recognised MSK and chronic pain as a major public health priority, and emphasised the importance of national real-time data for monitoring their prevalence, management, and adverse effects of medications [16]. More generally, increasing the scope and number of quality improvement activties has been recognised as being important for the Australian health care system and so the National Prescribing Service (NPS) MedicineWise was funded in 2011 to periodically collect longitudinal clinical and prescribing data from Australian general practices through MedicineInsight [17]. Utilising this large ongoing dataset, we aimed to investigate the prevalence of some MSK conditions (arthritis, chronic back pain, gout, osteoporosis, spondyloarthropathies, and rheumatoid arthritis) and consultations for chronic pain among adults attending Australian general practices, describe their distribution according to patients' sociodemographic characteristics and examine associations with other chronic non-communicable diseases (NCDs).

Methods

NPS MedicineWise was established in 1998 as an independent, evidence-based, not-for-profit organisation. It aims to promote the quality use of medicines. In 2011, NPS MedicineWise established MedicineInsight to drive quality improvement activities in general practice and improve primary health care and post marketing surveillance of medicine use in Australia [17]. MedicineInsight uses a data extraction tool (GRHANITE™) developed by the University of Melbourne and NPS MedicineWise, which weekly collects de-identified data from patients electronic medical records and securely transfers the information to NPS MedicineWise [17, 18]. Based on a unique identifying number attributed to everyone, patients within practices are tracked over time, allowing the development of an ongoing longitudinal database.

Patients' information collected by MedicineInsight include: demographics (gender, ethnicity, indigenous status, year of birth, postcode, suburb), diagnoses, reasons for consultations, medicines prescribed and reasons for prescription, known allergies or drug reactions, pathology test orders and results, imaging test orders, instances of referrals to other healthcare professionals (excluding referral documents), instances of patient assessment and management activities, clinical measurements (temperature, blood pressure, weight, height, waist circumference), and smoking status. For privacy reasons, a complete patient's listed past medical history (PMH considering the whole patient lifespan) is not collected by MedicineInsight [17]. However, by aggregating the information collected over several years at each general practice (46% of individuals with available electronic medical records prior to the launch of

MedicineInsight in 2011), the data extraction tool generates a "partial" clinical history for all active patients based on previous diagnoses, medications, laboratory results, and hospital admissions [17, 19–21].

Depending on the clinical information system available at each general practice, GPs used medical coding vocabularies (i.e. 'DOCLE', 'PYEFINCH' or 'ICPC') to register medical diagnosis, reasons for encounter, and reason for prescription into their systems. Although GPs are required to complete all these fields every time they see a patient, the use of the codes is not mandatory and clinicians can enter medical terms as free text [17].

By the end on 2016, MedicineInsight had recruited 557 Australian general practices. Although a non-random sampling process is used, the sample includes practices from all states/territories (New South Wales (NSW) = 29.5%; Victoria (VIC) = 22.7%; Queensland (QLD) = 20.1%; Western Australia (WA) = 12.2%; Tasmania (TAS) = 7.9%; South Australia (SA) = 3.6%; Australia Capital Territory (ACT) = 2.0%; North Territory (NT) = 2.0%), regions (major cities = 59.0%; inner regional = 24.5%; outer regional = 12.6%; remote/very remote =3.8%), and size (1 GP = 6.9%; 2 GPs = 11.6%; 3–5 GPs = 38.0%; 6–8 GPs = 24.0%; > 8 Gps = 19.5%) [17]. Following recommendations for improving data quality [20–23], only practices established for ≥2 years before the end of the analysis period (no interruptions > 2 months in practice), with recorded data (history item, reason for encounter, or reason for prescription) in ≥10% of encounters, and an average of ≥30 prescriptions/week were included in the analyses. Therefore, we used data collected by MedicineInsight from all active patients (three or more visits to the practice in the past 2 years) attending 4668 GPs (14.0% of the 33,275 GPs registered in Australia in 2014–15) in 329 general practices across Australia (4.7% of all 7035 practices in 2011) [24, 25]. All patients aged 18 and above, with information registered in a MedicineInsight practice between 10/2013 and 06/2016, and considered an active patient were eligible for inclusion [17]. The final dataset included a total of 1,544,303 individuals, who had encounters with general practice (including clinical and administrative face-to-face contacts and phone calls), and 7,411,945 different registered medical diagnoses during that period.

The available information from that three-year period was used to determine the percentage of individuals with (what we call) a "current" consultation for MSK, the percentage with a "current" consultation for chronic pain, and the average number of health contacts per year. However, to obtain more accurate data regarding (what we call) the "prevalence" of the investigated MSK (i.e. diagnosis of arthritis, chronic back pain, gout, osteoporosis, spondyloarthropathies, and/or rheumatoid arthritis) [20–23], all data available in MedicineInsight (including current data and past electronic health records going back to 2000 for most enrolled practices) was used to identify individuals with a history (i.e. "prevalence") of MSK.

Therefore, based in all available data, two different groups of binary variables were created for the investigated MSK: 1) general "prevalence", considering the diagnosis at any point since 2000 (i.e. past and current health records), and; 2) "current" diagnosis/encounter for the same disease occurring between 2013 and 2016 (i.e. current health records). Patients with some of the investigated MSK were identified from MedicineInsight databases (for both "prevalence" and "current" diagnosis/encounter) using an algorithm that included all diagnosis or reason for encounter (and their synonyms) related to arthritis ("osteoarthritis", "arthritis" "polyarthritis", "arthropathy", "polyarthralgia", "arthralgia", "osteoarthrosis", "arthrosis"), spondyloarthropathies ("spondyloarthritis", "spondyloarthropathy", "spondylolisthesis", "spondylolysis"), rheumatoid arthritis (including polymyalgia rheumatica), osteoporosis, gout, and/or "chronic back pain". Whenever a field specified the condition as unconfirmed (i.e. "suspected", "under investigation", "???"), acute (i.e. "suppurative", "bacterial", "infectious", etc.), or was just as a "family history" (or only a relative affected by these conditions), patients were considered as negative for that condition.

For "current" chronic pain consultations, only one binary variable (no/yes) was generated for data analysis, considering all consultations/diagnosis that occurred between 2013 and 2016. In that case, the terms used included "chronic pain", "pain treatment" and synonyms of these terms (e.g. "chronic -algia" and "chronic -ache"). Therefore, considering these terms, "chronic back pain" was included under "chronic pain", but also as a MSK, as this is consistent with clinical practice in Australia and with reports from the Australian Institute of Health and Welfare [6, 7, 26]. Patients were considered negatives for chronic pain whenever the condition was specified as recent/acute.

The total number of contacts with the general practice between 2013 and 2016 (independent of whether it was or not related to some of the investigated MSK or chronic pain) was also extracted from the database, as well as the date of the first and last consultation (past and "current" health records).

"Current" patient related information was obtained from the same database, including sex (male/ female), age (obtained as groups of 5-year categories), state of residence, rurality (major cities, inner regional, outer regional, or remote Australia), Australian Socio-Economic Indexes for Areas (SEIFA) Index of Relative Socio-economic Advantage and Disadvantage (IRSAD) deciles, pension (none, pensioner or health care card owner, Department of Veterans Affair (DVA)), ethnicity (Aboriginal and Torres Strait Islander yes/no), and smoking status (non-smoker, ex-smoker, current smoker). SEIFA-IRSAD is an indicator of relative economic and social advantage/disadvantage of people and households within an area [27]. The deciles were regrouped into quintiles (higher quintile indicating the respondent resides in a more advantaged area) for analysis.

Finally, the prevalence of some common NCDs and their risk factors were obtained following the same procedures used to identify the "prevalence" of the investigated MSK, considering medical registers since 2000 when available (past and current health records). These conditions included cardiometabolic risk factors (hypertension, diabetes mellitus, chronic kidney disease), cardiovascular diseases (ischaemic heart disease, stroke, heart failure), respiratory diseases (asthma, chronic obstructive pulmonary disease (COPD)), and mental health conditions (depression, anxiety).

Statistical analysis

Categorical variables were expressed as proportions (%), while median with interquartile range (p25-p75) were used to calculate the average number of health contacts, because of this variable's asymmetry. Confidence intervals of 95% (95%CI) were also estimated. The association between sociodemographic conditions and smoking status with the "prevalence" of the investigated MSK and chronic pain was expressed as prevalence and prevalence ratios (PR and their respective 95%CI estimated using Poisson regression). All associations with the investigated MSK diseases and "current" consultations for chronic pain were adjusted for sex and age, and *p*-values of heterogeneity were used to indicate those associations where the prevalence of the outcome was different across categories of the investigated sociodemographic variables and smoking status.

All analyses were performed in STATA 14.0 (StataCorp, Texas, USA), considering the clusters (general practices) and weighted to the inverse of the individual's probability of being in the sample (inverse of the average annual number of contacts with the general practice = 1/average number of contacts per year) [11, 12, 28].

The Human Research Ethics Committee of the University of Adelaide exempted this study of an ethical review, as it used existing and non-identifiable data.

Results

Of the total 1,544,303 active patients available in the MedicineInsight database, 2.8% ($n = 43{,}046$) were excluded because there was no recorded diagnosis or reason for encounter for the specified period (10/2013 to 06/2016). The percentage of individuals with missing data was up to 4% across categories of the investigated sociodemographic variables, although a higher frequency was observed in the NT (10.7%).

The final sample included for analysis consisted of 1,501,267 adults (57.6% females; 28.3% aged <35y and 22.5% ≥65y), and 65.2% of them had available records in the MedicineInsight database prior to 2013.

The combined "prevalence" of the investigated MSK (positive for arthritis, chronic back pain, gout, osteoporosis, spondyloarthropathies, and/or rheumatoid arthritis, considering past and "current" health records) in the whole sample was 16.8% (95%CI 15.9;17.7) with 21.3% (95%CI 20.2;22.4) of all patients consulting for chronic pain in the period between 2013 and 2016. Considering both variables together, 9.4% of the sample had some of the investigated MSK and also consulted for chronic pain (Additional file 1: Figure S1). For instance, chronic back pain could be both a MSK and a consultation for chronic pain.

Arthritis was the most "prevalent" of the investigated MSK (9.5%), followed by chronic back pain (6.7%), with 3.7% of the whole sample being affected by two or more MSK (Table 1). Among those with any of the investigated MSK, 67.0% consulted for the same reason in the period between 2013 and 2016, and this frequency was greater (86.1%) among those affected by three or more MSK. "Current" consultations for the same MSK were more frequent among those affected by chronic back pain (89.3%) or rheumatoid arthritis (57.7%). Table 1 also shows that 56.1% of the patients with any of the investigated MSK consulted for chronic pain in the period between 2013 and 2016, and this frequency was 46% higher among those affected by three or more MSK. A "current" consultation for chronic pain was also more likely among those affected by chronic back pain (96.7%), and less frequent among patients with gout (30.9%). The average number of health contacts per year was twice as high among those with any of the investigated MSK compared to those without these conditions, and this number increased progressively with the number of MSK's in the same individual.

Figure 1 shows that the "prevalence" of the investigated MSK and "current" consultations for chronic pain increased with age, but the last remained relatively stable for those aged 40 years or over, especially among males (Fig. 1). The "prevalence" of chronic MSK and "current" consultations for chronic pain were higher in males aged 20–39 years than in women of the same age, becoming both more frequent in women than in men after the age 60 years.

The distribution of arthritis and chronic back pain according to age and sex (Fig. 2) reflects the differences previously described for the "prevalence" of MSK and "current" consultations for chronic pain. The "prevalence" of chronic back pain was 20–53% more common in males aged 20–49 years than their female peers, while no sex differences were found for arthritis in this age. On the other hand, the "prevalence" of arthritis increased after the age 50 years, especially among women, who were up to 29% more likely to have this condition than men. Moreover, although the "prevalence" of chronic back pain remained relatively stable at around 9% in older adults, it was 25–33% more frequent in females.

Table 1 Prevalence of the investigated musculoskeletal diseases and characteristic related to the management of these conditions. Adults aged 18+ years ($N = 1,501,267$)

	Prevalence (2000–2016)[a] % (95%CI)	Current consultation for the same problem (2013–2016)[b] %	Current consultation for chronic pain (2013–2016)[b] %	Average number of health contacts per year (2013–2016)[b,c] Median [p25-p75]	Average time in the dataset (years) (2000–2016) [a] Median [p25-p75]
Positive for any musculoskeletal disease[d]					
No	83.2 (82.3;84.1)	0.0	14.3	1.0 [1.0–2.0]	3.3 [0.7–8.6]
Yes	16.8 (15.9;17.7)	66.7	56.1	2.0 [1.0–5.5]	6.0 [1.8–12.6]
Number of musculoskeletal diseases[d]					
1	13.1 (12.5;13.7)	67.0	54.9	2.0 [1.0–4.5]	5.5 [1.6–12.1]
2	3.1 (2.8;3.4)	62.5	54.8	3.0 [1.0–8.0]	7.3 [2.5–13.9]
3+	0.6 (0.5;0.7)	86.1	80.0	6.5 [2.0–12.5]	8.1 [3.0–14.7]
Type of musculoskeletal disease					
Arthritis	9.5 (8.8;10.3)	48.3	40.0	2.5 [1.0–6.5]	7.7 [2.9–14.0]
Chronic back pain	6.7 (6.4;7.1)	89.3	96.7	2.0 [1.0–5.0]	4.5 [1.3–10.3]
Gout	1.6 (1.5;1.7)	–[e]	30.9	1.5 [1.0–4.0]	4.2 [1.1–10.4]
Osteoporosis	1.2 (1.1;1.4)	–[e]	38.5	3.5 [1.0–9.0]	5.7 [1.3–13.1]
Spondyloarthropathies	1.1 (0.9;1.3)	8.4	46.5	3.0 [1.0–7.5]	9.2 [3.9–14.8]
Rheumatoid arthritis	0.9 (0.8;1.0)	57.7	35.0	2.5 [1.0–7.5]	7.2 [2.1–14.1]

[a] Considering the whole period since the first register available in the MedicineInsight dataset (2000–2016)
[b] Consultations between Oct/2013 and June/2016
[c] Number of registers on different dates when the patient received some diagnosis and/or some encounter occurred between the patient and the health service, including face-to-face visits and telephone contacts
[d] Positives for arthritis, chronic back pain, gout, osteoporosis, spondyloarthropathies, and/or rheumatoid arthritis
[e] No data available on diagnosis for these conditions before 2013

Table 2 presents the distribution of the overall prevalence of MSK and current consultations for chronic pain according to sociodemographic characteristics and smoking status. The overall "prevalence" of MSK ranged from 14.7% to 19.4% across states, except in NT where 10.2% had some of the investigated MSK. "Current" consultations for chronic pain oscillated around 20% in most states, but a higher frequency was observed in the ACT and the lowest in NT (26.1% and 8.8%, respectively). Consequently, "current" consultations for chronic pain among patients with some of the investigated MSK were more common in ACT (63.8%) and less frequent in NT (38.0%). Differences in the overall "prevalence" of MSK and "current" consultations for chronic pain were less evident for rurality or socioeconomic position (lower frequencies in remote Australia and in the highest SEIFA-IRSAD quintile), and a lower proportion of patients with some of the investigated MSK consulted for chronic pain in remote Australia. After adjustment for age and sex, the overall "prevalence" of MSK, "current" consultations for chronic pain, and proportion of patients with some of the investigated MSK consulting for chronic pain were higher in DVAs holders. Both, the overall "prevalence" of MSK and "current" consultations for chronic pain were more frequent in Aboriginal and Torres Strait Islander people. However, the proportion of consultations for chronic pain among those affected by some of the investigated MSK was similar in Aboriginals and non-Aboriginals. The overall "prevalence" of MSK and "current" consultations for chronic pain were similar in ex-smokers and current smokers, while among non-smokers these frequencies were lower.

Fig. 3 shows the overall "prevalence" of the investigated MSK and chronic pain among individuals affected by other chronic diseases. The investigated MSK were more frequent among those affected by heart failure or COPD, and less frequent among people with diabetes mellitus. On the other hand, "current" consultations for chronic pain among individuals with a chronic disease ranged from 25% to 29% for most diseases, with the highest values observed among those affected by ischaemic heart disease, heart failure, COPD, or anxiety.

Discussion

Four principal findings can be highlighted in this study. Firstly, the investigated MSK and consultations for chronic pain are common, and often related, reasons for

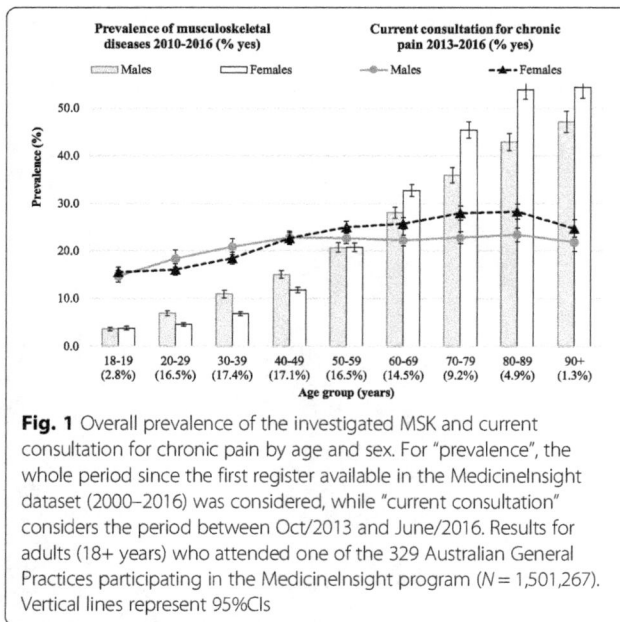

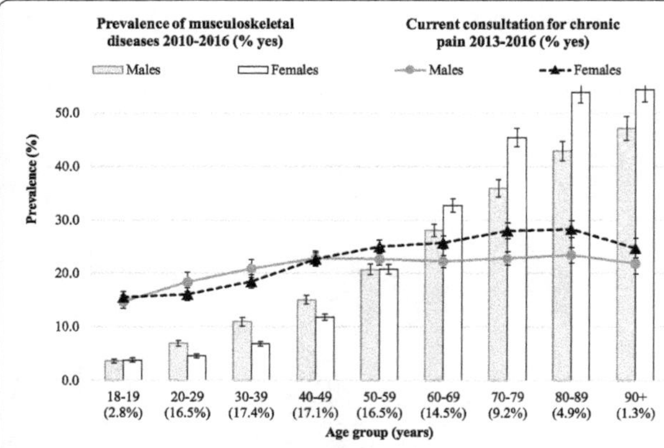

Fig. 1 Overall prevalence of the investigated MSK and current consultation for chronic pain by age and sex. For "prevalence", the whole period since the first register available in the MedicineInsight dataset (2000–2016) was considered, while "current consultation" considers the period between Oct/2013 and June/2016. Results for adults (18+ years) who attended one of the 329 Australian General Practices participating in the MedicineInsight program (N = 1,501,267). Vertical lines represent 95%CIs

presentation in Australian general practice. Secondly, patients affected by some of the investigated MSK attend general practice more frequently than those without these conditions. Thirdly, although the overall "prevalence" of the investigated MSK increases with age, the rate of "current" consultation for chronic pain remains stable once patients reach 40–49 years of age, especially among males. Finally, there appears to be some geographical and socioeconomic differences in the overall "prevalence" of the investigated MSK and "current" consultations for chronic pain in Australia that need to be explained.

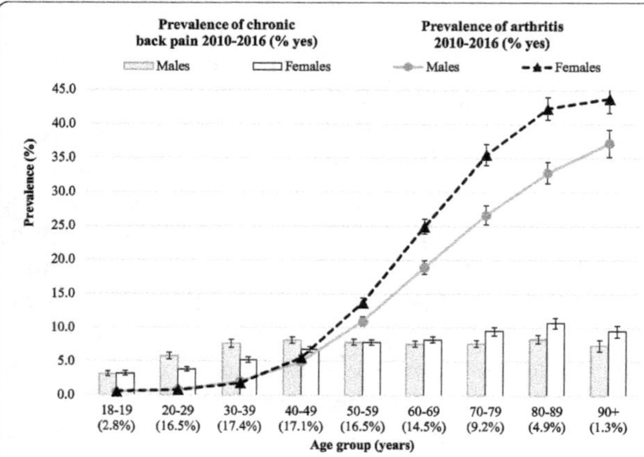

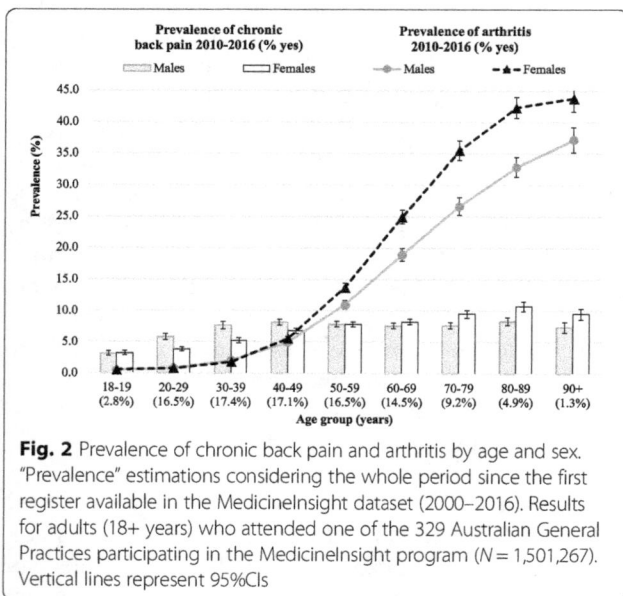

Fig. 2 Prevalence of chronic back pain and arthritis by age and sex. "Prevalence" estimations considering the whole period since the first register available in the MedicineInsight dataset (2000–2016). Results for adults (18+ years) who attended one of the 329 Australian General Practices participating in the MedicineInsight program (N = 1,501,267). Vertical lines represent 95%CIs

Previous estimates for the prevalence of MSK are similar to our "prevalence" obtained from MedicineInsight data [29], although we might expect a higher frequency in our study compared to community based surveys, because our participants are attending a doctor, which makes them less likely to be healthy than general population [17]. Using self-report data, the AIHW estimated that osteoarthritis affects 8.0% of all Australians adults, back pain 7.1%, osteoporosis 3.1%, and rheumatoid arthritis 1.9%. However, the use of self-reported information can undermine the ability to truly identify the scale of MSK within the population, especially for chronic pain, as the reliability of this information is also affected by question wording [15]. According to the BEACH program, chronic pain among Australian patients attending general practices changed from 18% in 2005 (N = 3211) to 19% in 2008–09 (N = 5793) [11, 26]. Therefore, the results obtained from MedicineInsight are similar to these previous estimates, with the advantage of providing results from a very large sample, which can be considered nationally representative of Australian adults (demographic distribution comparable to the census) [17, 30]. It is also based on medical diagnosis rather than self-report. Different countries have demonstrated that data from primary health care electronic records are accurate for the investigation of different diseases and their risk factors (sensitivity, specificity, and predictive positive values ranging from 70 to 95%) [19–23]. Programs like MedicineInsight are an excellent opportunity for governments to ascertain clinical outcomes on a large scale, at low cost, and with the potential to link to other data sources, thus facilitating monitoring and planning by heath policy makers [31]. Our findings also highlight the importance of these conditions in Australian health care because of their chronicity, rising health care costs, higher frequency among individuals affected by other chronic conditions, and adverse effects on patients' quality of life [6, 7, 32, 33].

It has been shown previously that MSK are a common reason for consultation in general practice, increasing with age and being more frequent in females [10, 34]. Chronic pain has also been reported to be more frequent among the less educated, those with lower family income, the physically inactive, smokers, and among those with depression [29], which is consistent with our results. Additionally, some studies have also found a higher frequency of chronic pain among women and a progressive increase with age, with a reduction after the age of 65 years, which is also consistent with our findings [11, 29, 35]. The reduction in the "prevalence" of chronic pain in the elderly may be a consequence of fewer work place related physical adverse effects post retirement [29, 35]. However, this could be also secondary to GPs recording MSK more frequently than chronic

Table 2 Prevalence of the investigated musculoskeletal diseases and consultations for chronic pain according to sociodemographic characteristics and smoking status. Adults aged 18+ years ($N = 1,501,267$)

	% of all data	Prevalence of chronic musculoskeletal disease (2010–2016)[a]		Current consultation for chronic pain (2013–2016)[b]		% of patients with a MSK that consulted for chronic pain (2013–2016)[b] %
		%[c]	PR (95%CI)[c]	%[c]	PR (95%CI)[c]	
State			$P < 0.001$		$P = 0.006$	
New South Wales (NSW)	28.2	17.6	Ref	22.7	Ref	57.5
Victoria (VIC)	25.5	16.5	0.94 (0.85–1.04)	22.2	0.98 (0.84–1.14)	58.1
Queensland (QLD)	18.7	16.9	0.96 (0.88;1.06)	19.8	0.87 (0.77–0.99)	53.4
Western Australia (WA)	13.3	14.7	0.83 (0.72–0.96)	19.1	0.84 (0.72–0.99)	55.9
Tasmania (TAS)	8.0	19.4	1.10 (1.01–1.21)	21.8	0.96 (0.83–1.12)	52.8
South Australia (SA)	3.4	17.3	0.98 (0.87;1.11)	22.3	0.98 (0.82–1.17)	54.9
Australia Capital Territory (ACT)	1.6	18.8	1.07 (0.73;1.58)	26.1	1.15 (0.77–1.71)	63.8
North Territory (NT)	1.3	10.2	0.58 (0.39;0.88)	8.8	0.39 (0.22–0.67)	38.0
Rurality			$P = 0.05$		$P = 0.07$	
Major cities	63.0	16.4	Ref	21.4	Ref	57.2
Inner regional	24.2	18.1	1.11 (1.02–1.20)	22.4	1.05 (0.93–1.17)	55.5
Outer regional	11.2	16.9	1.03 (0.95–1.12)	19.4	0.91 (0.80–1.02)	52.4
Remote Australia	1.6	14.6	0.89 (0.71–1.12)	16.6	0.78 (0.61–1.00)	49.0
Socioeconomic position (SEIFA-IRSAD quintiles)			$P < 0.001$		$P < 0.001$	
1 (Lowest)	17.3	18.9	Ref	23.8	Ref	57.1
2	15.7	19.1	1.01 (0.93–1.08)	23.5	0.99 (0.90–1.08)	57.2
3	20.5	16.5	0.87 (0.80–0.94)	20.2	0.85 (0.77–0.93)	54.2
4	20.1	16.5	0.87 (0.81–0.94)	21.2	0.89 (0.81–0.98)	56.3
5 (Highest)	26.4	14.6	0.77 (0.71–0.84)	19.6	0.83 (0.74–0.93)	56.0
Pension			$P < 0.001$		$P < 0.001$	
None	22.9	13.3	Ref	17.8	Ref	51.5
Pensioner or health care card	32.6	21.7	1.64 (1.52–1.76)	26.0	1.46 (1.32–1.63)	59.0
Department of Veterans Affair	1.3	24.1	1.82 (1.68–1.98)	29.6	1.66 (1.47–1.88)	60.8
Ignored	43.2	14.3	1.08 (0.98–1.19)	20.3	1.14 (1.00–1.31)	55.1
Aboriginal or Torres Strait Islander			$P < 0.001$		$P < 0.001$	
No	69.7	17.6	Ref	22.2	Ref	56.9
Yes	1.8	22.9	1.30 (1.22–1.39)	25.8	1.16 (1.08–1.24)	58.2
Ignored	28.6	14.7	0.83 (0.79–0.88)	19.0	0.85 (0.80–0.91)	53.8
Smoking status			$P < 0.001$		$P < 0.001$	
Non-smoker	50.3	16.8	Ref	21.3	Ref	54.8
Ex-smoker	20.1	19.8	1.17 (1.15–1.19)	24.4	1.14 (1.12–1.17)	57.2
Current smoker	14.5	20.5	1.22 (1.19–1.25)	24.8	1.17 (1.12–1.21)	59.4
Ignored	15.1	10.0	0.65 (0.61–0.70)	15.7	0.69 (0.64–0.75)	54.4

[a] Considering the whole period since the first register available in the MedicineInsight dataset (2000–2016), and including those positives for arthritis, chronic back pain, gout, osteoporosis, spondyloarthropathies and/or rheumatoid arthritis

[b] Consultation between 10/2013 and 06/2016

[c] Prevalence, prevalence ratios (PR) and p-values estimated based on Poisson Regression models, adjusted for sex and age. P-values of heterogeneity indicating differences across categories of each independent variable

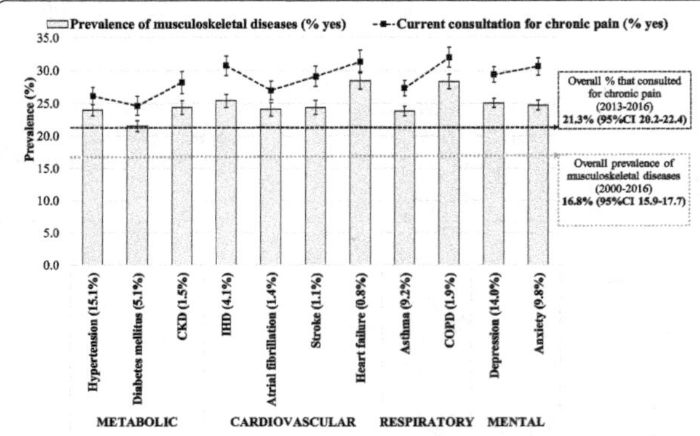

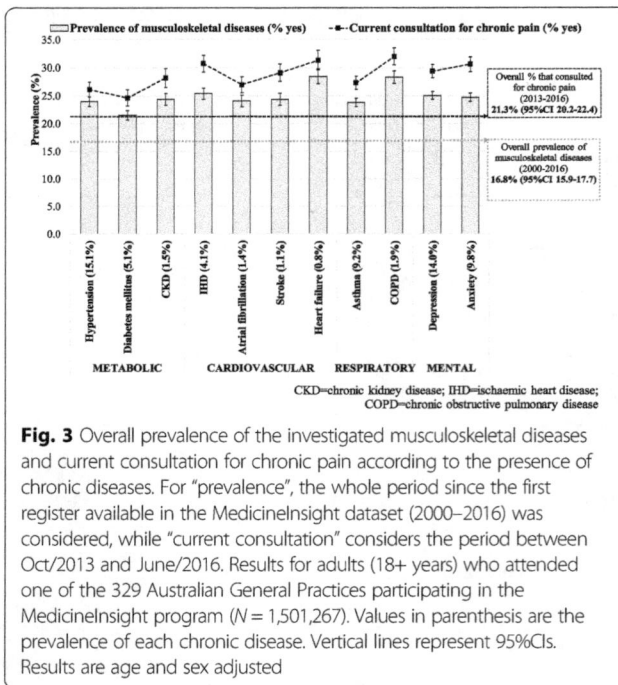

Fig. 3 Overall prevalence of the investigated musculoskeletal diseases and current consultation for chronic pain according to the presence of chronic diseases. For "prevalence", the whole period since the first register available in the MedicineInsight dataset (2000–2016) was considered, while "current consultation" considers the period between Oct/2013 and June/2016. Results for adults (18+ years) who attended one of the 329 Australian General Practices participating in the MedicineInsight program ($N = 1{,}501{,}267$). Values in parenthesis are the prevalence of each chronic disease. Vertical lines represent 95%CIs. Results are age and sex adjusted

pain as the reason for encounter once they confirm the diagnosis, or given the increase in comorbidity with age, the reporting of chronic pain may slip down the list of priorities compared to the other conditions older people have. However, some biological explanations are also possible. For instance, MSK developed later in life may be less painful due to a higher pain threshold associated with a loss of primary afferent fibres, reduction of pain receptors, or pain indifference resulting from a history of other chronic problems [36, 37].

More difficult to explain are the differences in consultation rates for chronic pain related to MSK between States, which has not been reported before in Australia [6, 11, 12, 32, 34], and may relate to differential access to general practice (i.e. poor access in non-urban locations) or recording of the reason for consultation, such as in the NT, where the percentage of excluded individuals due to missing data was 10.7%.

An advantage of using routinely collected morbidity data is the ability to examine the relationship between conditions. As expected, those with anxiety were more likely to consult for chronic pain [38]. Amongst comorbidities, the overall prevalence of the investigated MSK and chronic pain were particularly high among those affected by heart failure and COPD. This relationship has been reported previously [39–42] and attributed to abnormal inflammatory responses in extra-articular tissues, co-morbid depression and anxiety, insomnia, related symptoms (i.e. cough making pain worse, oedema), musculoskeletal fatigue, and restricted use of non-steroidal anti-inflammatory drugs for pain management.

In the absence of a disease register for MSK in general practice, MedicineInsight provides an alternative to population surveys. However, there are some limitations that should be highlighted. Firstly, not everyone with a MSK needs to see a GP regularly for diagnosis or management. For instance, most people over the age of 65 will have osteoarthritis or some other MSK, but not everyone will require regular medical care for these conditions [6, 7]. Secondly, depending on how critical information is recorded (e.g. missing data, non-mandatory fields, free-text for coding, different system coding vocabularies) or extracted (algorithms for data extraction), the accuracy of the information may be compromised [20–23, 43]. Although 2.8% of the individuals were excluded due to missing data on diagnosis or reason for encounter, it is very unlikely that it could have biased the results, as they were similar to the investigated sample according to sex, age, rurality, socioeconomic position, aboriginality or smoking status. Even though diverse methods were used to improve data quality (i.e. general practice characteristics, fields used for data extraction, variability of terms and synonyms), the algorithms used by MedicineInsight for data extraction have not been validated [28]. Furthermore, considering the non-random sampling process used for the enrolment of general practices and restrictions defined by MedicineInsight to get them included in the datasets, smaller practices are more likely to be underrepresented. However, the investigated sample seems to be representative of the Australian population, as the distribution in terms of gender, age, socioeconomic position, state, and rurality closely resembles figures from the last census [17, 30]. In any case, considering all these issues, MedicineWise is continuously expanding the number of recruited general practices and working towards the standardisation of its own data coding and extraction procedures [17]. Thirdly, diseases that are longstanding may only be recorded at initial diagnosis and a snapshot of GP attendance may not pick up the sentinel event. Including a longer period of data collection for the same patients and using a list of synonyms for the investigated conditions could improve the sensitivity to identify MSK cases and overcome these limitations.

Conclusions

The investigated MSK were an important and frequent reason for consultation in Australian general practice, especially among lower socioeconomic groups and the elderly. The distribution of these conditions differed according to other demographic characteristics and presence of comorbidities. Based on information collected from adults attending Australian general practices, MedicineInsight provided similar estimates to those obtained from population-based studies, with the advantage of being based on medical diagnosis and including a national sample.

Additional files

Additional file 1: Figure S1. Venn diagram for the combined frequency of the investigated musculoskeletal diseases and current consultation for chronic pain. Venn diagram for the combined frequency of the investigated musculoskeletal diseases and current consultation for chronic pain. For "prevalence", the whole period since the first register available in the MedicineInsight dataset (2000-2016) was considered, while "current consultation" considers the period between Oct/2013 and June/2016. Results for adults (18+ years) who attended one of the 329 Australian General Practices participating in the MedicineInsight program

Abbreviations

ACT: Australia Capital Territory; AIHW: Australian Institute of Health and Welfare; BEACH: Bettering the Evaluation and Care of Health Program; COPD: Chronic obstructive pulmonary disease; DVA: Department of Veterans Affair; GPs: General practitioners; MSK: Musculoskeletal conditions; NCDs: Chronic non-communicable diseases; NHS: National Health Survey; NPS: National Prescribing Service; NT: North Territory; PMH: Past medical history; PR: Prevalence ratio; SEIFA-IRSAD: Australian socio-economic indexes for areas index of relative socio-economic advantage and disadvantage; TAS: Tasmania; WA: Western Australia

Acknowledgements

The author acknowledges NPS MedicineWise for providing the necessary support for the completion of this study.

Funding

DAGC received a part fellowship from the NHMRC Centre of Research Excellence to Reduce Inequality in Heart Disease to conduct this study.

Authors' contributions

DAGC developed and designed the study, undertook the analysis and prepared the manuscript. SV and EH assisted with study design and commented on drafts of the manuscript. NS assisted with study design, reviewed the analysis, helped prepare the manuscript and commented on drafts. All authors read and approved the final manuscript.

Ethics approval and consent to participate

Medicinilnsight was approved by the Royal Australian College of General Practitioners (RACGP) National Research and Evaluation Ethics Committee on 10 January 2013. The program considers three different consent to participate levels before data collection. First, the general practice owner is provided with a comprehensive Practice Kit that includes information for them to make an informed decision to participate in the program. Second, GPs are informed by the general practice owner about the practice's participation in the program, and are given the opportunity to consent to receiving individual tailored reports. Finally, patients are made aware of the program through promotional material that is displayed within the waiting room of all participating practices, so they have the opportunity of verbally informing the practice about their choice not to participate. Verbal consent was obtained considering that MedicineInsight does not collect patients' identifiable information such as name, date of birth and address, thus representing a low safety risk for the participants. Additionally, all MedicineInsight data requests are approved by an independent Data Governance Committee that includes GPs, Statisticians and consumer representatives. Finally, the Human Research Ethics Committee of the University of Adelaide exempted this study of an ethical review, as it used existing and non-identifiable data.

Consent for publication

Not applicable.

Competing interests

There authors declare that they have no competing interests.

Author details

[1]Discipline of General Practice, Adelaide Medical School, NHMRC Centre of Research Excellence to Reduce Inequality in Heart Disease, The University of Adelaide, Adelaide, SA, Australia. [2]School of Public Health, The University of Adelaide, Adelaide, SA, Australia.

References

1. Briggs AM, Cross MJ, Hoy DG, Sanchez-Riera L, Blyth FM, Woolf AD, March L. Musculoskeletal health conditions represent a global threat to healthy aging: a report for the 2015 World Health Organization world report on ageing and health. Gerontologist. 2016(56 Suppl 2):S243–55.
2. Global Burden of Disease Study C. Global, regional, and national incidence, prevalence, and years lived with disability for 301 acute and chronic diseases and injuries in 188 countries, 1990-2013: a systematic analysis for the global burden of disease study 2013. Lancet. 2015;386(9995):743–800.
3. Cross M, Smith E, Hoy D, Nolte S, Ackerman I, Fransen M, Bridgett L, Williams S, Guillemin F, Hill CL, et al. The global burden of hip and knee osteoarthritis: estimates from the global burden of disease 2010 study. Ann Rheum Dis. 2014;73(7):1323–30.
4. Hoy D, March L, Brooks P, Blyth F, Woolf A, Bain C, Williams G, Smith E, Vos T, Barendregt J, et al. The global burden of low back pain: estimates from the global burden of disease 2010 study. Ann Rheum Dis. 2014;73(6):968–74.
5. Smith E, Hoy DG, Cross M, Vos T, Naghavi M, Buchbinder R, Woolf AD, March L. The global burden of other musculoskeletal disorders: estimates from the global burden of disease 2010 study. Ann Rheum Dis. 2014;73(8):1462–9.
6. Australian Institute of Health and Welfare 2014. Arthritis and other musculoskeletal conditions across the life stages. Arthritis Series no.18. PHE 173. Canberra: AIHW. Available at https://www.aihw.gov.au/reports/arthritis-other-musculoskeletal-conditions/across-life-stages/contents/table-of-contents. Accessed on 15/11/2016.
7. Australian Institute of Health and Welfare 2014. Health-care expenditure on arthritis and othermusculoskeletal conditions 2008–09. Arthritis series no. 20. Cat. no. PHE 177. Canberra: AIHW. Available at http://www.aihw.gov.au/publication-detail/?id=60129548392. Accessed on 17/11/2016.
8. Cooke G, Valenti L, Glasziou P, Britt H. Common general practice presentations and publication frequency. Aust Fam Physician. 2013;42(1–2):65–8.
9. Currow DC, Agar M, Plummer JL, Blyth FM, Abernethy AP. Chronic pain in South Australia - population levels that interfere extremely with activities of daily living. Aust N Z J Public Health. 2010;34(3):232–9.
10. March LM, Bagga H. Epidemiology of osteoarthritis in Australia. Med J Aust. 2004;180(5 Suppl):S6–10.
11. Henderson JV, Harrison CM, Britt HC, Bayram CF, Miller GC. Prevalence, causes, severity, impact, and management of chronic pain in Australian general practice patients. Pain Med. 2013;14(9):1346–61.
12. Brand CA, Harrison C, Tropea J, Hinman RS, Britt H, Bennell K. Management of osteoarthritis in general practice in Australia. Arthritis Care Res (Hoboken). 2014;66(4):551–8.
13. Hoy DG, Smith E, Cross M, Sanchez-Riera L, Blyth FM, Buchbinder R, Woolf AD, Driscoll T, Brooks P, March LM. Reflecting on the global burden of musculoskeletal conditions: lessons learnt from the global burden of disease 2010 study and the next steps forward. Ann Rheum Dis. 2015;74(1):4–7.
14. Dal Grande E, Fullerton S, Taylor AW. Reliability of self-reported health risk factors and chronic conditions questions collected using the telephone in South Australia, Australia. BMC Med Res Methodol. 2012;12:108.
15. Gill TK, Tucker GR, Avery JC, Shanahan EM, Menz HB, Taylor AW, Adams RJ, Hill CL. The use of self-report questions to examine the prevalence of musculoskeletal problems: a test-retest study. BMC Musculoskelet Disord. 2016;17:100.
16. Pain Australia, 2014. National Pain Strategy, Pain Managament for all Autralians, Australia. (Available at http://www.painaustralia.org.au/improving-policy/national-pain-strategy) Accessed on 08/09/2017.
17. MedicineInsight: MedicineInsight Data Book Version 1.2. Sydney; NPS MedicineWise, December 2016. (Available at http://www.nps.org.au/health-professionals/medicineinsight/interested-in-medicineinsight-data/medicineinsight-databook). Accessed on 15/01/2017. 2016.
18. Boyle DI. Middleware supporting next generation data analytics in Australia. Stud Health Technol Inform. 2015;216:1019.

19. Rubbo B, Fitzpatrick NK, Denaxas S, Daskalopoulou M, Yu N, Patel RS, Follow-up UKB, Outcomes Working G, Hemingway H. Use of electronic health records to ascertain, validate and phenotype acute myocardial infarction: a systematic review and recommendations. Int J Cardiol. 2015;187:705–11.
20. Tu K, Manuel D, Lam K, Kavanagh D, Mitiku TF, Guo H. Diabetics can be identified in an electronic medical record using laboratory tests and prescriptions. J Clin Epidemiol. 2011;64(4):431–5.
21. Woodfield R, Grant I, Group UKBSO, Follow-Up UKB, Outcomes Working G, Sudlow CL. Accuracy of electronic health record data for identifying stroke cases in large-scale epidemiological studies: a systematic review from the UK biobank stroke outcomes group. PLoS One. 2015;10(10):e0140533.
22. Horsfall L, Walters K, Petersen I. Identifying periods of acceptable computer usage in primary care research databases. Pharmacoepidemiol Drug Saf. 2013;22(1):64–9.
23. Marston L, Carpenter JR, Walters KR, Morris RW, Nazareth I, White IR, Petersen I. Smoker, ex-smoker or non-smoker? The validity of routinely recorded smoking status in UK primary care: a cross-sectional study. BMJ Open. 2014;4(4):e004958.
24. Primary Health Care Research & Information Service. PHCRIS Fast Fact: General practice numbers in Australia, 2000–01 to 2010–11. (Available at http://www.phcris.org.au/fastfacts/fact.php?id=6752). Accessed on 10/12/2016.
25. Australian Government, Department of Health. General Practice Statistics: GP Workforce Statistics – 2004-05 to 2014–15. (Available at http://www.health.gov.au/internet/main/publishing.nsf/content/General+Practice+Statistics-1). Accessed on 10/12/2016.
26. Australian Institute of Health and Welfare, Australian GP Statistics and Classification Centre, 2006. SAND abstract No. 82 from the BEACH program: Prevalence and management of chronic pain. Sydney: AGPSCC University of Sydney. ISSN 1444–9072. Available at https://sydney.edu.au/medicine/fmrc/publications/sand-abstracts/ Accessed on 10/11/2016.
27. ABS: Australian Bureau of Statistics. Census of Population and Housing: Socio-Economic Indexes for Areas (SEIFA), Australia. (Available at http://www.abs.gov.au/ausstats/abs@.nsf/mf/2033.0.55.001) Accessed on 01/03/2015. In., vol. cat. no. 2033.0.55.001 2011.
28. Benchimol EI, Smeeth L, Guttmann A, Harron K, Moher D, Petersen I, Sorensen HT, von Elm E, Langan SM, Committee RW. The REporting of studies conducted using observational routinely-collected health data (RECORD) statement. PLoS Med. 2015;12(10):e1001885.
29. McBeth J, Jones K. Epidemiology of chronic musculoskeletal pain. Best Pract Res Clin Rheumatol. 2007;21(3):403–25.
30. ABS: Australian Bureau of Statistics. Table Builder. (Available at http://www.abs.gov.au/websitedbs/censushome.nsf/home/tablebuilder) Accessed on 10/05/2016. In.; 2016.
31. Weber GM, Mandl KD, Kohane IS. Finding the missing link for big biomedical data. JAMA. 2014;311(24):2479–80.
32. Knox SA, Harrison CM, Britt HC, Henderson JV. Estimating prevalence of common chronic morbidities in Australia. Med J Aust. 2008;189(2):66–70.
33. van der Zee-Neuen A, Putrik P, Ramiro S, Keszei A, de Bie R, Chorus A, Boonen A. Impact of chronic diseases and multimorbidity on health and health care costs: the additional role of musculoskeletal disorders. Arthritis Care Res (Hoboken). 2016;68(12):1823–31.
34. Jordan K, Clarke AM, Symmons DP, Fleming D, Porcheret M, Kadam UT, Croft P. Measuring disease prevalence: a comparison of musculoskeletal disease using four general practice consultation databases. Br J Gen Pract. 2007;57(534):7–14.
35. Cimmino MA, Ferrone C, Cutolo M. Epidemiology of chronic musculoskeletal pain. Best Pract Res Clin Rheumatol. 2011;25(2):173–83.
36. Daoust R, Paquet J, Piette E, Sanogo K, Bailey B, Chauny JM. Impact of age on pain perception for typical painful diagnoses in the emergency department. J Emerg Med. 2016;50(1):14–20.
37. Lautenbacher S, Peters JH, Heesen M, Scheel J, Kunz M. Age changes in pain perception: a systematic-review and meta-analysis of age effects on pain and tolerance thresholds. Neurosci Biobehav Rev. 2017;75:104–13.
38. Dickens C, McGowan L, Clark-Carter D, Creed F. Depression in rheumatoid arthritis: a systematic review of the literature with meta-analysis. Psychosom Med. 2002;64(1):52–60.
39. Nannini C, Medina-Velasquez YF, Achenbach SJ, Crowson CS, Ryu JH, Vassallo R, Gabriel SE, Matteson EL, Bongartz T. Incidence and mortality of obstructive lung disease in rheumatoid arthritis: a population-based study. Arthritis Care Res (Hoboken). 2013;65(8):1243–50.
40. van Dam van Isselt EF, Groenewegen-Sipkema KH, Spruit-van Eijk M, Chavannes NH, de Waal MW, Janssen DJ, Achterberg WP. Pain in patients with COPD: a systematic review and meta-analysis. BMJ Open. 2014;4(9):e005898.
41. DeJongh B, Birkeland K, Brenner M. Managing comorbidities in patients with chronic heart failure: first, do no harm. Am J Cardiovasc Drugs. 2015;15(3):171–84.
42. Hall AJ, Stubbs B, Mamas MA, Myint PK, Smith TO. Association between osteoarthritis and cardiovascular disease: systematic review and meta-analysis. Eur J Prev Cardiol. 2016;23(9):938–46.
43. Stocks N, Fahey T. Labelling of acute respiratory illness: evidence of between-practitioner variation in the UK. Fam Pract. 2002;19(4):375–7.

Permissions

All chapters in this book were first published in MD, by BioMed Central; hereby published with permission under the Creative Commons Attribution License or equivalent. Every chapter published in this book has been scrutinized by our experts. Their significance has been extensively debated. The topics covered herein carry significant findings which will fuel the growth of the discipline. They may even be implemented as practical applications or may be referred to as a beginning point for another development.

The contributors of this book come from diverse backgrounds, making this book a truly international effort. This book will bring forth new frontiers with its revolutionizing research information and detailed analysis of the nascent developments around the world.

We would like to thank all the contributing authors for lending their expertise to make the book truly unique. They have played a crucial role in the development of this book. Without their invaluable contributions this book wouldn't have been possible. They have made vital efforts to compile up to date information on the varied aspects of this subject to make this book a valuable addition to the collection of many professionals and students.

This book was conceptualized with the vision of imparting up-to-date information and advanced data in this field. To ensure the same, a matchless editorial board was set up. Every individual on the board went through rigorous rounds of assessment to prove their worth. After which they invested a large part of their time researching and compiling the most relevant data for our readers.

The editorial board has been involved in producing this book since its inception. They have spent rigorous hours researching and exploring the diverse topics which have resulted in the successful publishing of this book. They have passed on their knowledge of decades through this book. To expedite this challenging task, the publisher supported the team at every step. A small team of assistant editors was also appointed to further simplify the editing procedure and attain best results for the readers.

Apart from the editorial board, the designing team has also invested a significant amount of their time in understanding the subject and creating the most relevant covers. They scrutinized every image to scout for the most suitable representation of the subject and create an appropriate cover for the book.

The publishing team has been an ardent support to the editorial, designing and production team. Their endless efforts to recruit the best for this project, has resulted in the accomplishment of this book. They are a veteran in the field of academics and their pool of knowledge is as vast as their experience in printing. Their expertise and guidance has proved useful at every step. Their uncompromising quality standards have made this book an exceptional effort. Their encouragement from time to time has been an inspiration for everyone.

The publisher and the editorial board hope that this book will prove to be a valuable piece of knowledge for researchers, students, practitioners and scholars across the globe.

List of Contributors

Tobias Schmidt, Tim Rolvien and Haider Mussawy
Department of Osteology and Biomechanics, University Medical Center Hamburg-Eppendorf, Lottestraße 59, 22529 Hamburg, Germany
Department of Orthopedic Surgery, University Medical Center Hamburg-Eppendorf, Martinistrasse 52, 20246 Hamburg, Germany

Katharina Ebert, Michael Amling and Florian Barvencik
Department of Osteology and Biomechanics, University Medical Center Hamburg-Eppendorf, Lottestraße 59, 22529 Hamburg, Germany

Nicola Oehler
Department of Orthopedic Surgery, University Medical Center Hamburg-Eppendorf, Martinistrasse 52, 20246 Hamburg, Germany

Jens Lohmann, Luca Papavero and Ralph Kothe
Clinic for Spinal Surgery, Schoen Klinik Eilbek, Denhaide 120, 22081 Hamburg, Germany

Jon Cornwall
Centre for Early Learning in Medicine, Otago Medical School, University of Otago, Dunedin, New Zealand

Ewan Kennedy
School of Physiotherapy, University of Otago, Dunedin, New Zealand

Rebecca Abbott
Department of Physical Therapy and Human Movement Sciences, Feinberg School of Medicine, Northwestern University, Chicago, USA

Rebecca J. Crawford
Faculty of Health Sciences, Curtin University, Perth, Australia

Tobias Lange, Georg Gosheger and Albert Schulze Boevingloh
Department of Orthopedics and Tumor Orthopedics, Muenster University Hospital, Albert-Schweitzer-Campus 1, 48149 Muenster, Germany

Tobias L. Schulte
Department of Orthopedics and Trauma Surgery, St. Josef-Hospital, University Hospital, Ruhr-University Bochum, Gudrunstrasse 56, 44791 Bochum, Germany

Raul Mayr and Werner Schmoelz
Department of Trauma Surgery, Medical University of Innsbruck, Anichstrasse 35, 6020 Innsbruck, Austria

Vivek A. S. Ramakrishna
Spine Service, Department of Orthopaedic Surgery, St. George & Sutherland Clinical School, University of New South Wales Australia, Kogarah, Sydney, NSW 2217, Australia
School of Biomedical Engineering, University of Technology Sydney, Ultimo, NSW 2007, Australia

Uphar Chamoli, Luke L. Viglione and Ashish D. Diwan
Spine Service, Department of Orthopaedic Surgery, St. George & Sutherland Clinical School, University of New South Wales Australia, Kogarah, Sydney, NSW 2217, Australia

Naomi Tsafnat
School of Mechanical and Manufacturing Engineering, University of New South Wales Australia, Kensington campus, Sydney, NSW 2052, Australia

Donghua Huang, Xiangyu Deng, Kaige Ma, Hang Liang, Deyao Shi, Fashuai Wu and Zengwu Shao
Department of Orthopaedics, Union Hospital, Tongji Medical College, Huazhong University of Science and Technology, 1277 JieFang Avenue, Wuhan 430022, China

Jinrong Xiao
Department of Epidemiology and Biostatistics, Ministry of Education Key Laboratory of Environment and Health, School of Public Health, Tongji Medical College, Huazhong University of Science and Technology, Wuhan 430030, Hubei, China
Pichitchai Atthakomol, Areerak Phanphaisarn and Sureeporn Phrompaet Department of Orthopaedics, Faculty of Medicine, Chiang Mai University, Chiang Mai, Thailand

Worapaka Manosroi
Division of Endocrinology, Department of Internal Medicine, Bangkok Chiang Mai Hospital, Chiang Mai, Thailand

Sawan Iammatavee
Department of Orthopaedics, Nakornping Hospital, Chiang Mai, Thailand

Siam Tongprasert
Department of Rehabilitation Medicine, Faculty of Medicine, Chiang Mai University, Chiang Mai, Thailand

Sarah M. Greising and Benjamin T. Corona
Extremity Trauma and Regenerative Medicine, United States Army Institute of Surgical Research, Fort Sam Houston, Texas 78234, USA

Gordon L. Warren
Department of Physical Therapy, Byrdine F. Lewis School of Nursing and Health Professions, Georgia State University, Atlanta, GA 30302, USA

W. Michael Southern, Anna S. Nichenko and Anita E. Qualls
Department of Kinesiology, University of Georgia, Athens, GA 30602, USA

Jarrod A. Call
Department of Kinesiology, University of Georgia, Athens, GA 30602, USA
Regenerative Bioscience Center, University of Georgia, Athens, GA 30602, USA

Peter David Clegg
Department of Musculoskeletal Biology, Institute of Ageing and Chronic Disease, University of Liverpool, William Henry Duncan Building, 6 West Derby Street, Liverpool L7 8TX, UK
School of Veterinary Science, Leahurst Campus, University of Liverpool, Chester High Road, Neston CH64 7TE, UK
The MRC-Arthritis Research UK Centre for Integrated research into Musculoskeletal Ageing (CIMA), Liverpool, UK

Eithne Josephine Comerford
Department of Musculoskeletal Biology, Institute of Ageing and Chronic Disease, University of Liverpool, William Henry Duncan Building, 6 West Derby Street, Liverpool L7 8TX, UK
School of Veterinary Science, Leahurst Campus, University of Liverpoo, Chester High Road, Neston CH64 7TE, UK

Elizabeth Gail Canty-Laird
Department of Musculoskeletal Biology, Institute of Ageing and Chronic Disease, University of Liverpool, William Henry Duncan Building, 6 West Derby Street, Liverpool L7 8TX, UK
The MRC-Arthritis Research UK Centre for Integrated research into Musculoskeletal Ageing (CIMA), Liverpool, UK

A. B. Ahrberg
Department of Orthopedics, Traumatology and Plastic Surgery, University of Leipzig, Liebigstr. 20, 04103 Leipzig, Germany
Translational Center for Regenerative Medicine (TRM), University of Leipzig, Leipzig, Germany

C. Horstmeier and W. Brehm
Translational Center for Regenerative Medicine (TRM), University of Leipzig, Leipzig, Germany
Saxon Incubator for Clinical Translation (SIKT), University of Leipzig, Leipzig, Germany
University Equine Hospital, University of Leipzig, Leipzig, Germany

D. Berner
Department of Clinical Science and Services, The Royal Veterinary College, University of London, London, UK

C. Gittel
University Equine Hospital, University of Leipzig, Leipzig, Germany

A. Hillmann
Translational Center for Regenerative Medicine (TRM), University of Leipzig, Leipzig, Germany
Saxon Incubator for Clinical Translation (SIKT), University of Leipzig, Leipzig, Germany

C. Josten
Department of Orthopedics, Traumatology and Plastic Surgery, University of Leipzig, Liebigstr. 20, 04103 Leipzig, Germany

G. Rossi
School of Biosciences and Veterinary Medicine, University of Camerino, Camerino, Italy

S. Schubert
Translational Center for Regenerative Medicine (TRM), University of Leipzig, Leipzig, Germany
Saxon Incubator for Clinical Translation (SIKT), University of Leipzig, Leipzig, Germany
Institute of Veterinary Physiology, University of Leipzig, Leipzig, Germany

K. Winter
University Equine Hospital, University of Leipzig, Leipzig, Germany
Institute of Anatomy, Medical Faculty, University of Leipzig, Leipzig, Germany

J. Burk
Translational Center for Regenerative Medicine (TRM), University of Leipzig, Leipzig, Germany
Saxon Incubator for Clinical Translation (SIKT), University of Leipzig, Leipzig, Germany
Institute of Veterinary Physiology, University of Leipzig, Leipzig, Germany
Department of Biotechnology, University of Natural Resources and Life Sciences, Vienna, Austria

James M. Elliott
Faculty of Health Sciences, The University of Sydney, Northern Sydney Local Health District, St Leonards, Australia 75 East Street Lidcombe NSW, Sydney 2141, Australia
Department of Physical Therapy and Human Movement Sciences, Feinberg School of Medicine, Northwestern University, Chicago, USA
Honorary Fellow School of Health and Rehabilitation Sciences, The University of Queensland, St. Lucia, Australia

Jae-Ang Sim
Department of Orthopaedic Surery, Gil Hospital, Gachon University of Medicine and Science, Inchon, South Korea

Jin-Kyu Lim and Byung Hoon Lee
Department of Orthopedic Surgery, Kang-Dong Sacred Heart Hospital, Hallym University Medical School, 134-701, Gil-dong, Seoul, South Korea

S. A. Dingemans
Department of Surgery, Trauma Unit, Academic Medical Centre, University of Amsterdam, 1100 DD Amsterdam, The Netherlands

M. P. J. van den Bekerom
Department of Orthopedic Surgery, OLVG, 1090 HM Amsterdam, The Netherlands

E. van Beeck
Department of Public Health, Erasmus MC, 3000 CA Rotterdam, The Netherlands

F. W. Bloemers
Department of Surgery, Trauma Unit, VU University Medical Centre, 1007 MB Amsterdam, The Netherlands

B. A. Twigt
Department of Surgery, BovenIJ Hospital, 1030 BD Amsterdam, The Netherlands

R. N. van Veen
Department of Surgery, OLVG, 1090 HM Amsterdam, The Netherlands

A. H. van der Veen
Department of Surgery, Catharina Hospital, 5602 ZA Eindhoven, The Netherlands

J. Winkelhagen
Department of Surgery, Westfries Hospital, 1620 AR Hoorn, The Netherlands

B. C. van der Zwaard
Department of Orthopaedics, Jeroen Bosch Hospital, 5200 ME's-Hertogenbosch, The Netherlands

Jing Zhang, Yuxuan Wei, Yang Dong and Zhichang Zhang
Department of Orthopaedic Surgery, Shanghai Jiao Tong University Affiliated Sixth People's Hospital, Shanghai 200233, China

Yue Gong
Department of Breast Surgery, Key Laboratory of Breast Cancer in Shanghai, Fudan University Shanghai Cancer Center, Fudan University, Shanghai 200032, China

Takashi Hirai
Department of Orthopedic Surgery, Tokyo Medical and Dental University, 1-5-45 Yushima, Bunkyo-ku, Tokyo 113-8519, Japan
Japanese Organization of the Study for Ossification of Spinal Ligament (JOSL), 1-5-45 Yushima, Bunkyo-ku, Tokyo 113-8519, Japan

Narihito Nagoshi
Department of Orthopedic Surgery, School of Medicine, Keio University, 35 Shinanomachi, Shinjuku-ku, Tokyo 160-8582, Japan

Kazuhiro Takeuchi
Department of Orthopedic Surgery, National Hospital Organization Okayama Medical Center, 1711-1 Tamasu, Okayama, Okayama 701-1154, Japan
Japanese Organization of the Study for Ossification of Spinal Ligament (JOSL), 1-5-45 Yushima, Bunkyo-ku, Tokyo 113-8519, Japan

Kanji Mori
Department of Orthopedic Surgery, Shiga University of Medical Science, Tsukinowa-cho, Seta, Otsu, Shiga 520-2192, Japan
Japanese Organization of the Study for Ossification of Spinal Ligament (JOSL), 1-5-45 Yushima, Bunkyo-ku, Tokyo 113-8519, Japan

Haruo Kanno
Department of Orthopaedic Surgery, Tohoku University School of Medicine, 1-1 Seiryomachi, Aoba-ku, Sendai, Miyagi 980-8574, Japan
Japanese Organization of the Study for Ossification of Spinal Ligament (JOSL), 1-5-45 Yushima, Bunkyo-ku, Tokyo 113-8519, Japan

Kei Ando
Department of Orthopedic Surgery, Nagoya University Graduate School of Medicine, 65 Tsurumaicho, Showa-ku, Nagoya, Aichi 466-0065, Japan
Japanese Organization of the Study for Ossification of Spinal Ligament (JOSL), 1-5-45 Yushima, Bunkyo-ku, Tokyo 113-8519, Japan

Shunsuke Fujibayashi
Department of Orthopedic Surgery, Graduate School of Medicine, Kyoto University, 54 Kawaharacho, Shogoin, Sakyo-ku, Kyoto, Kyoto 606-8507, Japan
Japanese Organization of the Study for Ossification of Spinal Ligament (JOSL), 1-5-45 Yushima, Bunkyo-ku, Tokyo 113-8519, Japan

Masashi Yamazaki
Department of Orthopedic Surgery, Faculty of Medicine, University of Tsukuba, 2-1-1 Amakubo, Tsukuba, Ibaraki 305-8576, Japan
Japanese Organization of the Study for Ossification of Spinal Ligament (JOSL), 1-5-45 Yushima, Bunkyo-ku, Tokyo 113-8519, Japan

Albert Tan, Joanne Protheroe and Kate M. Dunn
Arthritis Research UK Primary Care Centre, Research Institute for Primary Care & Health Sciences, Keele University, Keele, Staffordshire ST5 5BG, UK

Victoria Y. Strauss
Centre for Statistics in Medicine, Oxford Clinical Trial Research Unit, Nuffield Department of Orthopaedics, Rheumatology and Musculoskeletal Sciences, University of Oxford Botnar Research Centre, Windmill Road, Oxford OX3 7LD, UK

Francesco Bozzao, Stella Bernardi and Fabio Fischetti
Department of Medical Sciences, University of Trieste, Cattinara Teaching Hospital, Strada di Fiume 449, 34149 Trieste, Italy

Franca Dore and Lorenzo Zandonà
ASUITS, Cattinara Teaching Hospital, Strada di Fiume 449, 34149 Trieste, Italy

Jigang Lou, Beiyu Wang, Tingkui Wu, Ziyang Liu and Hao Liu
Department of Orthopedics, West China Hospital, Sichuan University, 37 Guoxue Road, Chengdu, Sichuan 610041, China

Wenjie Wu
Department of Orthopedics, Southwest Hospital, the Third Military Medical University, Chongqing, China

Huibo Li
Department of Orthopedics, Qianfoshan Hospital, Shandong University, Jinan, Shandong, China

Manayesh Delele, Balamurugan Janakiraman and Abey Bekele Abebe
Department of Physiotherapy, School of Medicine and Health Sciences, University of Gondar and Gondar University specialized comprehensive hospital, Gondar, Ethiopia

Ararso Tafese
Department of Public Health, School of Medicine and Health Sciences, University of Gondar, Gondar, Ethiopia

Alexander T. M. van de Water
Department of Physiotherapy, School of Medicine and Health Sciences, University of Gondar and Gondar University specialized comprehensive hospital, Gondar, Ethiopia
School of Physiotherapy, Academy of Health, Saxion University of Applied Sciences, Enschede, The Netherlands

Sebastian Lotzien
BG University Hospital Bergmannsheil, Bochum, Germany
Department of General and Trauma Surgery, Ruhr University Bochum, Bürkle-de-la-Camp-Platz 1, 44789 Bochum, Germany

Valentin Rausch, Thomas Armin Schildhauer and Jan Gessmann
BG University Hospital Bergmannsheil, Bochum, Germany

Michael J. Fischer
Vamed Rehabilitation Center Kitzbuehel, Kitzbuehel, Austria
Department of Rehabilitation Medicine, Hanover Medical School, Hanover, Germany
Department of Orthopedics, Medical University Innsbruck, Innsbruck, Austria

Gergo Horvath
Department of Medical Biochemistry, Semmelweis University, Budapest, Hungary

Martin Krismer
Department of Orthopedics, Medical University Innsbruck, Innsbruck, Austria

Erich Gnaiger
D. Swarovski Research Laboratory, Department of Visceral, Transplant and Thoracic Surgery, Medical University Innsbruck, Innsbruck, Austria

Georg Goebel
Department of Medical Statistics, Informatics and Health Economics, Medical University Innsbruck, Innsbruck, Austria

Dominik H. Pesta
Institute for Clinical Diabetology, German Diabetes Center, Leibniz Institute for Diabetes Research, Heinrich-Heine-University, Düsseldorf, Germany
German Center for Diabetes Research (DZD), München-Neuherberg, Germany
Department of Sport Science, University of Innsbruck, Innsbruck, Austria

Andreas Lenich
Helios Clinic Munich West, Department of Orthopedic Sports Medicine, Trauma Surgery and Hand Surgery, Steinerweg 5, 81241 Munich, Germany

Christian Pfeifer
Regensburg University Medical Center, Department of Trauma Surgery, Franz-Josef-Strauß-Allee 11, 93053 Regensburg, Germany

Philipp Proier, Roman Fleer and Jonas Pogorzelski
Department of Orthopedic Sports Medicine, Technical University of Munich, Klinikum rechts der Isar, Ismaninger Str. 22, 81675 Munich, Germany

Coen Wijdicks and Martina Roth
Department of Research & Development, Arthrex GmbH, Munich, Germany

Frank Martetschläger
German Center for Shoulder Surgery, ATOS Clinic Munich, Effnerstraße 38, 81925 Munich, Germany

Zhen Zhang
Department of Orthopedics, West China Hospital, Sichuan University, No. 37, Guoxue Lane, Wuhou District, Chengdu 610041, Sichuan Province, China
Department of Biologic and Materials Sciences, School of Dentistry, University of Michigan, Ann Arbor, USA

W. Benton Swanson
Department of Biologic and Materials Sciences, School of Dentistry, University of Michigan, Ann Arbor, USA

Yan-Hong Wang
Department of Neonatology, Beijing Gynecology & Obstetrics Hospital, Capital Medical University, Beijing, China

Wei Lin
Department of Gynecology, West China Second Hospital, Sichuan University, Chengdu, China

Guanglin Wang
Department of Orthopedics, West China Hospital, Sichuan University, No. 37, Guoxue Lane, Wuhou District, Chengdu 610041, Sichuan Province, China

David Alejandro González-Chica, Simon Vanlint and Nigel Stocks
Discipline of General Practice, Adelaide Medical School, NHMRC Centre of Research Excellence to Reduce Inequality in Heart Disease, The University of Adelaide, Adelaide, SA, Australia

Elizabeth Hoon
School of Public Health, The University of Adelaide, Adelaide, SA, Australia

Index

www.ingramcontent.com/pod-product-compliance
Lightning Source LLC
Chambersburg PA
CBHW082038190326
41458CB00010B/3400

* 9 7 8 1 6 3 9 2 7 4 0 0 0 *